Philosophy and Psychopathology

Manfred Spitzer   Brendan A. Maher
Editors

Philosophy and Psychopathology

Springer-Verlag
New York Heidelberg Berlin
London Paris Tokyo Hong Kong

Manfred Spitzer, M.D., Ph.D.
Visiting Associate Professor
Department of Psychology
Harvard University
Cambridge, MA 02138, USA

Brendan A. Maher, Ph.D.
Edward C. Henderson Professor of the
  Psychology of Personality
Department of Psychology
Harvard University
Cambridge, MA 02138, USA

Library of Congress Cataloging-in-Publication Data
Philosophy and psychopathology / Manfred Spitzer, Brendan A. Maher,
    editors.
        p. cm.
    Papers presented at a meeting at the Dept. of Psychology, Harvard
University, In Oct. 1989.
    Includes bibliographical references.
    Includes index.
    ISBN-13: 978-0-387-97303-6
    1. Mental illness—Philosophy—Congresses. 2. Schizophrenia—
Philosophy—Congresses. 3. Self—Congresses. I. Spitzer,
Manfred. II. Maher, Brendan A. (Brendan Arnold), 1924-
    [DNLM: 1. Philosophy, Medical—congresses. 2. Psychopathology—
congresses. 3. Psychotic Disorders—congresses. 4. Schizophrenia—
congresses. WM 202 P568 1989]
    RC437.5.P437 1990
    616.89'001—dc20
    DNLM/DLC
    for Library of Congress   90-9755

Camera-ready copy provided by the editors.

9 8 7 6 5 4 3 2 1

ISBN-13: 978-0-387-97303-6   e-ISBN-13: 978-1-4613-9028-2
DOI: 10.1007/978-1-4613-9028-2

Preface

Philosophy and psychopathology have more in common than philosophers, psychiatrists and clinical psychologists might think. Three fields of inquiry come to mind: (1) Questions about the scientific status of psychopathological statements and claims, (2) ethical questions, and (3) problems regarding the question of how to account for something like a disordered mind. While the first two domains have frequently been addressed in articles and debates (think of the mind–body problem and the problem of institutionalization versus self–determination as examples of issues in the two fields), the question of how the mind should be conceived in order for psychopathology to work best has seldom been discussed. The present volume focuses on this question.

Perception, thought, affect, will, and the like are terms which made their way from philosophy into psychology, and into present psychiatry, where disturbances of these "faculties" or "functions" are believed to form the most basic part of symptomatology. While these terms and many others that are used to refer to symptoms of mental disorder (such as "self", "consciousness", "drive", and "identity") may seem to be purely descriptive and theoretically "innocent", they are packed with implicit assumptions, theoretical concepts, and sometimes dogmatic postulates.

To be aware of those assumptions, to reflect upon them, and to rephrase them or even rethink them has always been the task of the philosopher. Interestingly enough, in order to push a concept to its limits, philosophers occasionally used phenomena of pathology as their examples, referring to hallucinations in the attempt to clarify perception, or to delusions in the attempt to clarify the degree to which we can be sure about different forms of knowledge. Thus, as the psychopathologist uses concepts derived from philosophy to deal with pathology, and as the philosopher uses pathology to derive arguments for the clarification of the very same concepts, a rich and mutually fruitful dialogue should be expected.

As a matter of historical fact and may be for other reasons as well (economic, psychological, political), such a dialogue hardly ever took place. Philosophy certainly is not the thing that the psychiatrist or clinical psychologist likes to do or feels that she or he should do. Without any special training in philosophy and lacking a clear idea of what it is all about, he or she may rather only feel anxious or embarrassed by the fact that other specialties claim to have something to say about psychopathological matters. Philosophers, on the other hand, tend to follow a trend that has long been present in the sciences: they tens to specialize and to become increasingly technical in their language so that the philosophical layman, the psychiatrist or psychologist, may not be able to understand what they say. The virtually omnipresent push 'away from psychopathology, towards biology' scarcely needs to be added to the picture in order to show that a dialogue between philosophers and psychopathologists seems to be even more unlikely at present than in the past.

However, people who do clinical work are more than ever before strongly opposed to biological reductionism and psychological operationalism. They feel a strong need to say and to think more about the patient, but they desire to do so neither only in terms of "objective" scales and scores, which seem to sacrifice meaning for reliability, nor in terms of biological markers, which seem to largely reduce the patient to a "piece of biological machinery" which happens to be somehow malfunctioning. While we are far from being opposed to measurement or biological research, we see that neither field adequately construes what is happening clinically. Matters of clinical psychopathology must not be regarded as fundamentally irrational (i.e., as rational *only insofar* as they can be translated into scoresor as yet undiscovered biological markers), and they should not be left as a subject only for those obscure, mystic and mystifying theories which are always ready to fill the gap. Moreover, philosophical clarification may not only be the desire of clinicians but also could soon become a more common goal among biologically oriented researchers. Certainly, as long as there seems to be an inverse correlation between the degree of sophistication of the methods applied to the brain and the degree of sophistication of the methods by which the pathology of the mind (which still defines what the research as a whole is about) is assessed, biological research is stuck with data that seem not to mean very much.

Yet, there are several signs on the horizon for a stronger mutual interest, and even a dialogue. Whereas in the fifty year period from approximately 1880 until 1930, during which psychiatry was shaped into the form it still largely holds, some version of phenomenology was the only philosophy that was recognized as concerned with "the mental", and as a fertile source for psychopathology. This is no longer the case. At present, in addition to phenomenology, there is a variety of theoretical frameworks to account for the mental, including "philosophy of mind", "transcendental philosophy", and "philosophy of subjectivity", to name but a few. Moreover, the approaches are no longer totally separated; parallels are discovered and discussed, and the general approach is undogmatically pluralistic.

This volume contains articles about philosophy and psychopathology that were presented at a meeting at the Department of Psychology, Harvard University, in October 1989. Philosophers, clinical psychologists, and psychiatrists from West–Germany and the United States met to discuss *Philosophical Issues in Psychopathology*, as the meeting was titled. It was the second meeting of this kind; the first took place at the Philosophy

Department of the University of Freiburg in July 1988.[1] Both meetings represented efforts to facilitate a discussion between specialists of different fields on topics of common interest.

That there are such topics and that such a discussion is needed is beyond question. Nevertheless, a cross–national comparison shows striking differences in the typical approach to, and reception of, such efforts at cross–fertilization. While such exchanges have some tradition in German psychiatry, they are of a more pioneering character in the United States. Further, whereas interest in philosophical matters in German psychiatry tends now to be regarded as an outmoded and non–rewarding enterprise that is mainly concerned with historical questions and hardly at all with clinical problems, and whereas the already limited number of philosophically interested psychiatrists in Germany is decreasing, interest in philosophy among American psychiatrists seems to be growing and to be extending to an increasing number of individuals. In fact, the *Group for the Advancement of Philosophy and Psychiatry* was initiated in the United States last year, and our meeting took place in an optimistic and encouraging spirit. We hope that this volume conveys some of that spirit to the reader.

We would like to thank a number of people who helped in the preparation of this symposium and this book: Wilma Koutstaal, Philip Daly, and especially Beatrix Spitzer M.D. The Springer Verlag Heidelberg gave good advice in recommending Springer New York for the publication of this volume. This work was supported in part by a Feodor Lynen grant from the Alexander–von–Humboldt Foundation.

Cambridge MA
January 1990

Manfred Spitzer
Brendan A. Maher

---

1 The contributions of the 1988 meeting have been published in a previous volume, entitled *Psychopathology and Philosophy* (M. Spitzer et al., eds., Springer, Berlin, Heidelberg, New York, London, Tokyo, 1988).

Contents

Contributors

Hector–Neri Castañeda, Ph. D.
The Mahlon Powell Prof. of Philosophy
Department of Philosophy
Indiana University
Bloomington, Indiana 47405, USA
The 1989 Tinbergen Prof. of Philosophy
Erasmus Universiteit Rotterdam
The Netherlands

Frank Döring
Department of Philosophy
Princeton University
Princeton, New Jersey 08544, USA

Hinderk M. Emrich, Prof. Dr. med.
Max–Planck–Institut für Psychiatrie
Kraepelinstraße 10
8000 München 40, FRG

Mathias Fünfgeld, Dipl. Psych.
Psychiatrische Universitätsklinik
Hauptstraße 5
7800 Freiburg, FRG

Anne Harrington, Ph. D.
Assistant Professor
History of Science Department
Science Center 235
Harvard University
Cambridge, Massachusetts 02138, USA

Paul Hoff, Dr. med. Dr. phil.
Psychiatrische Klinik der Universität
Nußbaumstraße 7
8000 München 2, FRG

Edward Hundert, M. D.
Director of Postgraduate and
Continuing Medical Education
McLean Hospital
Mill Street 115
Belmont, Massachusetts 02178, USA

Julian Jaynes, Ph. D.
Prof. of Psychology
Department of Psychology
Princeton University
Princeton, New Jersey 08544, USA

Peter Klein, Prof. Dr. phil.
Fachbereich Erziehungswissenschaft
der Universität
Von–Melle–Park 8
2000 Hamburg 13, FRG

Brendan A. Maher, Ph. D.
Edward C. Henderson Prof. of the
Psychology of Personality
William James Hall
Harvard University
Cambridge, Massachusetts 02138, USA

Alfred Margulies, M. D.
Director of Out Patient Services and
Director of Medical Student Education
The Cambridge Hospital
Department of Psychiatry at the
Harvard Medical School
1493 Cambridge Street
Cambridge, Massachusetts 02139, USA

Steven Matthysse, Ph. D.
Mailman Research Center
McLean Hospital
Mill Street 115
Belmont Massachusetts 02178, USA

Christoph Mundt, Prof. Dr. med.
Direktor
Psychiatrische Klinik der Universität
Voßstraße 4
6900 Heidelberg, FRG

Georg Northoff
Universities of Essen and Bochum
Bredebgrund 6
2104 Hamburg 92, FRG

Godehard Oepen, PD Dr. med.
Harvard Medical School
Metropolitan State Hospital and
Cambridge Hospital
475 Trapelo Road
Waltham, Massachusetts 02254, USA

Joseph F. Rychlak, Ph. D.
Department of Psychology
Loyola University of Chicago
6525 Sheridan Road,
Chicago, Illinois 60626, USA

Michael Alan Schwartz, M. D.
Clinical Professor of Psychiatry
St. Vincent's Hospital
New York Medical College
153 West 11th Street, 3E
New York, New York 10011, USA

Manfred Spitzer, Dr. med. habil. Dr. phil.
Visiting Associate Professor
Department of Psychology
William James Hall 1520
Harvard University
Cambridge, Massachusetts 02138, USA

Friedrich A. Uehlein, Prof. Dr. phil.
Philosophische Fakultät II
Bismarckplatz
8520 Erlangen, FRG

Osborne P. Wiggins, Ph. D.
Department of Philosophy
University of Louisville
Louisville, Kentucky 40292, USA

Introduction

Why Philosophy?

Manfred Spitzer

1. Problems in Contemporary Psychiatry

For at least two and a half thousand years, philosophers have thought about the mind and its functions. If we are to say anything reasonable about disorders of the mind and its functions, we cannot disregard philosophy.

This may be the shortest way of saying why it makes sense for the psychiatrist and clinical psychologist to take a philosophical stance, i.e., to apply philosophical reasoning to their field. By "philosophical reasoning" we do not mean any particular philosopher or philosophy, but rather a critical attitude towards one's concepts and (often unspoken) assumptions, an attitude that might thus be characterized by both the mirroring and the thinking connotations of the term *reflection*: thinking critically about what one is thinking and doing.

That psychiatry needs such philosophical reflection can easily be shown by pointing to a sample of contradictions, misconceptions, and obvious faults, in short, by pointing to "cracks" in what appears to be the nicely polished theoretical surface of present day psychiatry. On a large scale, examples of such issues are:

—While internal medicine has realized that myocardial infarction is more than a disease of blood-vessels in a muscle (i.e., that the diagnosis and prognosis of this disease cannot be adequately accounted for in only these physiological terms), psychiatry, on the contrary, turns from the schizophrenic person to the "broken brain".[1]

—While philosophers of science have pointed out convincingly that no science can be conceived as being just about pure data and theoretical accounts of such data (i.e., that logical empiricism, the idea that science is nothing but empirical facts and logic, is wrong), nonetheless psychiatry tries to become such a science.

—While in psychology the idiographic approach, and especially in neuropsychology, the case study is one of the most powerful means by which to arrive at new hypotheses about the mind and the way it functions,

1 I am indebted to Michael Schwartz, M.D., not only for this suggestion, but also for a critical reading of a previous version of this paper and his suggestions for improving it. Deficiencies that remain are entirely my own responsibility. This work has been supported by a Feodor Lynen grant from the Alexander–von–Humboldt foundation.

such approaches have been dismissed dogmatically as "unscientific" in the field of psychiatry.[2]

On a more intermediate scale, the following shortcomings of present day psychiatric theory may be stated:

—The criterial approach to diagnosis, as it is implemented in the *Diagnostic and Statistical Manual of Mental Disorders, revised third edition* (DSM–III–R) does not correspond to the way that clinicians actually make diagnoses (cf. Schwartz and Wiggins 1987a,b).

—In addition, the DSM–III–R's approach to personality disorders seems to be inadequate (what does it mean, for instance, to suffer from three different personality disorders?).

—The wide use of "rating scales" and "scores" implies a kind of scientific exactness that is simply not present when a person is "rated" by another person. Thus, while psychologists have long recognized that the mere number denoted by an IQ (although being the result of several tests rather than of one rating) says very little about an individual person, mere numbers are called for in the assessment of life-events or global functioning in the DSM–III–R. This approach fails to do justice to the complexity of human life, and while we agree that whatever can be measured, should be measured, we also claim that it is potentially harmful to pretend to be able to measure the unmeasurable.

Finally, on a small scale, a look at the way psychopathological phenomena—i.e., the very matter psychiatrists deal with all the time—are conceived and defined, reveals even more notable pitfalls:

—Delusions are defined as "false beliefs", yet their truth sometimes can never be determined, sometimes is in practice not determinable, and, even in rare cases is determinable, but such that the state of affairs to which the delusion refers is in fact true. Religious delusions in some textbooks are defined as "false religious beliefs"—an obvious nonsense. Delusions are further defined as "based on incorrect inference". However, whether delusions are the result of any kind of inference has yet to be determined; in addition, making "incorrect inferences" is a matter of formal thought, and the types of delusions that are common in schizophrenia seem not to deal with the external world but with (internal) experiences of control or reference. The inconsistencies are striking.

—Thought disorder is defined in many ways which not only are confusing but also point to many different mechanisms that might be involved but can hardly be assessed by the use of the actual concept.

—Hallucinations are defined as perceptions without adequate stimuli although most patients can distinguish their perceptions from their hallucinations. Furthermore, it is left unclear what "inadequate stimuli" might be, and it is questionable whether it is appropriate to refer to stimuli when talking about perception in the absence of any experimental framework

---

2 On scientific grounds, this is completely incomprehensible. Only political and historical reasons can possibly account for this state of affairs (see below).

("stimulus" is a highly theoretical construct that makes sense only in a specific framework; there are no stimuli as such).

—In short, the definitions of delusions, hallucinations and thought disorder, i.e., of some of the core symptoms in psychiatry, make little sense clinically. Needless to say, the definitions of other symptoms are questionable as well.

We could go on enumerating examples on the various levels, but we think that by now it is clear that there is something wrong with present day psychiatry, something that is not just a minor issue that could be resolved by introducing some changes here and there, but something rather serious and profound. Let us therefore turn to some of the reasons for a number of the misconceptions and pitfalls, and examine them more closely.[3]

2. The Cradle of Psychopathology

Many authors have pointed out that the beginning of scientific psychopathology is marked by the appearance of Karl Jaspers' *General Psychopathology* in 1913.[4] Although Kraepelin had shaped the *nosological* distinctions in a way that has stood the test of time up to the present, and although Freud is generally given credit for the first comprehensive *psychological* account of pathological phenomena, both authors did not greatly concern themselves with the very nature of those phenomena itself. In other words: the question of what disorder is characterized by specific symptoms (e.g. hallucinations and delusions) had been addressed by Kraepelin; the question of how hallucinations and delusions might originate from the interaction of intrapsychic entities had been addressed by Freud. But the remaining question of how symptoms in the mental realm can be established at all, i.e., of how to define properly such symptoms as hallucinations and delusions, was addressed by Jaspers.

The contribution of Karl Jaspers to psychiatric theory can easily be shown by the fact that many concepts of present day psychiatry, such as the concepts of hallucinations and delusions, mood–congruent versus mood–incongruent symptoms, to name but a few, can be traced back to his ideas, as we will show briefly in the following sections.

---

3 What follows is an elaboration of parts of my introductory remarks to the volume which contains the contributions of the first conference of this kind (cf. Spitzer 1988b), where further references to the present topic can be found.

4 See the comments on his *General Psychopathology* by Bumke (1914), Kurt Schneider (1938) and Kunz (1948). More recently Schmitt (1979, 1983) has stressed the same topic. The *General Psychopathology* appeared in 9 editions, the last of which has been issued in 1973. An English translation appeared in 1963. It must be emphasized that the authors did not use the term "scientific" to indicate that Jaspers carried out experiments in the tradition of German Psychology, that had been established by Wilhelm Wundt. The authors rather had in mind that Jaspers was the first to question the basic concepts of psychiatry such as disturbed perception and thought, and tried to provide a more basic reason for their use in psychiatry.

2.1 Hallucinations

Before 1838, the term "hallucination"—originally meaning "to wander in mind"—did not have any clear meaning. That is why the French psychiatrist Esquirol was able to redefine the concept in a technical way that could be used by psychiatrists from then on. "Anyone who is convinced of having perceived a sensation, although no outer object which could have excited this sensation was within the reach of the sense, is in a state of hallucination: he is a visionary" (Esquirol 1838, 159, transl. by the author, M.S.). Note that Esquirol does not talk about *a* hallucination, but rather of a "state of hallucination", i.e., he does not refer to a single symptom, *a* perception without an object. Moreover, the resemblance of hallucinations to perception was the subject of debate among the psychiatrists of the last century. It was Jaspers who established the view that there are individual mental symptoms, and that hallucinations are like perceptions.

He did this in coining the term "corporeality" ("Leibhaftigkeit"), which he defined as the "immediate sense of reality" (Jaspers 1963a, pp. 199ff), and which he used to characterize perception as opposed to mere imagery. According to Jaspers, "hallucinations proper", like perceptions, are to be characterized by their corporeality. Thus, Jaspers claimed that the sense of reality that is conveyed by hallucinations is not a result of judgement, but of the immediate impression of the hallucination itself, which "feels" entirely like a true perception. As can be seen by referring to the definition of hallucinations that can be found in the glossary of the DSM–III–R, his ideas were completely adopted: "Hallucination. A sensory perception without external stimulation of the relevant sensory organ. A hallucination has the immediate sense of reality of a true perception..." (DSM–III–R, p. 398).

2.2 Delusions

As with hallucinations, the DSM–III–R definition of delusions can easily be traced back to Jaspers, whose three famous "criteria" of delusions— certainty, incorrigibility, and falsity—are mentioned in its very first sentence: "Delusion. A false personal belief based on incorrect inference about external reality and firmly sustained in spite of what everyone else believes and in spite of what constitutes incontrovertible and obvious proof or evidence to the contrary" (DSM–III–R, p. 395). Although these criteria can be found in the writings of authors preceeding Jaspers, he was the first who stated (and also critisized) these criteria, who defined delusions as judgements and as some form of meaning, and who distinguished delusions clearly from other phenomena of mental ilness such as hallucinations, uncontrollable imagery and the like.

2.3 Mood–Congruence

In the DSM–III–R, mood-congruent psychotic features are defined as "delusions or hallucinations whose content is entirely consistent with either a depressed or manic mood", while "inconsistency" is the mark of "mood-incongruent" psychotic features (DSM-III-R, pp. 401, 402). This distinction not only directly reflects a distinction made by Jaspers in his *General Psychopathology*, but it also was originally stated more clearly by him.

The issue in question is the relation of different aspects of the mental to one another, in this case between perception and thought on the one hand, and affect or emotion (or mood) on the other hand. Jaspers rightly points out, that it is a specific way of understanding that is going on if we are to relate these aspects. Whenever we attempt to come to grips with the emergence of certain perceptions and thoughts from the basis of certain emotions, we try to understand the *genesis* of the perceptions and thoughts in terms of underlying affect. Therefore we think that Jaspers is right in calling the action that is performed by the psychiatrist who assesses those relations *genetic understanding*. "In some cases ... we understand directly how one psychic event emerges from another" (Jaspers 1963d, p. 27). "Psychic events 'emerge' out of each other in a way which we understand... The way in which such an emergence takes place is understood by us, *our understanding is genetic*" (Jaspers 1963d, p. 302, his italics).

The problem with the terminology as found in the DSM–III–R is that—contrary to Jaspers' efforts—it does not make clear how "congruence" is assessed. Although the glossary seems to solve this problem by simply defining which contents are "consistent" with depression and with mania, respectively, in clinical practice the problem is not that easy. In many cases, determining what the prevailing theme of delusions or hallucinations is, remains a matter of interpretation, and serious attempts to "understand" the relations between mood and the content of thought have to be made. Thus the notion of "congruence"—otherwise familiar from the geometry of triangles—to us seems to be either the wrong, or at least a misleading, metaphor for what is going on or should go on clinically. To conclude: Mood–congruence is not only an issue that had been emphasized by Jaspers for the first time, it is also obvious that Jaspers was well ahead of DSM–III–R in terms of clarity and clinical practicability.

3. The Problems Jaspers had to Face

Jaspers wanted to make *the patient and his symptoms* the center of interest rather than biological theories about the function of the brain—as much a fashion in the days of Jaspers as at present.[5] He strongly opposed attempts to

---

5 Again, it should be stressed that Jaspers neither aimed at a new classification (as Kraepelin did) nor at a theory of intrapsychic entities and their interaction (as Freud did). Nevertheless, both theories (of

reduce mental symptoms to speculations about brain structures or functions and called for conceptual strictness in psychopathology. As he was
also critical of psychoanalysis, when he entered psychiatry, he perceived that
the choice was only "between 'brain mythology' and the 'mythology of
psychoanalysis'" (Spiegelberg 1972, p. 181). In his autobiography, Jaspers
describes the situation of psychiatry as he saw it as follows:

"Frequently, the same things were discussed in different terms, in most cases in a
very obscure manner. Several schools had each its own terminology. It seemed as if
several languages were being spoken... There seemed to be no such thing as a common
scientific psychiatry uniting all those engaged in psychiatric research. During the
regular demonstrations of patients and the discussions among physicians I sometimes
had the impression as if we were always beginning all over again; then again that we
merely subsumed the particular facts under a few miserable generic types; whereas at
other times it would seem to me that what had already been said was constantly being
forgotten. As often as I was pleased with what I had learned, just as often it seemed to
me that no progress was being made. I felt as if I were living in a world of an insur-
veyable variety of ways of looking at things, which were at our disposal in chaotic
disorder, yet each one of which individually was of an intolerable simplicity. Psychiatrists must learn to think, I once opined in a group of physicians. 'Jaspers ought to be
spanked,' Ranke remarked with a friendly smile" (Jaspers 1957/1981, p. 17).

With this background—a background that sounds remarkably similar
to the current state of affairs—Jaspers set out to clarify the field of psychiatry: "In my psychopathology the object was to bring to conceptually clear
consciousness what one knows, how one knows it, and what one does not
know" (Jaspers 1957/1981, p. 19). Jaspers adopted phenomenology as an
empirical method and described in detail various symptoms of mental
disorder. "Not only hallucinations, but also delusions, modes of ego-
consciousness, and emotions could, on the basis of the patient's own
descriptions, be described so clearly that they became recognizable with
certainty in other cases. Phenomenology became a method for research"
(Jaspers 1957/1981, p. 18). From these quotations it is clear what
phenomenology was for Jaspers and what it was not. It was *not* Husserlian
phenomenology which (in the *Logical Investigations*, i.e., the part of
Husserl's work Jaspers is referring to) aims at general features of consciousness and its intentional acts, such as their objectifying, unifying, relating
and constituting functions in intending objects.

Phenomenology, rather, was an "empirical method", implemented to
counter the many "theories" about the mental which had been found to be
largely useless, and to be an obstacle to clarity and truth in the field. Here
we see the motivation for the goal of mere and pure description:
"Everywhere I fought against mere talk without real knowledge, especially
against the 'theories' which played such a big role in psychiatric language"
(Jaspers 1957/1981, p. 18). This is—in short—the origin of the notion of

Kraepelin and Freud) presuppose (although this is denied by some Freudians) a clear understanding of
what the symptoms of the patient are: We can neither classify a patient (i.e., make a diagnosis) nor
speculate concerning intrapsychic mechanisms, if we do not know what is wrong with him in the first
place. At the beginning of this century, Jaspers certainly was the psychiatrist who saw this problem
most clearly and devoted much of his work to its solution.

"phenomenology" in psychopathology. To most psychiatrists up to the present time, the term means nothing but *detailed description*. In fact, the "phenomenologists"—i.e., various (mainly) German speaking psychiatrists—have little in common with each other apart from the fact that they all sought to describe patients in detail; their success in this endeavour is evidenced by their case descriptions which, even today, are amongst the best available.[6]

There remains a problem, however, if one is to describe something: any description makes use of concepts; when I describe the piece of paper in front of me, for example, as white and rectangular, I have to have the notions of color and angle as well as notions of specific types of color and angle "at hand". We hardly see a problem here, because these notions seem so familiar to us that we do not wonder where they came from. If we are to describe in a scientific way what is going on in the mind of another person, however, we cannot simply rely on ordinary language and its expressions, because it may be vague or inappropriate, and full of misconceptions or hidden theories. The problem that Jaspers faced, therefore, was this: we have to find a way to develop concepts that can be used to describe the mind of other people without falling back on all the "theories" about the mind; in Jaspers' own words: "how do we get to the isolation, characterization and conceptual determination of mental phenomena?" (Jaspers 1963, p. 318). One thing seems to be clear: You cannot do this by description because what you are actually looking for are the very means you use to describe.

Jaspers saw this problem and combined it with another, related one: At his time medicine, which was based on the description of bodily symptoms, was quite advanced and had made considerable progress, visible to everyone in the field. Psychiatry, on the other hand, seemed to suffer from the fact that in the realm of the mental there were no clear–cut symptoms. In order to have (what at present is called) the "medical model" work in psychiatry, symptoms had to be established as in organic medicine. For both problems—(1) how to get to the concepts to describe other minds and (2) how to get to something like symptoms in psychiatry—Jaspers offered a solution: phenomenology. Of course, this had to be something other than "mere description of symptoms", as the very concept of a symptom as well as the variety of the distinct symptoms had to be derived. We have already pointed out that Husserlian phenomenology is more than "mere description" but rather aims at generalities (at "the essence of things", in Husserlian terms). Nevertheless, when Jaspers stated that "as method I adopted Husserl's phenomenology..." (Jaspers 1957/1981, p. 18),

---

6 Case studies are in no way unscientific or useless, as many present day psychiatrists may think. One does not have to refer to neuropsychology, which obviously relies heavily on case studies, but can also point to psychiatric knowledge that has been acquired by case studies. We know, for example, that cases of paranoid disorder do not necessarily deteriorate into "dementia" (as was supposed by Kraepelin) due to the detailed description of the Wagner case (cf. Gaupp 1914/1974a, 1938/1974b). Even if we only knew of that one case (though needless to say, there are other cases), we still would know that there is no *necessary* connection between paranoia and schizophrenia.

he meant just description and nothing else.[7] He rejected any phenomeno-logical aim of generalities while he still faced the task of finding the general concepts he wanted to use for description. Therefore, the problem was set up in a way that had to lead into difficulties. These can clearly be shown by looking at Jaspers' actual solution, namely, the way he carried out a phenomenological *analysis*, which was, for him, the main tool of his kind of phenomenology.

4. Phenomenological Analysis—Claims and Reality

"The task of phenomenology is to clearly bring to mind the mental states that are really experienced by the patients, to see what aspects they might have in common, to differentiate and to distinguish them and to denote them with fixed terms" (Jaspers 1973, p. 47).

In his article on *The Phenomenological Research Strategy in Psychopathology*[8], Jaspers rightly delineated, what phenomenology is *not*: (a) It is not about "personal, immediate experience which cannot be formulated in words" (Jaspers 1963c, p. 316), not about the "psychiatrist with empathy, who becomes absorbed in the patient without any concepts", because "knowledge only consists in psychological determina-tion". (b) Jaspers points to negative effects that theories about brain func-tioning may have on the description of mental activities: "We have to dis-regard... traditional theories, psychological constructs and materialistic myths about brain processes". (c) "Phenomenology does *not* have anything to do with the question of how mental phenomena come into being" (Jaspers 1963c, p. 317).

In his attempt to answer positively the question of how to get to symp-toms in the realm of the mind Jaspers mentions the concept of *analysis*. "The intended use of the resulting elements of an analysis is merely to enable the psychiatrist to *definitely characterize and securely differentiate* mental processes as they really are" (Jaspers 1963b, p. 194, his italics). Jaspers very clearly distinguishes between *analysis* and *explanation*: we explain how perceptions come into being physiologically; the products of an analysis of perception, however, are aspects or components which are of no use in explaining the origin of a perception. The components of perception, rather, have a justificatory function: If I am asked whether I am sure that I see a red rose, I may refer to sensations of red to justify my claim. In doing so, I do not explain how this perception came into being. By the same token, I may refer to those aspects in order to describe perceptions. In this case I also do not refer to the question of how they came into being.

---

7 One can only speculate about the reasons, why Jaspers did that. Maybe it was because Husserl himself was not so clear about his method in the first edition of his *Logical Investigations*.
8 *Die Phänomenologische Forschungsrichtung in der Psychopathologie*, first published in 1912, reprinted in Jaspers 1963.

"Explanation is totally different from analysis. Explanation operates with theoretical processes which are not conscious... What analysis separates did not originate out of the constituents that had been the results of analysis" (Jaspers 1963b, pp. 193-194).

However, Jaspers does not explicitly say how an analysis should be carried out.[9] Therefore, the meaning of this term may best be understood by looking at the way Jaspers carries out such an analysis. He does so in his article *On the Analysis of False Perceptions*[10], where he attempts to analyze perception phenomenologically in order to get to the means he needs to describe perception and its disorders, i.e., hallucinations, illusions, and pseudohallucinations. He uses various rather unexpected concepts such as "corporeality", "act", "character of objectivity", "subjective space", "sensory element" etc. when he portrays these symptoms (see § 1 of chapter 1 of the *General Psychopathology*, pp. 60–79). How does Jaspers analyze perception? How does he arrive at the concepts he needs to describe perceptual disorders in detail?

He starts as follows: "At first there is the old and familiar knowledge that each perception can be analyzed into final elements which are called sensations" (Jaspers 1963b, p. 194). Jaspers says that sensations are "the most simple things in the world" (p. 205), distinguishing "primary" sensations (caused by external stimuli) and "secondary" sensations (not caused by external stimuli), and thus obviously has in mind a concept that was in fashion in the German psychology of his time (i.e. the beginning of the 20th century). In addition to "the group of sensations... we may mention spatial and temporal qualities as a second group of phenomenologically final elements of perception" (Jaspers 1963b, p. 195). Here Jaspers also speaks of the intuition [Anschauung] of space and time and thus refers to Kant. A third element of perception for Jaspers are the acts, which he specifies as "ways of intending" [Weisen des Meinens].

The discrepancies between the claims made in, and the actual status of, Jaspers' analysis are obvious: *Sensations* do not have the status of an "old and familiar knowledge"; the concept is rather subject to a ongoing debate (see Gregory 1987; Neumann 1972). Moreover, in mentioning sensations, Jaspers simply adopts what was fashionable in his time and thus does not clarify how he arrived at these "elements". Nevertheless, Jaspers means this to be the analysis. In addition, he says that he has found sensations within perception "phenomenologically" and by "immediate observation". This contradicts what he said about the components of perception, as they are "not given as isolated". He also would not have needed an analysis if the elements of perception had been perceivable (which by his own definition they are not). A further contradiction between his analysis, and what he

---

9 Jaspers negatively determines how an analysis is not carried out: "We analyze perception. What does analysis mean? It does not mean that we look for the elements in perception which bring perception into being. We cannot really divide perception in these elements or find isolated elements which somehow interact and produce perception. These isolated elements are never given to us, given to us is the whole complete perception" (Jaspers 1963b, p. 193).
10 *Zur Analyse der Trugwahrnehmungen*, first published in 1911, reprinted in Jaspers 1963.

says of that analysis can be shown in his distinction between primary and secondary sensations: this distinction is made with respect to cause and genesis, which had been explicitly excluded as matters of phenomenological analysis. The second group of elements of perception—spatial and temporal qualities—is introduced by the words "we may mention" (p. 195). Again, no "analysis" had been carried out, not even a short comment had been made. All we can say is that the second element is brought forward by an allusion to Kant (who referred to the spatial and temporal material of intuition, whereas Jaspers speaks of the spatial and temporal material of sensation). The acts or "ways of intending" are also just mentioned and are taken from Husserl's Phenomenology but are in no way the result of an analysis.[11]

The use that Jaspers makes of the acts in dealing with false perceptions gives further clues to his approach. In order to distinguish perception from imagery, he introduces the term "corporeality", saying that it meant a "way of objectively intending" (Jaspers 1963b, p. 214). He does not clarify this concept[12], and a close look at the way he introduces it instead reveals that he is *defining arbitrarily* (while still pretending to phenomenologically analyze). He does so in making use of an ambiguity of the German word "erklären" which means "to explain" (etwas *durch* etwas erklären: to explain something by means of something), but also "to declare" (etwas *für* etwas erklären: to declare something as something). When he says that perception can be *declared* as a way of objectively intending, the German reader who is not aware of what is going on may overlook (and many have in fact overlooked) the definitional rather than explanatory character of his account.

It is by definition that every hallucination comes with "the immediate sense of reality of a true perception" (DSM–III–R, p. 398), and by definition perception itself comes with that.—But does it?

As Kurt Goldstein already pointed out in 1908 (and as has been noted since then by many psychologists) there is no intrinsic quality in a perception that qualifies it as a perception (as opposed to mere imagery). Many such features have in fact been proposed (vividness, clarity, uncontrollability, passivity, etc.), but none proved to be flawless. Moreover, it has been shown by experimental psychology, that perception and imagery may easily

---

11 It might be argued that Jaspers did not mean to fully carry out an analysis but rather only pointed out the results. One passage in his *On the Analysis of False Perceptions* (Jaspers 1963b, p. 194) may be read in favor of that view: "Our analysis of perception which is to follow now necessarily is a very brief and rough review of psychological results, which we think are true. The reasons we give obviously can only make plausible our claims." In a footnote, he adds: "The real and mandatory reasons for [the assumption of] sensation–elements can be found in Wundt's Physiological Psychology, for the acts and the whole idea of the analysis [Zergliederung] the reasons can be found in Husserl's phenomenological analyses (*Logical Investigations*, Halle 1901). A comprehensive and clearly organized Account is given by Messer, *Sensation and Thought*, Leipzig 1908." From the two quotes it can be seen clearly that our argument is still valid: Jaspers again refers to physiology (Wundt) although he had ruled out physiology as an issue of analysis. His reference to Husserl is hardly anything but "lip service", and the reference to Messer's "armchair psychology" confirms our view that Jaspers was just referring to concepts that had been in fashion in those days.
12 For being unclear in this respect, Jaspers has already been criticized by Goldstein in 1913 and by Schröder in 1915.

be confused by normal subjects. Additionally, physiology has shown that both, perception and imagery make use of basically the same mental processes and functions (not to mention some structures). In short: There are no scientific grounds to justify the assumption that "true perception" provides any "immediate sense of reality". The fact that this assumption can be found in the DSM–III–R glossary, however, shows the still strong influence of Jasperian thought.

It is obvious that Jaspers is confused by his own terminology, especially by the two meanings of "phenomenology": On the one hand he distinguishes between (1) "detailed description" and (2) "finding the concepts in order to do so", but on the other hand he does not have a clear idea of the second meaning. For that reason, he does not succeed in providing the necessary concepts to describe false perceptions. Moreover, his characterization of his own analysis is inconsistent with what he actually does. The lack of a clear notion of phenomenology also led him to overlook the problems of his "analysis".

To summarize: Jaspers claims to perform a phenomenological analysis of perception, but instead, he

—refers to physiology and to the genesis of perception,

—refers to questionable, popular theories,

—defines arbitrarily, while maintaining that he is describing free of any theory.

On a second level of interpretation, a further contradiction has to be added to the contradictions between the claims and facts of his analysis. Jaspers would insist on (and has been given much credit for) methodological clarity. He blamed other psychopathologists for "hovering between the actual experience, theory and philosophy and the penetrating as well as exasperating character of such confusions" (Jaspers 1963d, p. 779), yet in the case of our example, it is clear that he was not aware of his method when he was carrying out a phenomenological analysis. He was *not* aware of his actual method when he purportedly was undertaking a phenomenological analysis.

Notice that we do *not* criticize Jaspers for making presuppositions and referring to theories. We rather criticize that he, *contrary to what he really does, claims to proceed without presuppositions and without theories.* Furthermore, because Jaspers emphasizes method and requires a full appreciation and awareness of one's own method and procedure, this criticism has even to be made *on two levels.*

5. The Legacy of Karl Jaspers

Why do we bother about a German philosopher who has practiced psychiatry for only seven years at the very beginning of his career? The answer is: Our way of thinking in psychiatry is still heavily influenced by his ideas and concepts. In order to show this, we will look at some examples.

Prior to Jaspers, *hallucinations*—although defined as disorders in the realm of perception—had not been totally identified with perceptions. This identificationwas done by Jaspers, and remains part of out understanding of hallucinations up to the present. Nevertheless, this definition not only makes little sense in clinical settings[13], it also has been found to be nearly useless by almost any researcher who has investigated hallucinations empirically, whether in the field of experimental psychosis, sensory deprivation, electrical brain stimulation, hypnosis or whatever (cf. Spitzer 1988). Why, we must ask, can it be, that such an obviously useless definition "survived"? The answer is simple, because it is for the same reason that already led Jaspers to establish such a definition: hallucinations are defined as they are for the sake and simplicity of the medical approach to mental disorder. That is to say, the need for symptoms in the field of psychiatry generated and still maintains concepts that cannot withstand close scrutiny. (In fact, the scrutiny does not even have to be very close.)

Delusions have *not* been defined by Jaspers. This is important to note because almost all definitions that can be found in current textbooks can be traced back to Jaspers and his famous three criteria: (1) certainty, (2) incorrigibility, and (3) falsity.[14] Nevertheless, Jaspers did not mean these features to be defining, he rather referred to them as "external characteristics" (Jaspers 1963d, p. 95).[15] The reasons he gives are mainly concerned with the third criterion: as delusions sometimes cannot be called false (because the issues in question are religious or metaphysical ones), as falsity may sometimes be not an issue in diagnosing delusions (in cases where empirical counterevidence cannot be provided), and as delusions sometimes are true (Jaspers gave the example of delusions of jealousy which should not depend on the behavior of the spouse), falsity cannot be a defining criterion of delusions. Jaspers does not make any attempt to solve the problem. He calls delusions a "primordial phenomenon" (Urphänomen) and leaves us in the dark as to what to think about that. However, the reasons Jaspers gives against using falsity as a defining criterion aremain valid, and we still, therefore, have to search for an adequate definition.

Up to the present Jaspers has been criticized for his distinction between primary and secondary delusions, the former being not genetically related to any affect of the patient while the latter are conceived as derivable from some affect. It has been said that the distinction impedes

---

13 Jaspers had to invent another concept—pseudohallucinations—in order to account for most of the clinical phenomena. He borrowed the term from Hagen and gave it the meaning of "vivid imagery, almost like perception". Schröder (1915) was right in pointing out that little is gained by replacing a term that has been used for certain phenomena (i.e.: "hallucinations") by another term. Needless to say, almost all patients can distinguish their perceptions from their hallucinations, although not all can state how they do so (cf. Spitzer 1988a for a detailed discussion).

14 Cf. Jaspers 1973, p. 78, 1963d, pp. 95–96. The third criterion is also referred to as impossibility of content, but the context makes it clear that it was falsity (which is a weaker notion than impossibility), that Jaspers had in mind.

15 Moreover, we find: "To say simply that a delusion is a mistaken idea which is firmly held by the patient and which cannot be corrected gives only a superficial and incorrect answer to the problem. Definition will not dispose of the matter" (Jaspers 1963d, p. 93). The view that delusions cannot be defined is still to be found in most of the German psychiatric textbooks.

empirical research on the role of affect in the formation of delusions and therefore should be abandoned. If this criticism is valid then it is also true of the mood–congruent versus mood–incongruent opposition, because this distinction reflects the same basic idea. At any rate, a solution by definition, as implied by the DSM–III–R definition of mood–congruence, seems to be the wrong way to settle the issue.

A *purely descriptive approach to psychopathology* was Jaspers' goal. As we have stated above, Jaspers thought of phenomenology as a method of description free of any theory. He *dismissed*—contrary to what he says elsewhere and contrary to what he is famous for—*philosophical* (and not only psychological and physiological!) theory as a means of psychopathological research: "Phenomenology cannot gain anything by theory but only lose" (Jaspers 1963b, p. 327). The "theories" he had in mind were speculations about brain malfunctioning ("brain myths", as he called them) and psychoanalysis, which he criticized for providing only "pseudounderstanding" of mental disorders.[16] In his attempt to get rid of any theory, Jaspers confused two different meanings of the concept of phenomenology, the philosophical meaning and the "ordinary medical language" meaning. It should have been clear to him that "pure description" cannot provide the means which pure description has to use.

6. Karl Jaspers and the DSM–III–R

By now it should be clear that the problems Jaspers was facing are the problems of psychiatry still. The reader who is not convinced may compare what Jaspers had said about the different languages of psychiatric theory in his account of the situation of psychiatry when he entered the field, with a short quote from the Introduction to the DSM–III–R (p. xxiii):

> "For example, Phobic Disorders are believed by many to represent a displacement of anxiety resulting from the breakdown of defense mechanisms that keep internal conflicts out of consciousness. Others explain phobias on the basis of learned avoidance responses to conditioned anxiety. Still others believe that certain phobias result from a dysregulation of basic biological systems mediating separation anxiety."

As we have pointed out, the DSM–III–R relies heavily on concepts that were first introduced, or at least refined, by Karl Jaspers. We also saw the shortcomings of his approach, which basically consisted of a radical dismissal of any theoretical concepts disguised as what he called "phenomenology".

What may be even more important to state is the fact that the DSM–III–R obviously relies on the same solution to the problems as Jaspers. It not only defines basic concepts along his lines (hallucinations as perceptions, delusions in terms of falsity, etc.), it also claims to be purely descrip-

---

16 Jaspers was not, as often wrongly stated, totally opposed to psychoanalysis but rather had a sophisticated view on Freud (see Jaspers 1963d, pp. 306f, 359–363, 373–378, 537–540, 773–775).

tive. Historically, that may be understood as a reaction to the quite uncritical application of Freudian ideas to psychiatry after the works of Freud had been translated and became widespread in the 1940s and 1950s. However, in pursuing its goal of pure description, and minimizing inference, respectively, the DSM–III–R—like Jaspers—is throwing out the baby with the bathwater.

Compared to Jaspers, who explicated his basic ideas in the 1910s, we are in a much better position to criticize any proposal for a purely descriptive approach because we can look back at the most outstanding and profound attempts to do so ever made, consisting in the contributions of *logical empiricism.* It has been shown that even such a "hard" science as physics cannot be understood just in terms of fact and logic. In respect to psychiatry and along the lines of arguments first made by positivists, several authors (cf. Faust and Miner 1986) have pointed out that the objective of pure description can neither be achieved, nor is it a desirable goal.

7. Why Philosophy?

How the mind should be conceived for the purposes of psychopathology, what its faculties, functions or elements are (if there are any), how these can be distinguished, and how mental disorders can be comprehended by an application of these concepts are philosophical questions. Issues like "types versus categories", "continua versus discrete entities" do not only denote methodological difficulties but also—and in the first place—philosophical problems. If there are no pure facts and if minimal inference is not necessarily a goal, how can we integrate psychopathology as a science with the other sciences that are applied in medicine? How can we avoid reductionistic views that always endanger psychiatry, especially young psychiatrists (who spend most of their time in the biochemical lab) and their relation to patients?

As we have seen, these problems are far from solved. From the general approach to specific symptoms, we need to rethink our presuppositions and unspoken assumptions. As we still use concepts that were mainly coined at the beginning of this century, we must not forget their historical roots in order not to make the same mistakes as our "conceptual ancestors", among whom Karl Jaspers is one of the most outstanding. Present psychopathology is shaped by Jaspers to a great extent, but we cannot rest on the shoulders of Jaspers if we want to avoid the traps that are necessarily lurking in the framework that was set up by him. This means that we have to take him seriously, as a philosopher and as a psychopathologist.

"If anyone thinks he can exclude philosophy and leave it aside as useless, he will be eventually defeated by it in some obscure form or another" (Jaspers 1963d, p. 770). The problems that Jaspers tried to solve are still our problems, but we can learn from his mistakes. In order to understand better than we do now, what hallucinations and delusions are, what psychopathology is about and how it can be the bedrock for psychiatry, not only since Jaspers, but for now and the future, philosophical thinking is inevitable for us. We have to take the burden!

Summary and Conclusion

We still use the concepts invented and clarified by Karl Jaspers, and the framework of psychopathology as it was set up by him. However, we not only profit from his achievements, but we also suffer from his mistakes. Only by a thorough examination of the assumptions we share with Jaspers, their criticism and—if necessary—their careful replacement, can we overcome the difficulties and problems we face. This goal can only be achieved by philosophical reasoning, which has to be carried out more carefully and more extensively than ever before in psychiatry.

References

American Psychiatric Association: Diagnostic and Statistical Manual of Mental Disorders, Third Edition, Revised. American Psychiatric Association, Washington, DC, 1987.

Bumke O: Allgemeine Psychopathologie (1914). In: Saner H (ed): Karl Jaspers in der Diskussion, pp. 11-13. Piper, München, 1973.

Esquirol, J: Des maladies mentales. Paris, 1838.

Faust D, Miner RA: The Empiricist and His New Clothes: DSM–III in Perspective. Am J Psychiat 143: 962–967, 1986.

Gaupp R: The Scientific Significance of the Case of Ernst Wagner (1914). In: Hirsch SR, Shepherd M, Kalinowsky LB (eds): Themes and Variations in European Psychiatry, pp. 121–133, 1974a.

Gaupp R: The Illness and Death of the Paranoid Mass Murderer, Schoolmaster Wagner:A Case History (1938). In: Hirsch SR, Shepherd M, Kalinowsky LB (eds): Themes and Variations in European Psychiatry, pp. 134–150, 1974b.

Goldstein K: Zur Theorie der Halluzinationen. Archiv für Psychiatrie 44: 584–655, 1036–1106, 1908.

Goldstein K: Weiter Bemerkungen zur Theorie der Halluzinationen. Zeitschrift für die Gesamte Neurologie und Psychiatrie 14: 502–544, 1913.

Gregory RL: Sensation. In Gregory RL (ed): The Oxford Companion to the Mind, pp. 700-701. Oxford University Press, Oxford, New York, 1987.

Husserl E: Logische Untersuchungen. Niemeyer, Tübingen, 1901 (2nd ed, 1913).

Jaspers K: Gesammelte Schriften zur Psychopathologie, Springer, Berlin, Göttingen, Heidelberg, 1963.

Jaspers K: Zur Analyse der Trugwahrnehmungen, (first published in 1911), reprinted in: Jaspers K: Gesammelte Schriften zur Psychopathologie, pp. 191–251, 1963a.

Jaspers K: Die Trugwahrnehmungen, (first published in 1912), reprinted in: Jaspers K: Gesammelte Schriften zur Psychopathologie, pp. 252–3313, 1963b.

Jaspers K: Die Phänomenologische Forschungsrichtung in der Psychopathologie, (first published in 1912), reprinted in: Jaspers K: Gesammelte Schriften zur Psychopathologie, pp. 314–328, 1963c.

Jaspers K: General Psychopathology (transl. Hoenig J, Hamilton MW), Manchester University Press, The University of Chicago Press, Manchester, Chicago, 1963d.

Jaspers K: Allgemeine Psychopathologie, 9th ed, Springer, Berlin, Heidelberg, New York, 1973.

Jaspers K: Philosophical Autobiography (1957). In: Schilpp PA (ed): The Philosophy of Karl Jaspers (The Library of Living Philosophers), augmented edition, pp. 3–94, Open Court, La Salle, Illinois, 1981.

Kunz H: Allgemeine Psychopathologie (1947). In: Saner H (ed): Karl Jaspers in der Diskussion, pp. 17-20. Piper, München, 1973.

Messer A: Empfindung un Denken (1908). Quelle und Meyer, Leipzig, 1924.

Neumann O: Empfindung. In: Ritter J (ed): Historisches Wörterbuch der Philosophie, Vol. 2, pp. 456–474, Wissenschaftliche Buchgesellschaft Darmstadt, 1972.

Schmitt W: Karl Jaspers und die Methodenfrage in der Psychiatrie. In: Janzarik W (ed): Psychopathologie als Grundlagenwissenschaft, pp. 74-82, Enke, Stuttgart, 1979.

Schmitt W: Die Psychopathologie von Karl Jaspers in der modernen Psychiatrie. In: Peters UH (ed.): Psychiatrie, Bd. 1, pp. 36-52, Beltz, Weinheim, 1983.

Schneider K: 25 Jahre 'Allgemeine Psychopathologie' von Karl Jaspers (1938). In: Saner H (ed): Karl Jaspers in der Diskussion, pp. 13-16. Piper, München, 1973.

Schröder P: Von den Halluzinationen. Monatsschrift für Psychiatrie und Neurologie 37: 1–11, 1915.

Schwartz MA, Wiggins, OP: Diagnosis and Ideal Types. A Contribution to Psychiatric Classification. Comprehensive Psychiatry 28: 277–291, 1987a.

Schwartz MA, Wiggins OP: Typifications. The First Step for Clinical Diagnosis in Psychiatry. J Nerv Ment Dis 175: 65-77, 1987b.

Spiegelberg H: Phenomenology in Psychology and Psychiatry. Northwestern University Press, Evanston, 1972.

Spitzer M: Halluzinationen. Springer, Berlin, Heidelberg, New York, London, Paris Tokyo, 1988a.

Spitzer M: Psychiatry, Philosophy, and the Problem of Description. In Spitzer M, Uehlein FA, Oepen G (eds): Psychopathology and Philosophy, pp. 3–18. Springer, Berlin, Heidelberg, New York, London, Paris Tokyo, 1988b.

Experience and Its Disturbances

Toward a Husserlian Phenomenology of the Initial Stages of Schizophrenia

Osborne P. Wiggins, Michael A. Schwartz, Georg Northoff

Dedicated to the memory of R.D. Laing

> *...the ontologically insecure person is preoc-*
> *cupied with preserving rather than gratifying*
> *himself: the ordinary circumstances of living*
> *threaten his low threshold of security.*
> Ronald D. Laing (1960, p. 42)

1. Introduction

Schizophrenic patients confront the psychiatrist with a wide array of extraordinary experiences. Such patients may assert that other people make their thoughts, actions, and desires. They can hallucinate voices which talk about them, commenting on their actions, praising and condemning them. They may complain that their thoughts and feelings are transparent to the world or insist that their bodies incarnate seemingly random features from the surrounding world. In order to explain experiences like these, psychiatrists have invoked terms and formulations such as ego weakness, ego boundary disturbance, ego pathology, depersonalization and derealization, and the breakdown or violation of the unity of the self (Spitzer 1988, pp. 167-183).

What, however, do these terms and formulations mean? We shall attempt to clarify the underlying features of these schizophrenic experiences by drawing on the phenomenology of Edmund Husserl. His philosophy contains, we think, analyses of human life that are rich enough to illuminate these remarkable experiences.

Husserl's phenomenology assigns primacy to *the constitutive functioning of mind* (Husserl 1973a, 1982). Mental life, for Husserl, constitutes both the world and itself as a part of the world (Husserl 1969, pp. 232-266). These constituted objects, the world and the worldly self, always refer back to something more fundamental, namely, a constituting subject which imputes meaning and being to them (Gurwitsch 1966, pp. 89-106). Husserl's philosophy then allows us to view early schizophrenia as a radical erosion of this constituting subject. As a result of the erosion of the constituting self, the entire constituted world begins to splinter and dissolve. And with the dissolution of the constituting self, the constituted self loses its cohesiveness and identity. The self-pathology that characterizes schizophrenia must be conceived from both of these perspectives: it consists in a disorder of the *constituting* self and, consequently, in a disorder of the *constituted* self. In our essay we shall briefly describe how the self constitutes itself. This will allow us to indicate how the self-disorders of schizophrenia reside in disorders of the self-constituted self.

In normal mental life, changes occur all the time, changes in the world and in oneself. What is constituted, then, is a continuously changing self and world. But these changes occur within limits; certain aspects of self and world do not change. In normal mental life certain aspects of self and world are experienced as invariant, as necessary for the very existence of self and world. We shall maintain that in the early stages of schizophrenia these invariant and necessary constituents of self and world are experienced as crumbling and evaporating. The invariant starts to vary; the impossible becomes actual; and the necessary grows deeply contingent. This is why we shall describe the early phases of schizophrenia as involving an "ontological crisis" for the patient: even the most fundamental components of self and world grow uncertain and unreliable.

We shall now sketch Edmund Husserl's view of the self. Our discussion will focus upon the ways in which mental life "constitutes" itself and things.

2. The Constitutive Function of Mental Life

As is well known, Husserl maintained that every mental process is *an awareness of something*. And he claimed, correlatively, that in order to understand fully an object of any sort, we must explicate the kinds of mental processes through which we are aware of the object (Gurwitsch 1964, pp. 280-306). This necessary relationship between mental processes and objects and between objects and mental processes Husserl called "intentionality" (Husserl 1982, pp. 171-235).

Intentive processes fall into two basic kinds: (1) active mental processes, and (2) passive or automatic mental processes. (1) Active mental processes are those which have an ego living in them. (2) Passive mental processes are those which have no ego living in them (Husserl 1973a pp. 77-81).

(1) An *active subject*, an *ego*[1], lives in *some* of the processes of mental life (Husserl 1973b, pp. 71-101).[2] Most of the intentive processes of mental life have no active subject living in them; the ego inhabits only a *part* of an individual mental life. The ego is the agent who attends to, focuses on, or

---

1 Throughout this abstract and our paper we employ the term "ego" exclusively in the Husserlian sense. The Husselian use of "ego" should in no way be associated with Freud's use of the same term.
2 We are here translating Husserl's German term *"Bewusstsein"* with the English phrase "mental life" rather than the more common "consciousness." We are doing so in order to avoid arousing in the reader's mind a contrast between "consciousness" and the "unconscious" or "unconsciousness." In Husserl's philosophy, a contrast between consciousness and the unconscious makes no sense (Husserl 1970, pp. 385-387).

thematizes objects (Husserl 1982, pp. 75-78). Thus those mental processes in which the ego is living are precisely the *thematizing* processes, those processes which *attend to* the "theme" of consciousness (Gurwitsch 1966, pp. 175-286). To call this subject "active" is to say that it voluntarily chooses to produce its mental processes. There are, therefore, certain intentive processes which would never arise in mental life if an ego did not choose to generate them. Examples of such necessarily egoic processes are our acts of speaking, reading, and reasoning. When Husserl uses the word "ego," he uses it only this sense. Husserl does not employ the term "ego" to refer to an individual mental life as a whole. In other words, "ego" and "mental life" *(Bewusstsein)* are not synonymous terms in Husserl's vocabulary (Husserl 1982, pp. 190-192). We shall henceforth employ the term "ego" exclusively in this strict Husserlian sense.

(2) Most of the intentive processes of mental life, however, have no active subject living in and producing them (Husserl 1982, pp. 199-201). An individual mental life is largely composed of ego-less mental processes. These mental processes simply occur "on their own"; they are not produced by any ego (Husserl 1966b). Because they are not actively generated by an ego, Husserl labels these processes "passive"; we prefer to call them "automatic." Because automatic processes are ego-less and because it is the ego who chooses the themes of mental life, automatic processes are non-thematizing ones. Automatic processes intend objects in the *field* or *horizon* of consciousness (Gurwitsch 1964, pp. 340-354). For example, as I am now reading this paper, my ego is focused on the meanings of the words I am reading. My mental life, however, is automatically co-intending the whiteness of the paper, the way it feels between my fingers, the floor touching the soles of my feet, my own body posture, and so forth.

An individual mental life, then, is composed of both active and automatic intentive processes. An ego lives in and voluntarily generates some of the processes of mental life, viz., the active and thematizing processes of mental life. The remainder of mental life intends manifold objects, but it does so "on its own," i.e., automatically and non-egoically.

According to Husserl, three different levels of intentive life must be distinguished (Husserl 1982, pp. 211-303). The first level is that of doxic intentionality. With the word "doxa" Husserl wishes to signify "belief." The second level is the stratum of emotional intentionality. The third level is the conative. We shall not depict these three strata further at this time. They shall be addressed, however, at different points in the essay.

Multiple intentive processes are combined together in a way that Husserl called "synthesis" (Husserl 1982, pp. 283-287). A "synthesis" occurs when multiple mental processes intend manifold features of an identical object (Husserl 1973a, pp. 39-55). Each mental process intends its own feature; and when many mental processes are synthesized together, they intend manifold features of the same object. Thanks to these synthesizing processes of mental life, there exists a world composed of objects with their various features, including myself as one synthetically unified object that is related to others.

By being synthesized together as features of one object, the features of an object come to have a special relationship to one another: the relationship that Aron Gurwitsch has called "Gestalt-coherence" (Gurwitsch 1964, pp. 132-153; 273-279). In a Gestalt, each part is what it is by virtue of its relationship to other parts of the whole. Each part shapes and qualifies the significance of the others, and the other parts shape and qualify it. The redness of the wool rug is not the redness of the plastic cup. The redness of the wool rug is a "woolly" redness. The wooliness of the rug shapes and qualifies the redness. The wooliness and the red of the rug are *interdependent* and interrelated parts: each shapes and qualifies the other. Each feature thus takes on the significance it has only by virtue of its relatedness to other features of the whole. If any part were separated from the whole, it would lose its significance; it would no longer be the definite and determinate feature it is (Gurwitsch 1966, pp. 332-349).

For example, as I look at this sheet of paper in my hands, the white color of the side facing me is directly given to me. On the basis of the direct givenness of this aspect, other aspects of the object are synthetically co-intended by my mental life. For example, my mental life is now co-intending the other side—the unseen side—of the sheet of paper and its whiteness. This side of the sheet now seen refers to and qualifies the unseen side of the sheet. Any perceived object thus has an "inner horizon" of manifold aspects, and these manifold aspects depend on and qualify one another in the manner of Gestalt-coherence (Gurwitsch 1964, pp. 235-245).

In addition to intending the sensory properties of the object, my mental life experiences these properties as real, unreal, possibly real, possibly unreal, etc. In other words, my mental life automatically ascribes "ontic statuses" to objects and their properties.[3] This is what Husserl means by the "doxic positionality" of mental life: mental life automatically "takes a position" toward the ontic statuses of its intended objects (Husserl 1982, pp. 251-272).

The ontic status of an object-property can change when that property is experienced as incompatible with another property that the object is also intended as having. Such experienced contrarieties will cancel the ontic status of one property and impute a status to the other property. Suppose, for example, that when I do turn the sheet of paper over, I directly perceive a green backside rather than the protended white one. In that case my mental life will automatically cancel the protended reality of the white backside, and it will henceforth intend the green backside as real (Husserl 1973b, pp. 87-101).

---

3 Notice that reality and unreality are not the only possible ontic statuses that objects may be experienced as having. Objects can in fact display indefinitely many degrees of reality and unreality, such as very probably unreal, certainly real, uncertainly real, etc.

These alterations in the ontic statuses of objects occur on the basis of *the unalterable ontological status of the world*. My perception of the whiteness of the paper may change from certainty of its whiteness, to doubt of its whiteness, to a new certainty of its greenness. But beneath such common-place doxic changes in my mental life lies what Husserl called an *Urdoxa, a primordial, unshakable certainty* in the fundamental features of myself and the world (Husserl 1973b, pp. 28-31). For example, the paper may turn out to be green rather than white. Indeed, the "paper" may prove to be a thin piece of white metal as I examine it further. Subsequent experiences can correct earlier ones, and yet throughout these corrections of belief some features of objects and myself remain invariant and necessary. The object does have a backside of some sort, even if it turns out to be black rather than the protended white. The object has a location in world space, even if the spatial object is inflexible metal rather than flexible paper. The thing cannot come alive and begin speaking to me in an unknown but strangely familiar language. The object may prove to be different, but there are onto-logical limits to this possible difference. At a fundamental level the object *must* remain the same. Of course, *this* phenomenon may prove not to be an object at all; *it* may not exist. But object-hood remains invariant; and there continue to be objects in the world.

It is this *Urdoxa*, this primordial certainty in the primordial features of things, that is shaken in the early stages of schizophrenia. This is why we have said that in schizophrenia the impossible becomes actual: not only the contingent attributes but also the essential and necessary attributes of things grow uncertain and dubious.

3. The Constituted Self

Mental life, in addition to constituting objects that are transcendent to it, synthetically intends itself. Through these active and passive self-in-tendings, mental life as constituting subject constitutes itself as object.

The ego can actively reflect upon that mental life of which it forms a part. But prior to such egoic self-reflection, mental life is already automati-cally intending its own processes. Each mental process intends its own ob-ject. But in addition each mental process also "protends" future mental processes of the same mental life. And furthermore, each mental process "retends" past phases of this same mental life. Indeed, what makes these manifold processes processes of "the same" mental life is the fact that they, in addition to intending their own objects, protend and retend one another. Mental processes do not simply cease to exist once they occur. They are rather retended as past by the present phase of mental life. And similarly, the future processes of mental life, even before they occur, are protended by the present phase of mental life as "coming." Through this "inner time," then, mental life *unifies* itself; it experiences itself as con-tinuously the same over time (Husserl 1966a). This synthetic unification of mental life through its own self-intendings are what constitute personal identity.

These protending and retending processes are all passive processes. No ego is actively living in them, and no ego is thematizing anything through them. Thus the synthetic unification of mental life that is achieved through "inner time" is exclusively a "passive" or "automatic" unification. This unification is simply going on all the time, without requiring the activities of the ego. That is to say, the ego need not and indeed cannot actively unify its own mental life. The unification of mental life is achieved "behind the back" of the thematizing ego which inhabits mental life.

Husserl has said that an individual mental life as a whole is "anonymous" (Husserl 1966a). By this he means that mental life as a whole is not produced by the active ego. The ego rather inhabits and actively produces only a part of a more encompassing "anonymous" mental life. But once we comprehend Husserl's point here, we can set it aside and say that this individual mental life as a whole is "mine" in the sense that it is the mental life in which "I" (ego) am living. This unified totality of experiences is "mine" in the sense that "I" am a part of it; it is a unified whole, and "I" am integrated into it as a part of this whole. There is thus both a narrower and a broader sense of "mineness." In the narrower sense only my actively produced mental processes, i.e., the acts produced by my ego, are "mine." But in a broader sense the total individual mental life in which my ego lives is "my" mental life.

In addition to unifying itself through these processes of inner time, however, mental life synthesizes its own being with that of a body. Mental events are synthesized with various bodily phenomena that are given through perceptual intendings, visual, auditory, tactual, kineasthetic, olfactory, and gustatory. Thus my *decision* to move my arm is conjoined with the *kineasthetic* experiences of moving my arm and hand and with the *visual* perception of my moving arm and hand. Through these complex syntheses, "my" mind is integrated with "my" body; indeed, only thanks to this synthetic integration is "a" body experienced as "my" body. In this manner I experience myself as a psychosomatic being who is continuous through time. We wish to emphasize that these syntheses of mind and body occur completely *automatically*.

4. Phenomenological Interpretation of the Delusional Mood

In the earliest stages of their illness, schizophrenics often experience what is called "a delusional mood" *(Wahnstimmung)* (Jaspers 1963, pp. 98-99, Slater and Roth 1969, pp. 273, 289). In this delusional mood the person feels that reality in its entirety, including him- or herself, is fundamentally different, bewildering, dubious, or strange. The change that occurs is experienced as a radical one. Furthermore, the schizophrenic is certain that this change has some important connection with him- or herself. We shall try to capture this extreme alteration in the being of oneself and the world by calling it an "ontological change." By employing the term "ontology" here, we again mean *the essential features* of things in contrast to their *contingent or accidental* features. In a normal condition I experience some of the features of myself and of things as in principle *transformable* or as (in the ultimate analysis) *unnecessary* to my and their being. Other features of myself and things, however, are experienced as *invariant* and *necessary* to our being, as those features without which I and they would not exist. In the delusional mood even these essential features of myself and of worldly things are experienced as dissolving or unreliable.

This is why we can adopt R.D. Laing's phrase "ontological insecurity" and apply it to the delusional mood (Laing 1960). Ontological "insecurity," as we understand it, is a condition in which I become radically uncertain of my essential self. When one is "ontologically insecure," one's being as physical or non-physical, mental or non-mental, existent or non-existent, temporal or supratemporal, spatial or aspatial, mechanical or organic, human, divine, or demonic, male or female, real or unreal, alive or dead, or animate or inanimate—to mention just a few!—becomes dubious and indeterminate.

In the delusional mood the synthetic processes which normally constitute objects as unified objects and as interrelated networks of objects are seriously weakened. The constitution of world and self is profoundly attenuated. Because of this weakening of the constitution of self and world, they are no longer experienced as inviolably different from one another. The synthesizing function of mental life, we have claimed, is what constitutes things and myself as identical through time. If intentive syntheses constitute identity, they also constitute difference. In normal mental life I experience the table and the chair as different from one another because I experience each as having a firm and continuous identity in itself. With the weakening of syntheses in schizophrenia, then, there is a weakening of identity. But with the weakening of syntheses, there is also a weakening of difference. In schizophrenia my mental life might synthesize itself with the voice on the radio because my mind no longer firmly identifies itself with itself nor does it identify the voice with the unseen radio announcer. Because identity is weakened, objects and myself may appear splintered, inchoate, and fragmented. But because difference is weakened, features of different things may be synthesized with one another or with features of myself. In this way even the essential features of things and other people can forfeit their "otherness" and become "self." And likewise, aspects of myself can lose their "mineness" and become "other." The "ontological insecurity" of the early stages of schizophrenia consists in this fluidity and changeableness of the self-other difference.

Let us focus at first on the schizophrenic's experience of fragmentation and disunity. James Chapman provides us with a patient's report on this kind of experience: "Everything I see is split up. It's like a photograph that's torn in bits and put together again. If somebody moves or speaks, everything I see disappears quickly and I have to put it together again" (Chapman 1966, p. 29).

With the weakening of synthetic processes, the Gestalt-coherence of objects dissipates. The features of an object no longer qualify and refer to one another. Remember that it was precisely this interdependence and interrelatedness of the features that rendered each definite and determinate in significance. If the Gestalt-coherence of the features now diminishes, the features, if they are intended at all, will be intended as unrelated to one another. And when the features forfeit their placement within the whole, they also lose their definite and determinate significance for mental life. The fragmented and separate features of things, then, are intended, not only as separate, but also as *indeterminate* and *indefinite*. The intended features of the splintering objects become highly *ambiguous:* the "whatness" of objects grows extremely opaque and elusive.

But, as we have indicated, schizophrenic experience, in its initial phases, is not only characterized by this splintering of the self and the world into indeterminate fragments. It is also marked by certain fragmented aspects of the self being synthetically conjoined with aspects of what has previously been intended as the other, the not-me, the world. In the midst of this delusional mood unusual and unexpected syntheses will occur transiently and momentarily. Hence the schizophrenic may perceive a red dress and momentarily intend having sexual intercourse with this woman who is seen as an alien from the red planet, Mars. Yet this experience will then rapidly dissipate. The weakened *Gestalten* will thus be replaced by such fleeting and inventive ones.

The doxic positionality of the person's experience is that of extreme uncertainty or doubt. The uncertainty is a profound one because it is not only individual objects that have become dubious and unreliable. It is the fundamental ontology of reality that has grown unclear and uncertain. The very being of the self and of the world are suspect. Everything is experienced as more or less unreal.

In the delusional mood the schizophrenic lives in a state of anxious expectancy: the person is caught in the *midpoint* of an all encompassing Gestalt-shift. The prior organization of reality has dissolved, but no new synthetic reality has yet emerged to replace it. The person now senses the imminent emergence of a new world and a new self. Things are even intended as somehow related to one another, but as related to one another in an as yet *extremely* unclear and indefinite fashion.

This new relatedness of things thus becomes an urgent problem for the ego to *actively* solve. This problem is so important and urgent that all other concerns must be ignored. The ego thus devotes its attention solely to deciphering this mystery. What can normally be taken for granted, namely, that my world and myself are basically familiar, can no longer be taken for granted. The ego is thus overburdened with the enormous task of having to constitute the entire world. It was normally *automatic* mental life that had constituted reality as a whole. But this automatic unification has grown profoundly weak. Consequently, the ego must *actively* decipher the fundamental nature of things and him- or herself.

For example, one of the patients studied by Chapman reported the following: "I have to put things together in my head. If I look at my watch I see the watch, watchstrap, face, hands, and so on, then I have got to put them together to get it into one piece" (Chapman 1966, p. 229). Chapman himself says of this kind of experience: "[The patients] are unable to interpret the whole, as a meaningful gestalt, until they have taken sufficient time to coordinate its different elements, *and this has to be done in a conscious deliberate fashion"* (Chapman 1966, p. 230, italics ours).

Let us now see how this weakening of the constituting syntheses affects mental life's constitution of itself. The syntheses involved in the constitution of a continuous self are, as we claimed above, those of inner time. In the delusional mood these syntheses of inner time, too, are seriously attenuated. This means that the present phase of intentional life will only weakly protend coming future phases of itself and only weakly retend past phases of itself. Mental life will then reside primarily in a *present* awareness; and this present awareness will *not* be experienced as, on the one hand, having arisen from earlier intendings which are now regressing into the past or, on the other hand, as about to give way to oncoming future intendings. In other words, the present awareness will be experienced as simply *enduring*—and as enduring without being bounded by a receding past or an approaching future. This extreme attenuation of the syntheses of inner time accounts for the experience of a "prolonged" or "distended present" which many schizophrenics report.

Out of this ontological disunity can arise the primary features of acute schizophrenia. The fundamental Gestalt-shift for which the schizophrenic ego is anxiously and actively seeking emerges passively and automatically. Novel syntheses become stabilized, and new Gestalt-contextures crystallize. Features of the world take on new and interdependent significances. Multiple Gestalt-shifts occur, and these may even involve radical transformations in self-other differentiations: what was previously a feature of the other now becomes an abiding feature of the self. Various transformations of this kind have been enumerated by Kurt Schneider as the "first-rank symptoms" of schizophrenia (Schneider 1959, Mellor 1970, 1982). For example, Julian Leff reports one of his patients as saying, "I have tingling feelings in my legs caused by electric currents from an alternator" (Leff 1982, p. 11). Another of Leff's patients describes how the thoughts in his own mind are the thoughts of another person: "Thoughts are put into my mind like 'Kill God'. It's just like my mind working, but it isn't. They come from this chap, Chris. They're his thoughts" (Leff 1982, p. 10).

Conversely, the patient may experience a feature of him- or herself as an enduring component of the other. Guilty feelings, for example, can come to be regularly experienced by the schizophrenic as voices speaking about her in a critical manner. Or, as one patient has reported, "My thoughts go into other people's minds. It's telecommunication between people" (Leff 1982, p. 10).

Thanks to these new organized wholes, the ontological insecurity of the delusional mood finally relaxes. A measure of ontological security and certainty returns. The new Gestalt-contextures now call forth activities which more favorably adapt the schizophrenic to his or her environment—but at the expense of a psychotic condition.

5. A Note on the Conative Dimension of Schizophrenia

We would like to conclude with a brief description of schizophrenia as a conative disorder. Kraepelin appreciated the conative dimension of dementia praecox early on (Kraepelin 1904). Since Bleuler, however, cognitive aspects of this disorder have been emphasized while conative features have been neglected. We contend that the conative features of the illness remain crucial.

In normal mental life my strivings are experienced by me as primarily produced by me. Even when I act in response to some demand placed on me from outside, I experience my response as originating with my agency. My automatic strivings too are experienced as more or less "under my control." This means that if I should catch myself automatically performing some activity that is somehow undesirable—e.g., embarrassing or unseemly—I can try to change it, often with success. Of course, with deeply entrenched patterns of behavior I may have to struggle hard and even then I may fail to alter them. But I do nonetheless experience these behaviors as "my" behavior; they emanate from something that is part of me.

In schizophrenia, the strivings of the person are frequently experienced less as produced by the self and more as produced by the other—whether the "other" here be an object or another person, an animate or an inanimate other. These strivings are experienced as not originating from me, or, once they have begun, as not being determined in their ongoing course by me.

The schizophrenic does strive to do things: the schizophrenic may be as "active" as any normal person. But the goals of these strivings are often experienced by the subject as produced by something other than him- or herself. This discloses the "weakness" of the ego that is so prominent in schizophrenia. But this weakness of the ego is manifest even in sometimes frantic activities because these activities are experienced as not emanating from the ego but rather from some "other."

A schizophrenic, for example, may be preoccupied with a movie star. This preoccupation may lead the person to engage in many activities directed toward the object of his concern. But these activities are experienced by him as determined by the movie star, the preoccupying object. The weakness of the ego is manifested precisely in the preoccupation: it is not the schizophrenic who has decided that he will focus on this movie star. It is rather something in the movie star's being that *compels* the schizophrenic to focus on her.

The projects of the schizophrenic are, therefore, not experienced as primarily chosen by him or her. These projects are rather *responses to demands* of objects in the field of awareness. These "objects" may be delusional objects, of course. But because they are intended—even if delusionally so—they, too, can compel the ego to turn to them and focus on them. The schizophrenic, too, has his or her dominant projects, then; the schizophrenic need not be projectless. It is rather that these projects are often experienced as set, not at the schizophrenic's own initiative, but rather by the object or goal of the project.

Strictly speaking, therefore, the schizophrenic does not engage in actions but rather in *reactions.* Some important event occurs in the schizophrenic's world, and this event delineates a range of possible responses to itself. The schizophrenic must then choose from among these possibilities or invent further possibilities (of response). The event cannot be simply ignored or dismissed; it is too important. The schizophrenic's choices, however, must provide an adequate response to the important event.

Of course, normal people regularly find themselves "compelled to respond" to demands in their environment. Schizophrenic experience does not differ so much in kind from this normal "need to react" as it differs in degree: the schizophrenic's strivings remain *far more* at the mercy of powerful requirements emanating from outside than the normal person's do.

Another example can further illustrate the conative dysfunction in schizophrenia. In normal experience my strivings are synthetically unified with my other mental and bodily processes. When I lift my arm, my decision and striving to do so are synthesized with my kineasthetic experiences of feeling my arm move and with my visual experience of seeing my arm and hand move. These three components—and more—are experienced by me as interdependent constituents of a Gestalt-whole which is my deliberate action of moving my arm. But in schizophrenia, we have claimed, there occurs a weakening of all synthesizing processes, including those processes which automatically synthesize my own being as a psychosomatic unity. Consequently, the felt and seen movements of my arm may not be synthetically conjoined with my decision to move it. In such cases I would not experience myself as the agent moving my arm. I would rather experience my arm as simply moving on its own, independently of my own agency. And if these felt and seen movements of my arm were synthetically unified with something else—something *other* than my own decision to move it— then I could experience this "other" as the agent moving my arm. In this way my own striving would be experienced by me as produced by something other than myself.

In this example, we have spoken of an egoic decision to move my arm. But this same problem could arise in purely automatic strivings. I may be casually sitting with my legs crossed, gently swinging one leg. Usually this action occurs completely habitually, i.e., automatically. In schizophrenia, however, my mental life might synthetically unify this kineasthetic and visual experience of feeling and seeing my leg swinging with some "other" agent or thing. In this case I would experience my leg as being moved by something other than myself, and the strangeness of this experience would in all probability motivate my ego to focus on my swinging leg and the "alien" cause of it.

Of course, in intending this "other" as somehow producing my own movement, I may not intend it as having any "definite" nature. It may remain quite unclear to me just what this causal "other" is; it may be intended as highly indefinite and indeterminate. All that may be experienced, then, is that it *is* producing my movement and that it is "not-me." On the other hand, this "other" may be intended as having a very precise nature as a part of an elaborate delusional schema.

6. Conclusion

We have sought to appropriate central concepts of Husserlian phenomenology in order to explicate the delusional mood of schizophrenia and some of its conative dysfunctions. In this way, we think that a better understanding of the self-pathology as well as other important aspects of schizophrenia can be developed.

Summary

Husserl's phenomenology provides basic concepts of normal mental life in the light of which schizophrenic experience can be better understood. Husserl's distinction of intentional syntheses into automatic (passive) and active kinds leads to a further distinction between an individual mental life as a whole and the ego who lives and acts in that mental life. Relevant here is Husserl's phenomenology of the synthetic unification of mental life itself that is automatically achieved through inner temporality (*Zeit-bewußtsein*). These notions will allow us to clarify further the profound disturbances of self and world which are so frequently encountered in schizophrenia.

The earliest phase of schizophrenia, the phase of the "delusional mood," is then explicated in Husserlian terms. Pervasive in this phase is a severe weakening of the normal intentive syntheses of mental life. The self of the schizophrenic experiences itself as at the center of a bewildering, confusing, and dubious transformation of itself and of its world. The unity of the self splinters, and the identity of objects and the networks among objects grow disordered. The most basic features of the world and of the self become deeply strange and opaque. Because the syntheses which constitute a continuous and unitary self have become seriously weakened, the self disintegrates and begins to be experienced as conjoined with aspects of the non-self. The automatic processes of mental life no longer sufficiently constitute wordly objects or the self, and thus the ego must actively thematize and devote itself to topics that could normally be taken for granted. This need to actively (egoically) constitute what could normally be passively (non-egoically) constituted finally overwhelms the ego. The ego thus grows extremely weak or withdraws into its own self-constituted world, or both. Finally we discuss the conative dysfunction of the ego: it experiences its own strivings and projects as determined less by itself and more by the "other," the non-ego—whether this determining "other" be a thing or a person.

References

Chapman J: The Early Symptoms of Schizophrenia. British Journal of Psychiatry 112: 225-250, 1966.

Gurwitsch A: The Field of Consciousness. Duquesne University Press, Pittsburgh, 1964.

Gurwitsch A: Studies in Phenomenology and Psychology. Northwestern University Press, Evanston, 1966.

Husserl E: Zur Phanomenologie des inneren Zeitbewusstseins, Husserliana X, herausgegeben von R. Boehm. Martinus Nijhoff, The Hague, 1966a.

Husserl E: Analysen zur passiven Synthesis, Husserliana XI, herausgegeben von M. Fleischer. Martinus Nijhoff, The Hague, 1966b.

Husserl E: Formal and Transcendental Logic (transl. Cairns D). Martinus Nijhoff, The Hague, 1969.

Husserl E: The Crisis of European Sciences and Transcendental Phenomenology (transl. Carr D). Northwestern University Press, Evanston, 1970.

Husserl E: Cartesian Meditation: An Introduction to Phenomenology (transl. Cairns D). Martinus Nijhoff, The Hague, 1973a.

Husserl E: Experience and Judgment: Investigations in a Genealogy of Logic (rev. and ed. Langrebe L, transl. Churchill JS, Ameriks K). Northwestern University Press, Evanston, 1973b.

Husserl E: Ideas Pertaining to a Pure Phenomenology and to a Phenomenological Philosophy, First Book, General Inroduction to a Pure Phenomenology (transl. Kersten F). Martinus Nijhoff, The Hague, 1982.

Jaspers K: General Psychopathology (transl. by Hoenig J, Hamilton MW), University of Chicago Press, Chicago, 1963.

Kraepelin E: Lectures on Clinical Psychiatry (rev., ed, transl. Johnstone T). Bailliere, Tindall and Cox, London, 1904.

Laing RD: The Divided Self: An Existential Study in Sanity and Madness. Tavistock Publications, London, 1960.

Leff JP: Acute syndromes of schizophrenia. In: Wing, JK, Wing L (eds): Psychoses of Uncertein Etiology. Handbook pf Psychiatry 3, pp. 8–13, Cambridge University Press, Cambridge, London, New York, New Rochelle, Melburne, Sydney, 1982.

Mellor CS: First rank–symptoms of schizophrenia. Br. J. Psychiatry 117: 15–23, 1970

Mellor CS: The present status of first–rank symptoms. Br. J. Psychiatry 140: 423–424, 1982.

Schneider K: Clinical Psychopathology (transl. by Hamilton MW), Grune and Stratton, New York, London, 1959.

Slater E, Roth M: Clinical Psychiatry. Williams and Wilkins Company, Baltimore, 1969.
Spitzer M: Ichstörungen: In Search of a Theory. In: Spitzer M, Uehlein FA, Oepen G (eds): Psychopathology and Philosophy, pp. 167-183, Springer, Berlin, Heidelberg, New York, London, Paris, Tokyo, 1988.

Concepts of Intentionality and Their Application to the Psychopathology of Schizophrenia—A Critique of the Vulnerability Model

Christoph Mundt

1. Introduction

At present, the vulnerability model (Zubin and Spring 1977) or the diathesis–stress model (Nuechterlein 1987) are widely accepted disease models of schizophrenia, especially in English speaking countries. Both propose that there is a threshold in an individual vulnerable or predisposed to emotional stress. In these models it is hypothesized that information processing in vulnerable individuals is slowed down and distorted so that an information load above the threshold makes the system break down. At a first glance these models seem to be convincing because they are simple, clear–cut and based on replicated empirical findings. They have guided research for years in many fields. Nevertheless there are some shortcomings.

Before discussing these we have to ask why conceptual tools are needed at all for the interpretation of the psychopathology of schizophrenia. What is it that has to be interpreted, what is the "Explicandum" of schizophrenia?

Four points shall be raised:

1) The heterogeneity of clinical symptoms.

So far there are no biological findings that are able to define the syndrome schizophrenia by its etiology. The definition of the syndrome remains based on psychopathology and on convention. The clinical psychopathology of schizophrenia, however, is heterogeneous. Consequently, attempts have been made to split up the syndrome into subgroups. In empirical investigations employing operationally defined symptom catalogues such as the *Inpatient Multiple Psychopathology Scale* (IMPS) three factors were found that govern the organization of the following single symptom items: paranoid projection, disorganization and apathy or retardation (Mundt 1985). What do they have in common, what is the supra-symptomatological structure that could explain these subsyndromes as different expressions or variants of one common basic disturbance?

2) The stages of the illness and the defect outcome.

Modern research on probands at high risk for schizophrenia and long-term studies of course and outcome describe three stages of the illness: premorbid microsymptoms, manifest psychosis, and the defect state. Despite the enormous variability of the long–term course certain rules can be derived from the findings. Roughly two thirds of the patients already show premorbid emotional irritability and instability at an early school age. These characteristics seem to evolve later in adolescence into schizoid or other abnormal personality traits (Huber et al. 1979, Marcus et al. 1981). After the onset–peak of 22 years for male and 29 years for female patients, stabilization at a defect level is usually achieved after 5 to 10 years of illness. In 5% of cases a definite improvement occurs in later life. Because the deterioration comes to a standstill and even improvements occur, Ciompi (Ciompi and Müller 1976) argued against Huber's (1966) hypothesis of a systematized loss of brain tissue such as is the case, for example, in multiple sclerosis. We also know that ventricular and fissural enlargements exist already before the onset of the illness. But what else, what pathogenetic mechanism is it, that governs the course of the illness through these stages?

3) Precipitating and protective factors.

In both, the vulnerability and diathesis–stress model emotional stress, as it has been elaborated by Selye, is considered a precipitating factor. Overstimulation and understimulation are presumed to be responsible for positive and negative symptoms. Findings suggesting this restricted interpretation come from life–events research, from expressed–emotion studies and from investigations of autoprotective mechanisms. But we do encounter some first episodes and relapses without precipitating dramatic life–events. On the other hand, some life events have no impact on the patient. Is it possible to come to a more specific and individual understanding of these factors, which are of great significance for therapy?

4) Findings in experimental psychopathology, neurophysiology, biochemistry and cerebral morphology demonstrate a great variety of nonspecific microsymptoms. These are not always present in all patients but can consistently be found in large samples. Moreover, these findings seem to be unsystematic. Is it conceivable that, even within the biological basis of the syndrome, one unitary common pathogenetic mechanism mediates the sequence from a predisposing biological substrate to the manifestation of the illness? This question is of great importance to modern geneticists, for example, who need a reliably defined phenotype of the illness.

Despite all the heterogeneity of these findings and their considerable variance in patients, cross–cultural psychiatry provides a strong argument in favour of a unitary syndrome model of schizophrenia. The WHO schizophrenia studies (Sartorius et al. 1987) show an impressive consistency concerning incidence in different countries and at different times, at least with regard to the narrowly defined schizophrenic syndrome. Thus, it can be assumed that its psychopathology is really a syndrome in the original meaning of the term; single symptoms run together. The search for a transsymptomatological structure seems to be justified; it may even be given preference to attempts to deal with heterogeneity by subdividing the syndrome.

2. Concepts of Intentionality

At the beginning of the century attempts were already being made to utilize the term "intentionality" and its different conceptualizations for the description of a basic pathogenetic mechanism in schizophrenia. Although some authors did not use this specific term, they employed terms with identical meaning: for example Janet spoke of "abaissement du niveau mental" and Stranski of "intrapsychic ataxia". Berze even offered a kind of neologism for the whole syndrome which he called Hypophrenia, by which he denoted the low level of a basic psychic activity underlying the performance of concentration, rational thinking, and volition (cf. Mundt 1985). One disadvantage of these terms and metaphors was that they did not make a clear distinction between simple activity level or general drive which makes up a person's temperament on the one hand, and a more specific sort of activity which was claimed to be at too low a level in schizophrenics on the other. It was Beringer (1924, 1926) in the 1920s who came closer to such a specification. He used the term intentionality when working on formal thought disorders in schizophrenia. Beringer found that in schizophrenic language there was a lack of hierarchical organization such that the importance of certain components would be emphasized while other ones would be diminished. Sentences were sequentially additive and did not, as usual, elaborate their meaning around one central message. Beringer tried to pinpoint the underlying disturbance when he proposed that schizophrenics suffer a "reduced intentional span". Gruhle (Berze and Gruhle 1929) called this at the same time "lack of teleological discipline".

A clearer elaboration of the term intentionality designed to specify the basic pathogenetic mechanism in schizophrenia was given by Blankenburg in the 1960s. He (Blankenburg 1971) examined hebephrenic patients by means of the phenomenological reduction, called epoché. Blankenburg emphasized a deficiency in constituting the self, the world, and inter-subjective relations in these patients, which leads to a loss of interconnectedness in all the subtle meanings and purposes of everyday–life. This was called by Blankenburg "lack of transcendental organization" thereby making use with this expression of Husserl's philosophy with special reference to his term 'intentionality'. According to Blankenburg such a lack of entangledness in the meanings and purposes of everyday life is not per se abnormal, but does typically constitute a stimulus and need for striving for a closer and safer position in a framework of common sense and societal references. What is disturbed in schizophrenics, according to Blankenburg, is the balance between connectedness and disconnectedness, a balance that is tipped in favour of disconnectedness; this condition he called anthro-pological disproportion.

For some time such an approach to a basic disturbance was also pursued by psychoanalytic ego–psychology, although the actual term inten-tionality did not play a paramount role here. Moreover, this term was in a sense spoiled as it was contaminated with different meanings, among them the meaning of mere drive or volitional aspects of psychic life, as for exam-ple in the work of Schultz–Hencke (1927), and Dührssen (1985). Closer to our concept of intentionality, however, is David Rapaport's (1967) construct of attention cathexis. By means of attentional overcathexis a person should be able to actualise any content of the kind that Rapaport called psychical representatives. For Rapaport basic disturbance meant that this attention cathexis is no longer available. One of the factors that contribute to its loss is affective overstimulation. Rapaport made use of Freud's old metaphor of the ego as the rider governing the instinctual drives. In this sense in terms of ego–strength one could speak of a person's specific capacity to bind affects by structure.

Psychoanalytic structuralism and their linguistic schools took up the construct of psychic representatives. Lang (1986), who introduced de Saussure's and Lacan's work to German psychoanalysis hypothesized that in schizophrenics the world of representatives is deficient , which means that opening up from a protected and guided dyadic mode of relations towards a basically less secure and less determined triadic one, which challenges the individual's intentional activities, must fail.

One of the criticisms of the phenomenological approach is the diffi-culty that arises when trying to operationalize its descriptions and to submit them to empirical research. This demand seems to be met more adequately by changing the point of view from the empathetic inner perspective to a more objective outer behavioural perspective.

This latter perspective is taken by Daniel Dennett, the analytical philosopher. He examined reactions and acting strategies that refer to a supposed intention in the addressed person. Interesting examples from animal psychology prove, that intentional systems, as Dennett calls behaviour of this type, are able to operate without having the intentions reflected rationally or even without their being represented in conscious-ness at all. Intentional systems may be looked at as a hierarchy of schemes for communicative behavior perhaps acquired on an operant basis. These schemes make individuals understandable, in a sense even calculable, for each other. For Dennett intentionality is a prerequisite for communica-tion. Its quality and complexity is determined by reciprocity. There are three degrees of reciprocity which are distinguished by the multitude of back and forth references between the communication partners: the intention which deals with the other as an unintentional object represents the intentional system of the first order, the intention which addresses the other's intention that of the second order, and the intention, which takes into account the reference of the other's intention to mine, the system of third order. Only this third order system can be subject to false pretenses and deceptions, perhaps it is also the only one which is prone to suffer alienation.

There is an interesting equivalence between Dennett's hierarchy of intentional systems of growing reciprocal complexity and Piaget's (1975) observation of the circular reactions between assimilation and accomodation in developing infants. Primitive reflex actions with only vague directions like hand–to–mouth movements become more and more refined. This is accomplished by a circular causal mechanism: When the infant tries to assimilate the object's position, the object's resistance to this attempt necessitates the accomodation of the sensori motor scheme. Then in turn a new attempt to assimilate the object's position can be made. Assimilation and accomodation, however, can be considered as essentials of reciprocity and thus intentionality in Dennett's sense. Piaget's observations describe the growth of hierarchies and nets of such sensori-motor schemes into a representation of the infant's objectal world. Since in recent years minor disturbances in the sensori-motor development of schizophrenics have been reported consistently, these concepts are of great interest for our purpose.

Which concept of intentionality is best suitable for the interpretation of the syndrome of schizophrenia?

Apparently all the authors who used the term 'intentionality' and similar constructs for discussing the psychopathology of schizophrenia show remarkable convergence in their selection of the same few aspects for definition. The term intentionality denotes the ability to build up and maintain a coherent subjective world of patterns of meanings and purposes. These have to be kept in permanent exchange and adjustment with the objective world and with the referential society. Thus, the term intentionality does not merely describe drive, impetuousness, or general volitional activity. Intentionality in the sense of intent, motive, motivation, ethical responsibility represents a reduced or partial aspect of intentionality, which is, however, suitable for operationalization. Consciousness and rational elaboration do not seem to be essential for intentionality but reciprocity is essential either with the objective world if sensori-motor schemes are concerned or with the referential society if mental representations are concerned. There is a controversial discussion whether mood and feelings are of intentional character. Bieri denies Brentano's ontological dualism to them. But studies on hypochondriasis and pain after amputation demonstrate that body schemes and the emergence of pain as gestalt from neuronal afferences need an intentional elaboration. Many other definitorial aspects of the term may remain unresolved. Nevertheless an interpretation of the psychopathology of schizophrenia ought to be attempted now and a clarification of the term's concept may go along with it.

3. Conclusions

Looking at the four points which were raised at the beginning and which need interpretation, the following statements can be made:

1) In terms of intentional performance two elements can be distinguished in the clinical symptomatology of schizophrenia: disorganization of patterns of meaning as shown in loosening of associations and incoherence; and structured alienation as shown in delusional experiences. Volition, movements, thinking, language, affective reactions and rapport can be affected. It seems that both elements are equivalent since some microsymptoms as, for example, blurring or exchange of a single word's meaning (called *Wortfeldstörung*) can be looked at as alienation or disorganization.

Other clinical symptoms, however, represent reactions to instable intentionality. In terms of intentionality the development of systematized delusions, for example, can be interpreted as a repair mechanism which restructures meanings and purposes, be it after an initial gliding of meanings in a delusional mood (Conrad) or be it after a sudden change of meaning, for example by developing a delusional idea. The re-establishment of patterns of meaning sustains a feeling of wholeness and experiential continuity. The same function, a sort of desperate, helpless search for lost structures can also be seen in echo-phenomena, other repetitive movements, ruminating thinking and in obsessive compulsive symptoms before the schizophrenic break-down. On the other hand, stressful emotional complexes, in the sense employed by Eugen Bleuler and C.G. Jung are projected into the delusion and thus excluded from intentional operations and from dealing with them. Symptoms of passivity can be considered as one possible consequence.

2) The hypothesis of compensatory mechanisms can also be applied to the psychopathology of the long-term course of the illness with its different stages. An already premorbidly fragile intentionality is hampered by increased irritability, for example due to strong affects which in turn is an obstacle for learning and maturational processes in puberty and adolescence. After the manifestation of the psychosis in the adult, the defect states then bring about a decline of or a retreat from intentional efforts. After some years a new balance is reached and patients live a reduced life with as little or just as much intentional reciprocity as is tolerable for their still minimally structured or deviantly restructured psychic life. Three types of retreat from or decline of reciprocity can be described: the autistic one with intentionality deflected into a private world; amorphous intentionality as in hebephrenia with shifting, unreliable patterns of meaning; and asthenic intentionality which protects itself from confrontation with the other's intentionality by withdrawel. One could say these three types concern direction, consistency and vigour of intentional efforts. All of them include a marked restriction of reciprocity.

This hypothesis that defect state acts as a balance between restricted intentionality and the maintenance of some bridge of reciprocity (for as much traffic as the bridge can bear) also sheds some light on precipitating and preventive factors for the manifestation of and relapses into the illness. There obviously are transitional phases in life history when intentional efforts are challenged in a special way, as for example when the individual is about to leave his/her structuring primary relations and educational institutions and has to live his/her life and to assert his/her secondary relations, his/her psychosexual and psychosocial identity in private and professional life. Both, the intentional vacuum of suddenly feeling alone and the overwhelming intentionality of the other in intense contacts can be understood as specific triggers for the precipitation of the illness. Examples of steps into an insecure situation which require increased definition by intentional reciprocity are, besides puberty and leaving parents' home mentioned above, entry into professional life, post–examination, exam or the birth of a child, which are well known as potential precipitators of psychotic break-down. An example for the possibly harmful overwhelming intentionality of the other person is the experience of schizophrenics in encounter groups. R.v. Held (1984) studied schizophrenic patients whose first episode occurred in such groups. He could demonstrate that intrusive interpretations of the patient offered in such groups, the questioning of the patient's integration into in everyday–life and common sense, can cause a devastating loss of intentional reciprocity damaging to the patient's position in the group, the elaboration of a subjective stand and view. Other examples are provided by expressed-emotion research.

With the onset of the illness the intentional outline of personality and biography usually breaks off. This means that the patient's development of personality structure comes to a standstill at this point because reduced intentionality does not suffice to deal with the highly affect–laden content which is being experienced. So the individual is not able to get through the conflictual tendencies up to a clear–cut gestalt. Thus, the person's future development has to do without, for example, the ability to achieve a certain degree of intimacy. Perhaps in some other fields a higher standard of reality-constituting reciprocity may be achieved and kept.

Schizophrenic psychology through the stages of his/her life and the illness, especially with regard to the development of defect states, seems to be better explicable by the intentionality concept than by the vulnerability model—which is best applicable selectively to the moderately ill chronic patient and his relapse risk.

3) The variegated and disparate biological findings in schizophrenics and high risk for schizophrenia probands may be considered as risk factors for developing a less integrated and stable hierarchy and net of functions, especially with respect to basic affect regulations and cognitions. This might be the nonspecific and heterogeneous substrate of fragile intentionality which is prone to develop a pre–schizophrenic personality structure with emotional instability and cognitive micro–deficits as

described in the high–risk studies. The nonspecifity of such a handicap accords well with genetic findings and the psychopathology of spectrum disorders in relatives of schizophrenics.

Thus, the intentionality model conceptualizes schizophrenia as the reaction type of idiopathic psychoses, which are characterized by structural deficiencies. The schizophrenic syndrome seems to be the final common pathway from very heterogeneous etiologies. Development, insufficiency, break-down and partial restitution and repair of intentionality follow intrinsic rules of the psychic life, which are no longer strictly determined by the biological origines of this unfavourable development.

Summary

Although in cross–cultural psychiatry schizophrenia appears as a unitary syndrome its clinical symptomatology is very complex. Psychopathological heterogeneity, the long–term course with defect states, the mechanisms of precipitating and preventive factors, and the multitude of disparate biological findings require interpretation. Concepts of intentionality as opposite to the vulnerability model focus on the schizophrenic's difficulty to constitute the self, the objectal world in psychic representatives and the difficulty to enter into the process of social reciprocity. The intentionality concept appears to be well suitable for the interpretation of the different stages of the illness, especially the pathogenetic mechanisms which govern the development of defect states. In the view of the intentionality concept they can be seen as repair mechanisms for insufficient constituting reality or eleviation for already premorbidly instable and overchallenged intentional efforts.

References

Beringer K: Beitrag zur Analyse schizophrener Denkstörungen. Zeitschr. f.d.ges. Neurol. u. Psychiat. 93: 55-61, 1924.
Beringer K: Denkstörungen und Sprache bei Schizophrenen. Ztschr. f. die ges. Neurol. u. Psychiat. 103: 185-197, 1926.
Berze J, Gruhle HW: Psychologie der Schizophrenie. Springer, Berlin, 1929.
Blankenburg W: Der Verlust der natürlichen Selbstverständlichkeit. Enke, Stuttgart, 1971.
Ciompi L, Müller C: Lebensweg und Alter der Schizophrenen. Eine katamnestische Langzeitstudie bis ins Senium. Springer, Berlin, Heidelberg, New York, 1976.
Dennett DC: Intentional Systems. The Journal of Philosophy 68: 87-106, 1971.
Dührssen A: Die "kognitive Wende" in der Verhaltenstherapie.—Eine Brücke zur Psychoanalyse? Nervenarzt 56: 479-484, 1985.
Held H-Rv: Umgang mit Psychosen in Encounter- und Therapiegruppen, Gruppenpsychother. Gruppendynamik 19: 231-242, 1984.
Huber G: Reine Defektsyndrome und Basisstadien endogener Psychosen. Fortschr. Neurol. Psychiatr. 34: 409-426, 1966.

Huber G, Gross G, Schüttler R: Schizophrenie. Eine verlaufs- und sozialpsychiatrische Langzeitstudie. Springer, Berlin, Heidelberg, New York 1979.

Lang H: Die Sprache und das Unbewußte. Jacques Lacans Grundlegung der Psychoanalyse. Suhrkamp, Frankfurt am Main, 1988.

Marcus J, Auerbach J, Wilkinson L, Burak C: Infants at risk for schizophrenia. The Jerusalem infant development study. Arch. Gen. Psychiat. 38: 703-713, 1981.

Mundt Ch: Das Apathiesyndrom der Schizophrenen. Springer, Berlin, Heidelberg, New York, 1985.

Nuechterlein KH: Vulnerability Models for Schizophrenia: State of the Art. In: Häfner H. Gattaz WF, Janzarik W (eds): Search for the Causes of Schizophrenia, Springer, Berlin, Heidelberg, New York, London, Paris, Tokyo, pp. 297-316, 1987.

Piaget J: Der Aufbau der Wirklichkeit beim Kinde, Gesammelte Werke 2, Klett, Stuttgart, 1975.

Rapaport D: The theory of attention cathexis. An economic and structural attempt at the explanation of cognitive processes. The collected papers of D. Rapaport. Basic Books, New York, London, 1967.

Sartorius N. Jablensky A, Ernberg G, Leff J, Gulbinat W: Course of Schizophrenia in Different Countries: Some Results of a WHO International Comparative 5-Year Follow-up Study. In: Häfner H. Gattaz WF, Janzarik W (eds): Search for the Causes of Schizophrenia, Springer, Berlin, Heidelberg, New York, London, Paris, Tokyo, pp. 107-113, 1987.

Schultz-Hencke H: Einführung in die Psychoanalyse. Fischer, Stuttgart, 1927.

Zubin J, Spring B: Vulnerability—a new view of schizophrenia. J. Abnorm. Psychol. 86: 103-126, 1977.

Kant on Schizophrenia

Manfred Spitzer

1. Introduction

Only in recent years has Kant's philosophy been considered relevant to psychiatric questions, especially to the understanding of some of the most puzzling phenomena of that most enigmatic disease in psychiatry, schizophrenia.[1] For the empirically minded Anglo-American psychiatrist or psychologist, it may be hard to understand why one should learn something about Kant in order to understand a mental disorder that had not even been conceptualized in Kant's time. Thus, the title of this paper seems to imply—to say the least—a categorical mistake: The term "schizophrenia" was introduced by Eugen Bleuler in the beginning of this century, i.e., about 100 years after Kant had died. Therefore, Kant could not have had any opinion about schizophrenia if you take the concept literally. However, there are *two ways* in which it makes sense—and in which it can be, according to my point of view, highly rewarding—to ask what Kant had to say about mental illness in general, and about what was later called "schizophrenia" in particular.

(1) Kant had a system of psychiatric diagnoses which proved to be quite advanced, especially taking into account what was known about the subject matter in his time.

(2) Kant's philosophy is relevant to the understanding of certain concepts that are used to describe the most important symptoms or syndromes[2] in schizophrenia. This thesis can be put forward in numerous versions that differ in strength, and we will examine a weak and a strong version of it.

To learn psychopathology from Kant, however, is difficult. One of the reasons is that his psychiatric system is contained in his *Anthropology*, a book that was not regarded as "scientific" when it was first published and

---

1 These ideas were proposed independently by German and American authors. For an example of a "transcendental" approach to medicine, see Diemer 1966. Psychiatric questions are discussed within the framework of a version of Kant's philosophy by Hoff (1988, 1989), Hundert (1989 and in this volume) and Spitzer (1985, 1988b). The present paper is an elaboration of themes developed in my *General Subjectivity and Psychopathology* (Allgemeine Subjektivität und Psychopathologie, 1985), and dealt with in two more recent papers (Spitzer 1988a,b).

2 Whether you refer to many psychopathological "phenomena"—to use a somewhat neutral term—as symptoms or syndromes is to some extent a matter of taste. Hallucinations, for example, are most often referred to as a symptom, yet, they may be called a syndrome because there are many different characteristics of a person who is in an "hallucinatory state". The same is true for delusions, and thought disorder frequently is split up into many categories (cf. Spitzer 1988d, 1989).

still is not regarded as "philosophy" either.[3] Kant's *philosophy*, however, is taken as a rational reconstruction rather than as a psychological analysis of knowledge. Thus it is often thought of as having little or nothing to do with *actual* (let alone *mentally ill*) human beings. Although Kant himself seems to have implied such a view by writing his most famous book on *pure* reason, we should note that the distinction between psychology and philosophy made by the present departmental organization of our universities scarcely existed in Kant's time. For him, psychology was part of philosophy, and therefore we should be careful in separating out philosophical and "merely" psychological statements in Kant's writings. Moreover, it is hard to believe that Kant inadvertently used the same terms with different meanings in philosophical and psychological writings. That is to say, taking into account his highly systematic style of writing it is hard to assume that he was *not* aware of the implications of the terminology he used. In this paper we will take Kant seriously, the philosopher *and* the psycho–(patho–) logist (for a more detailed discussion of methodological issues with regard to Kant, see below).

Although the focus of this article is on the impact of Kant's *philosophy* on psychiatric thinking we will, for systematic reasons, begin with a brief discussion of his psychopathology.

2. Kant and Psychopathology

2.1 General Remarks

For several reasons it is generally unknown, especially in the English-speaking world, that Kant had a considerably detailed psychiatric classificatory system, i.e., a type of what today is the *Diagnostic and Statistical Manual of Mental Disorders in its revised 3rd edition* (DSM–III–R). It is contained in his *Pragmatic Approach to Anthropology*, a book he published late[4] (1798) and later rewrote for a second edition which came out in 1800. As we have already mentioned, this book was regarded neither by philosophers nor by scientists as something worth studying, and this is probably the reason why it had to wait 180 years to be translated into the English language.[5] At

---

3 Heidegger, for example, thought of Kant's *Anthropology* as "merely" empirical, hereby implying that its content is not worth study by the philosopher (cf. Kisker 1957).
4 He must have been dabbling with the problem, though, for a long time since he held his first lectures on Anthropology in the fall term of 1772/73.
5 A note, however, has to be made about this translation: The thorough reader should in any case consult the German original as it contains many expressions with subtle meanings for which there is hardly an appropriate translation. Moreover, the German terminology is not strictly represented on a one-to-one basis: Some important German terms have more than one English representative, and some English terms stand for two different German terms. Sometimes there are simply mistakes: The English translation, to give an example, of the German term "stumme Verrücktheit" which describes some abnormal grief reaction and/or some reactive depressive psychosis, and which should be translated as "silent madness" is obviously mistranslated by the English term "stupid madness". "Witz" should not have been translated as "intelligence" but as "wit", and the "Grillenkrankheit" could have remained the "cricket-disease", and not been mistranslated as "melancholia", a term which is also used by Kant, but with a different meaning. (This list could be continued.)

present one may simply say that philosophers are not interested in, and psychiatrists do not know about, these writings. Moreover, the fact that Kant was ahead of his time with regard to his psychiatric classificatory system resulted in its sharing the most likely general fate of such work, that is to say, it was not taken seriously during his time and was forgotten.

One may argue that Kant did not actually have the clinical experience that is needed to provide a classification of mental disorders. Nevertheless, as the "mental" doctors at that time did not see patients to a great extent either (rather they "administrated" them)[6], the least one can say is that his "clinical" experience may not have been substantially less than the experience of his contemporary "psychiatrists". Moreover, as Kisker in his article on *Kant's Psychiatric System* (1957) pointed out, Kant was interested in medical problems, read medical journals, and knew the issues of contemporary medical investigation.[7]

Before we give an overview on Kant's system we shall concentrate on some general ideas and features. These features, rather than the actual nosological entities Kant proposed, according to our point of view, are of particular interest.

First of all, the only *general* feature of mental illness according to Kant is a *loss of the communal sense* (sensus communis), i.e., the loss of the ability of a person to be corrected by others.

"The only general characteristic of insanity is the loss of a sense for ideas that are common to all (sensus communis), and its replacement with a sense for ideas peculiar to ourselves (sensus privatus); for example, in broad daylight a man sees a light burning on a table, which, however, another person standing next to him does not see; or he hears a voice which no one else hears. It is a subjectively necessary touchstone of the correctness of our judgement and, consequently, of the soundness of our understanding that we relate our understanding to the understanding of others, and not merely isolate ourselves within our own experiences, and make public quasi judgements which are merely based on our own private ideas" (Kant, *Anthropology* § 53, p. 117).

This assumption of Kant's was almost neglected for the following 150 years, only to be revived in the recent decades under such headings as "social" or "interactional" psycho–(patho–)logy.

A second accomplishment consists of the idea that mental illness may be a result of various kinds of somatic illnesses and—in addition—that it may have a genetic component. Kant mentions psychotic states caused by fever or epilepsy, and he gives advice not to marry a person in whose family there have been members with a mental disorder.

Thirdly, with regard to what are presently called the "endogenous" psychoses, Kant remarks that some strange behavior is not the cause but rather the consequence of mental illness:

---

6 Cf. Ackerknecht 1968.
7 When, for instance, in Great Britain the Bedlam Hospital was reorganized, Kant wondered about the practical problems of free will in psychiatry (cf. Kisker 1957).

"'Love made him crazy,' people say of one; while of another they say, 'Pride made him crazy,' and of a third person they say, 'he has studied too hard.' Falling in love with a person of high social standing and to expect from that person the folly of marriage is not the cause but the result of derangement; and as far as pride is concerned, an insignificant person's demand that others bow and scrape before him, and the insinuation that others challenge his position presupposes mental derangement without which he would not have dared to make such demands in the first place" (Kant, *Anthropology* § 53, p. 115)[8]

Thus he emphasized the "endogenous" rather than the "psychogenous" nature of these illnesses.

Fourthly, Kant stresses the relevance of the form rather than content for the understanding of mental illness and he doubts that there is any difference between making mad statements in general and making mad statements about particular themes.

"Unreason (which is something positive and not just a lack of reason) is like reason, a mere form, to which objects [of thought] can be adapted; and both reason and unreason, therefore, concern themselves with the general" (Kant, *Anthropology* § 53, p. 116).

The almost unlimited variety of idiosyncratic themes is, fifthly, then explained as follows:

"However, what first comes into the mind at the (usually sudden) outbreak of a crazy disposition (the accidentally encountered subject matter about which the person will rave later) will be from then on the novelty of the impression, more firmly fixed in his mind than anything else occurring afterward" (Kant, *Anthropology* § 53, p. 116).

As these general remarks show, Kant reflected upon problems that are still subjects of discussion, and he did so in quite a sophisticated way.

2.2 The System

Kant generally distinguishes mental *weaknesses* from mental *disorders*. Under the heading "Mental weaknesses" he discusses different sorts of mildly pathological abnormalities and also some mere variations of normality. He mentions the "simpleton", "imprudent", and "stupid", the "coxcomb", "fool" and the "buffon". Kant argues about tutelage[9], the

---

8 Kant's remarks on "overstudying" seem to be rather up-to-date: "But, as to studying too hard, there is no need to warn young people. With regard to studying, youth needs spurs, rather than reins" (Kant, *Anthropology* § 53, p. 115). In a footnote he adds: "It is an ordinary thing to see a merchant overextend himself and dissipate his powers in vast schemes. Anxious parents, however, have nothing to fear from overtaxing the industriousness of young people (as long as their minds are otherwise sound). A student is protected by nature from such overloading with knowledge by finding subjects distasteful, over which he only broods and breaks his head to no avail" (Kant, *Anthropology* § 53, p. 115).

9 "Children are naturally minors and their parents are their natural guardians. The wife, whatever her age, is declared to be a minor in civil matters... Learned men usually allow themselves to be kept in a state of tutelage by their wives as far as domestic arrangements are concerned. When a servant shrieked

distinction between lack of judgement with and without "wit"[10], discusses cunning and slyness ("the art of deceiving")[11], the need for some distraction as a "necessary and partially artificial way of taking care of one's mental well being" (Kant, *Anthropology*, p. 102)[12], and a variety of other issues.

Mental disorders can be classified with regard to the mental faculty that is affected. So with regard to cognition, Kant describes "melancholia (Hypochondria)"[13], which may be characterized by loss of control over affective states, inhibition of thought, and a realization of being ill, distinguishing it from "mental disorder (mania)", which amounts to a loss of control of thought content, presumably without the realization of being ill. In order to gain just one impression of how nicely Kant was able to describe these states, consider the following example:

> "A melancholic man is well aware that the train of his thought does not move properly, but he has not sufficient control over himself to direct, restrain, or control the course of his thought. Unjustified joy and grief whimsically change in such a person like the weather which one has to accept as it comes" (Kant, *Anthropology* § 45, p. 97).

Disturbances of sense perception are "either irrationality or insanity"; "delirium or imbecility" are the terms for disturbed judgement and reason. "Daydreamers" who lack the capacity to compare their "imagination with the laws of experience" (Kant, *Anthropology* § 45, p. 97) are called "visionaries"; if this impairment of reality-testing—to use contemporary terminology—is due to "emotional excitement" (Kant, *Anthropology* § 45, p. 97) Kant's designation is that of an "enthusiast".

Thus Kant tries to give a comprehensive and systematic account of mental disorders with regard to what was known about the mental "faculties" in general. As we already have remarked above and in several footnotes, Kant's work seems to be rich in insights about human nature (though, occasionally, he merely states the prejudices of his days).

3. Kant and Understanding Schizophrenia

In the rest of this article we will discuss a thesis that may be stated briefly as follows:

---

that there was a fire in one of the rooms, a learned man, buried in books, answered, 'You know, things of that sort are my wife's affair" (Kant, *Anthropology*, pp. 105-106).

10 "Lack of judgement without wit is stupidity... But the same lack of judgement accompanied by wit is silliness" (Kant, *Anthropology*, pp. 99-100; translation corrected by the author, M.S.).

11 "The question is: Whether the deceiver must be smarter than the one who is easily deceived, and whether the latter is the stupid one" (Kant, *Anthropology*, p. 101; translation corrected by the author, M.S.).

12 "To be distracted in society is impolite, and often laughable as well. Women are ordinarily not subject to this impulse, unless they devote themselves to learning" (Kant, *Anthropology*, p. 101).

13 The terms before and in brackets are Kant's terms and the quotation marks indicate that he used the terms in exactly the way we do here.

Kant's theory of the transcendental subject provides a framework that is useful for understanding a variety of otherwise unrelated schizophrenic phenomena.

There are several versions of this thesis that differ in strength, and I shall discuss a weak version first but then argue for a strong version of the thesis. Before I do so, we first need to become acquainted with some of the phenomena that I have in mind.

3.1 Ichstörungen

The German term "Ichstörungen" does not have a proper English translation. Literally, it means "I-disorders", and as the *experiencing I* is meant, and *not* the idiosyncratic aspects of a person, *not* the character, *not* the personality, one may refer to the phenomena in question as *disorders of the form of experience in general*. Furthermore, we are not talking about the "ego" of psychoanalysis, although more recent developments in "object relations theory" show some similarities between psychoanalytic thinking and the phenomena to which I am referring.[14]

In order to give a rough picture of the kind of phenomena that can be frequently observed in schizophrenic patients, I quote some of their utterances. I am sure that the psychiatrist and clinical psychologist are quite familiar with these statements (taken from Spitzer 1988b).

(a) "I feel that it is not me who is thinking."
(b) "My thoughts are not thought by me. They are thought by somebody else."
(c) "Things are not seen by me, only by my eyes."
(d) "This thing directly refers to me."
(e) "There is an immediate relation between this object and me."
(f) "My thoughts can influence things. This event happens because I think of it."
(g) "To keep the world going, I must not stop thinking, otherwise it would cease to exist."
(h) "My experience has changed somehow. It is not real and I myself am not real."
(i) "Things do not feel real. There is something between me and the things and persons around me; something like a wall of glass between me and everything else."
(j) "Time has disappeared. Not that it is longer or shorter, it's just not there; there are bits and pieces of time, shaken and mingled; often there is no time at all."

The pathology in these statements is referred to in the Anglo-American literature by various concepts, the extension of which overlaps to some degree with that of the German concept of Ichstörungen. Thus, the statements might be classified as indicating "loss of control", "passivity

---

14 Some of these similarities (or analogies) are mentioned in Hundert (this volume).

phenomena", "depersonalization", "derealisation", "disturbance of ego-boundaries", to name but a few of a variety of technical terms. According to more recent developments in Anglo–American psychiatry, most the phenomena are simply classified as "delusions", and thus are lumped together with a large number of other phenomena (cf. DSM-III-R, pp. 188, 395–396). For reasons which I have discussed elsewhere[15], there are good reasons for trying to be more specific, and for giving a more "interpretive" account of such phenomena than saying merely that they are false beliefs about the external world, as stated in the DSM–III–R. Such statements—contrary to the explicitly stated DSM–III–R definition[16] of delusions—are *neither false* (but rather the patient's *valid* account of what is different in their experience) *nor about external reality* (but rather about *internal* feelings, thoughts, and so on).

We will discuss these ideas in more detail below, as they represent the strong version of our thesis. Nevertheless, there is a weak version of our claim of a relation between Kant's philosophy and the understanding of schizophrenia which we want to examine first.

3.2 Kant and Schizophrenia: The Weak Version

Several weak versions of our thesis, i.e., of a link between Kantian philosophy and the concept of schizophrenia or some of the core symptoms of this illness, respectively, are possible. One of these may run as follows: The men who gave contemporary psychiatry its imprint in the second half of the last century were influenced by the main cultural and philosophical movements or ideas of their time. As psychiatry was strongly influenced by German psychiatrists, it is not surprising that German philosophy (which happened to be Idealism) was "at work" when basic concepts were formed. This was certainly the case when the concept of "mental" was introduced to medicine, when distinctions such as those between hallucinations, illusions, pseudohallucinations, and delusions were made, and, moreover, when the concept of "Ichstörungen" was formed at the beginning of the century by Karl Jaspers in his famous *General Psychopathology*.[17]

In this particular case, Idealism was certainly "at work", i.e., *used*, but *not explicitly mentioned*: Jaspers refers to the I and its characteristic features of *activity, unity, identity*, and the *me-not-me distinction*. However, there is no reference to either Kant or to transcendental philosophy, respectively, to be found in Jaspers' *General Psychopathology* that would fit his account of the disturbed I.[18] Under the heading "Ichbewußtsein" (which has been

---

15 See the Introduction to this volume, as well as Spitzer 1988a, 1988d (chapter 11).

16 "Delusion. A false personal belief based upon incorrect inference about external reality..." (DSM-III-R, p. 395).

17 The book was first published in 1913 and appeared in several new editions until a final version was prepared by Jaspers in 1942/43, which also served as the source for the English translation which appeared in 1963.

18 Jaspers quotes Kant's *Anthropology* several times (pp. 36, 216, 420, 431, 452, 856), the *Critique of Judgment* is quoted twice (pp. 331, 454), and two minor works are quoted once each (pp. 387: *On the*

translated as "awareness of the self", the literal translation being "I-consciousness") Jaspers talks about these *formal characteristics* but does not explain how he arrived at these four characteristics, which obviously fit nicely into the clinical picture of many schizophrenic patients who serve as examples throughout the whole section about the "Ichbewußtsein". Although quite a few references to Kant can be found in this section[19], Jaspers does not mention Kant in this context. Jaspers seeks to convey the impression that he had derived the concepts by mere description without any form of interpretation. This is a self misunderstanding, as interpretation *has to be done* whenever the patients' utterances are schematized, categorized and labeled with certain concepts.[20]

Jaspers set the stage for the notion of "Ichstörungen" to become a well known issue in the psychopathology of schizophrenia in German psychiatry. Kurt Schneider, his most famous successor, for example, adopted his four characteristics and added a fifth one, the "experience of existence", but, like Jaspers, did not reflect on the origin of these characteristics of the I.[21] Neither did German psychiatric textbooks: Most of them deal with "Ichstörungen" in some detail along the lines of Jaspers and Schneider, but there is hardly any concept of the normal I, that underlies the notion of a disturbed one.[22] The famous ninth volume of the *Handbuch der Geisteskrankheiten (Handbook of Mental Disorders,* Bumke 1932), to take just one example, deals with "Ichstörungen" in detail (pp. 188-191, 302, 584), and rates their general diagnostic significance highly—ahead of delusions and second only to thought disorder (p. 584). However, no account can be found concerning the I, that explains what it is that is disturbed in I–disturbances.

Thus, a weak version of our thesis proceeds approximately as follows: It can be shown that Kant's philosophy—although officially disregarded by some psychiatrists[23]—had in fact an impact on the formation of some basic concepts of psychiatry. As the basic concepts in the field have not greatly changed since then, we would gain a better understanding of at least some concepts that are used for descriptive purposes in present day psychiatry if we become familiar with some of Kant's philosophical concepts. In other

---

power of mind...; 480: *De mundi sensibilis...*). Kant's name is mentioned together with the names of other philosophers twice (pp. 756, 821), and there is only one reference to the *Critique of Pure Reason* (on p. 560, consisting in a rather obscure reference to the notion of the "world in itself").

19 The four characteristics themselves are the best example as they are taken directly from Kant (Jaspers' notion of "activity" only has to be replaced by Kant's "spontaneity", meaning roughly the same thing) who used the same concepts. Jaspers' explanations further show strong similarities to Kant, although Jaspers tries to "psychologize" and to simplify Kant to a great deal. When Kant (*Critique of Pure Reason* B131/132), for example, says: "It must be possible for the 'I think' to accompany all my representations...", Jaspers simply states: "The 'I think' accompanies all perceptions, ideas, and thoughts" (Jaspers 1963, p. 101, translation corrected by the author, M.S.).

20 See my introductory article to this volume, *Why Philosophy?*.

21 Cf. Spitzer 1988b.

22 The only references one may find under the entry "Ich" in German textbooks are about Freud's "ego" and about the individual "person". A *formal* structure, as used by Jaspers and Schneider in order to describe some schizophrenic phenomena, is not mentioned (see also Spitzer 1985).

23 Many psychiatrists were very "antiphilosophically" minded (see Stransky 1923, for a remarkable example of how far this had gone).

words, the weak thesis asserts the *historical* importance of Kant's philosophy while leaving open the question of its *systematic* impact.

3.3 Kant and Schizophrenia: The Strong Version

The strong version of the argument about a link between Kant's philosophy and schizophrenia runs something like this: Kant's notion of the transcendental subject, i.e., the general structure of any (possible) experience, can serve as an interpretative framework for making sense out of many otherwise unrelated schizophrenic phenomena. His theory could lead us to discover the exact relations between such schizophrenic symptoms as disturbed identity, broken unity, blurred me–not–me distinction, and fragmentation of time. His theory, thus, may be used to get a clearer clinical picture in cases where there is doubt about which symptoms might actually be present.

In order to find out what the features of disturbed experience of *objectivity* are—to give another version of the strong thesis—we have to find out what the features of the subject are. To be more precise, we need to determine the features of the general structure of experience, of *general subjectivity* (as we might call it), and also find the supporting evidence for claims about such a structure.

One implication of the strong thesis is that reality is some result of *production*. This means that physical objects and all their properties are not presupposed as being "given" or "just there", but rather are conceived as the result of some active process. By "physical objects" or by "reality" we mean not just features like "of a certain color" and "having a specific shape" etc., but also "existing without being perceived", "existing independently of the subject", "not being related to the subject" and so forth.

The process may be exemplified by analogy: When I see this piece of paper in front of me, it looks white and rectangular. However, I know from physics that the light traveling from its surface into my eyes has some yellow bias and that the edges must consist of some non–rectangular angles because the surface of the paper is not parallel to my retina—leaving me with some tilted and colored retinal image. Nevertheless, what I *see* is a white rectangular piece of paper, and from physiology I know how this is achieved: There are "constancy–mechanisms" built into my visual system that eliminate not only my perspective and some general color of my visual field, but, even more so, also eliminate movements of my eyes or my body (although these lead my retinal image to change very quickly, the things that I see are quite stable).[24] The mechanisms that are involved in this construction of reality *as it really is*—the paper *is* in fact white and rect-

---

24 The famous drawing of Ernst Mach of his visual field which shows, among other things, his own nose, together with the fact that we hardly have ever noticed our own nose before having seen Mach's drawing, also shows that we do not perceive constant features of our retinal images.

angular[25]—can be studied to a great extent by investigating sense perceptions, which in most cases turn out to be the result of mechanisms which in the ordinary case provide us with a more adequate perception of reality (cf. Gregory 1974). As we rarely worry about the problem whether digestion is done *by* us or *for* us (by our digestive system) we may leave the question aside whether *I do* the "white-adjustment" and "perspective-adjustment" or whether all this (and much more) *is done for me.* What is most important to keep in mind here, however, is the fact that all the mechanisms mentioned[26] eliminate *subjective* features (*my* nose, *my* perspective, *my* movements, the color of *my* actual visual field) in order to make the result—i.e., what we actually perceive—as *objective* as possible. In other words, scientists have dealt at length with aspects of the subject in order to find out about what is objectively there.

We have only to push this idea a little further in order to see the relevance of Kant's synthetic unity of apperception—the transcendental I—to phenomena that frequently occur in schizophrenia. Kant's Copernicanian revolution in the manner of looking at reality consists of the idea that —to put the idea along the lines of our analogy—objectivity is not only achieved by disregarding my nose, perspective, movements, etc., but also by disregarding the very fact that *it is me who does all this disregarding.* Reality, i.e., the idea that "this object is there regardless of my perception of it, regardless of my idea of it, even *totally regardless of me at all*", thus becomes the *utmost achievement of objectivity* a subject can make. Reality, the objectivity of things, is not just given; objectivity rather is the achievement of a *subject*; and if we want to know how the objectivity of the external world can be (experienced as being) disturbed, we have to study the subject (i.e., *subjectivity* in general) whose accomplishment is nothing but objectivity.

Much has to be learned about disorders of experience as just described. We hold that our limited account, as given here, is simply a first conceptual step in a direction in which psychopathological research has to follow. Measures of validity have to be applied, and the way we interpret utterances of patients has to be studied very carefully to obtain a clearer picture of what schizophrenia is like, and how it can be treated for the good of the patient.

---

25 This is not a circular argument of the form "we perceive things as we perceive them". Once we start learning about perceptual processes we cannot help asking the question of how we perceive things as they are, for the simple reason that, within the process, things are represented differently from how they are. Like Berkeley who had to wonder why we see things upright because he had seen the upside-down image on the retina of an oxen's eye, we can wonder about the wavelength, shape and motion of what we can see and independently measure, about what the picture on our retina looks like, and about what our phenomenological experience is like.

26 It should be noted here that neither the odd representations nor the mechanisms proposed to compensate for them are merely postulated. They both can be shown empirically, and the whole explanation is *not*, as the philosopher might suspect, circular.

3.4 Objections and Refutations

There are some objections to what we just have said that seem to make the strong version of our thesis at least unlikely, or even more so, quite wrong. We want therefore to deal with some of these objections in the rest of this paper.

3.4.1 Experience versus Delusions

Kant refers to the structure of experience as the structure of *any possible* experience, but schizophrenics describe their experience in a way that seems to falsify Kant. To take an example:[27] Kant's famous notion that "it must be possible for the 'I think' to accompany all my representations" (Kant, *Critique of Pure Reason*, B131) simply seems to be wrong when we are confronted with a schizophrenic patient saying that his thoughts and feelings are *not his*. Our interpretation of this state of affairs is this. We have to have a firm notion of the default case of experience (as described by Kant) in order to understand, as clearly as possible, those cases of experience where something goes profoundly wrong. Of course, the schizophrenic patient refers to *his* experience as not being his and simply seems to make a confused (and confusing) statement. Nevertheless, the "I think" in some very deep sense does not accompany many of his thoughts. If we do not recognize the general feature of *mine–ness of experience* we will never be able to understand what the schizophrenic patient has to say about the changes in his experience. It will remain only "strange" to us, and we will only be able to classify such experiences as delusions, i.e., as plainly false statements about reality. So, while Kant obviously is talking about the default case of experience—in which it happens to be unified, mine, in a time–order, and of some identical object that is not identical with me—he is right in saying that these features are features of any possible experience *I* can think of. Nevertheless, we argue, that in the non–default case of schizophrenia it makes sense to apply Kantian concepts and use them to describe variations in experience that we normally do not think of as possible.

We claim that it seems very unlikely that almost all schizophrenics tell us something *wrong* when they tell about their experience. Moreover, why should about 70%[28] of all schizophrenics come up with approximately the same "delusions"?[29] This remarkable fact has not been reconciled and cannot be reconciled by a psychiatric classification which has no expression for the way in which the experience of patients suffering from the most

---

27 Cf. also Blankenburg 1988, Hundert 1989.
28 The number (cf. Murray 1986, p. 342) refers to delusions of reference, i.e., the reported experience that objects are not just as they are but somehow no longer independent of the experiencing subject. The former *achievement* of objectivity has been lost.
29 As the DSM–III–R (p. 188) states: "Certain delusions are observed far more frequently in schizophrenia than in other psychotic disorders." The phenomena that are referred to are precisely the phenomena in question here.

frequently occurring disorder in psychiatry is changed. Therefore, we claim that to label "Ichstörungen" as "delusions" is a serious mistake. What is overlooked in this case is the fact that many of the patients refer to the *same* topics, to similar features of their experience that have changed. These experiences might, over time, be elaborated further into delusions,[30] i.e, into statements and beliefs referring to something else,[31] but in and of themselves they are something totally different from delusions (which are, at least by the definition given in the DSM–III–R, *false* and about *external* reality). So if the patients refer to a change in the structure of their experience (of the kind: "not me", "no unity", "no identity", "fragmented time"), we should try to match their statements with appropriate concepts. And we can learn about them from Kant.

3.4.2 The Limitations of Kant's Actual Psychopathology

As Kant actually reflected on psychopathology, one question must be answered: Why don't we find a good account of disorders of experience as we just outlined in Kant's writings on psychopathology?—There are two explanations, a "philosophical" one, and a simple empirical one. Let us turn to the first: Among scholars of Kant, the view is widely held that Kant may sometimes have used the same terms to refer to different concepts, depending on whether he was discussing "pure" or "empirical" matters. Thus it is argued that when he talks about "reason" he might mean it "purely" in his most famous *Critique*, but not so when he discusses insanity as a disorder of reason in his *Anthropology*. Therefore, it is argued, he did not link his "psychopathology" to his philosophy.

Although this account may be true, it does not give a reason *why* he did what he did, i.e., why he used terms like "judgement" and "reason" with two totally different meanings. The ultimate and most simple reason for this, according to my point of view, is *his lack of relevant data*.[32] Even though we said in the beginning that Kant knew as much about mental illness as did the medical professionals of his time, this knowledge was, nonetheless, very limited. The following facts should especially be borne in mind when considering this issue: In Kant's time, chronic patients by far dominated the picture of the mentally ill in general.[33] Not until the middle of this century were comparatively more studies conducted on the

---

30 The experience of feeling that one is not thinking one's own thoughts, for example, may give way to the interpretation by the patient, that somebody else is thinking his or her thoughts. Thus, Ichstörungen might be the seeds out of which some delusions grow.

31 Cf. Spitzer 1988c, 1989.

32 Philosophers need to have the right data and, of course, do deal with some kind of data. I owe this insight to Professor Hector–Neri Castañeda. Although he holds a different view on the "nature" of the I, the discussions I had with him on various occasions helped me to substantially clarify my own thoughts on the issue.

33 Here it is important to relate this section of the paper to the previous one: We know what Kant knew concerning this subject and what kind of data he must have been familiar with in order to make his classification.

outbreak of a psychosis with its preceding changes of mind.[34] The symptoms we are talking about, however, are most clearly observable at the outbreak of psychosis but become increasingly confounded by the patients' "interpretations" the longer they persist. For example, it is not a large step from the immediate experience of one's own thought occurring passively, outside of one's own control, to the idea that "somebody else" might have taken over. In short, Kant may not have encountered pathological phenomena that reminded him of his philosophy, and therefore he did not relate the two to each other.

One observation may serve as a slight support of this view: In his *Anthropology*, he first discusses *Mental Weaknesses in the Faculty of Knowledge* (section B, §§ 46–49) and then goes on to discuss *Mental illnesses* (section C, §§ 50–52), leaving out the "faculty of knowledge", although the two chapters are conceived "symmetrically" and to be found under one . Thus, to Kant the concept of an *ill faculty of knowledge* seems to be either impossible or at least unlikely (although he allowed for weaknesses).

4. Conclusion

We cannot claim that Kant's philosophy is the only way to think generally about experience. Nevertheless, it provides one of the most sophisticated frameworks ever given for such enquiry. Philosophers and philosophies that regard experience, such as that of "objects" and "independent reality", as given cannot provide a solution to the problem of how to conceptualize disturbances of experience as they occur in schizophrenic patients. The very fact that in order to account for disorders of experience the concept of *Ichstörungen* (disorders of the experiencing I) was developed and used mainly by Continental psychiatrists, may well reflect not merely a historical coincidence but also constitute an advantage with regard to the appropriate conceptual framework.

Summary

In his *Anthropology*, Kant proposed a psychiatric system that was quite advanced relative to the standards of his day. Many features of mental disorder which we now know were already pointed out by Kant. This is one way in which Kant can be of interest to modern psychiatry. In addition, and much more relevant from a systematic point of view, we have tried to show that Kant's philosophy may be relevant to the understanding of some very common disturbances of schizophrenic patients. These disturbances refer to changes in their experience. Thus the idea of experience has to be appropriately conceived in order to provide psychiatrists with the con-

---

34 Cf. especially Conrad 1971.

ceptual framework they need to make sense out of such "crazy" statements as, for instance, "my thoughts and feelings are not mine". A weak version of our argument consists in saying that for historical reasons psychiatry relied upon some of Kant's notions to account for such statements. However, the strong version of the argument, which is the one that we favor, consists in the assumption that Kant's account of objective experience as the product of a general structure of the subject is, for systematic reasons, one way to conceptualize experience whereby the psychiatrist is enabled to make better sense out of disordered experience.[35]

References

Ackerknecht, EH: A Short History of Psychiatry, 2nd ed., transl. Wolff S, Hafner, New York, 1968.
American Psychiatric Association: Diagnostic and Statistical Manual of Mental Disorders, 3rd ed., revised (DSM–III–R). American Psychiatric Association, Washington DC, 1987.
Blankenburg W: Zur Psychopathologie des Ich–Erlebens Schizophrener. In: Spitzer M, Uehlein FA, Oepen G (eds): Psychopathology and Philosophy. Springer, Berlin Heidelberg New York London Paris Tokyo, pp. 184–197, 1988.
Bumke O (ed): Handbuch der Geisteskrankheiten, vol. IX (Die Schizophrenie), Springer, Berlin, 1932.
Conrad K: Die beginnende Schizophrenie. Thieme, Stuttgart, 1971.
Diemer A: Zur Grundlegung einer Philosophie der Medizin. Festvortrag anläßlich des 37. Fortbildungskurses für Ärzte in Regensburg am 13. Oktober 1966.
Gregory RL: Concepts and Mechanisms of Perception. Duckworth, London, 1974.
Hoff P: Der Krankheitsbegriff in der Psychiatrie aus transzendentalphilosophischer Sicht. Phil. Diss., Munich, 1988.
Hoff P: Erkenntnistheoretische Vorurteile in der Psychiatrie. Fundamenta Psychiatrica 3: 141–150, 1989.
Hundert EM: Philosophy, Psychiatry and Neuroscience. Three Approaches to the Mind. Clarendon, Oxford, 1989.
Hundert EM: Are Psychotic Illnesses Category Disorders? Proposal for a New Understanding and Classification of the Major Forms of Mental Illness. This volume, 1990.
Jaspers K: General Psychopathology (1913), transl. Hoenig J, Hamilton MW, Manchester University Press, Manchester, 1963.
Kant I: Critique of pure reason (1781/1787), transl. Kemp Smith N, St Martin's Press, New York, 1965.
Kant I: Anthropology (1798), transl. by Dowdell, VL, rev. and ed. by Rudnick HH, Southern Illinois University Press, Carbondale and Edwardville, 1978.
Kisker KP: Kants psychiatrische Systematik (Kant's Psychiatric System). Psychiatria et Neurologia 133: 17–28, 1957.
Mach, E.: Contributions to the Analysis of Sensations (Die Analyse der Empfindungen), Open Court, Peru Publ. IL,
Murray R: Schizophrenia. In: Hill P, Murray R, Thorley A (eds): Essentials of Postgraduate Psychiatry, Grune and Stratton, London, Orlando, New York, San Diego Boston, San Francisco, Tokyo, Sydney, Toronto, pp. 339–379, 1986

35 This work has been supported by a *Feodor Lynen* grant from the *Alexander–von–Humboldt Foundation*, West–Germany.

Spitzer M: Allgemeine Subjektivität und Psychopathologie (General Subjectivity and Psychopathology). Hagt & Herchen, Frankfurt a.M., 1985

Spitzer M: Psychiatry, Philosophy, and the problem of Description. In: Spitzer M, Uehlein FA, Oepen G (eds): Psychopathology and Philosophy. Springer, Berlin Heidelberg New York London Paris Tokyo, pp. 3-18, 1988a.

Spitzer M: Ichstörungen: In Search of a Theory. In: Spitzer M' Uehlein FA, Oepen G (eds): Psychopathology and Philosophy. Springer, Berlin Heidelberg New York London Paris Tokyo, pp. 167-183, 1988b.

Spitzer M: Karl Jaspers, Mental States, and Delusional Beliefs. In: Spitzer M, Uehlein FA, Oepen G (eds): Psychopathology and Philosophy. Springer, Berlin Heidelberg New York London Paris Tokyo, pp. 167-183, 1988c.

Spitzer M: Halluzinationen. Springer, Berlin Heidelberg New York London Paris Tokyo, 1988d.

Spitzer M: Was ist Wahn? Untersuchungen zum Wahnproblem. Springer, Berlin Heidelberg New York London Paris Tokyo, 1989.

Stransky E: Psychiatrie und Philosophie. Monatsschrift für Psychiatrie und Neurologie 53: 251–262, 1923.

Are Psychotic Illnesses Category Disorders?

Proposal for a New Understanding and Classification of the Major Forms of Mental Illness

Edward M. Hundert

> *Psychopathology does not need philosophy because the latter can teach it anything about its own field, but because philosophy can help the psychopathologist so to organise his thought that he can perceive the true possibilities of his knowledge.*
> Karl Jaspers (1923, pp. 46-7)

1. Philosophical Background

At least since Aristotle, philosophers have been aware that human experience only becomes possible when specific instances of things are brought under more general concepts relating to them. For many years, this was discussed in terms of the relationship between "particulars" and "universals." I can only experience *this* piece of paper as *a* piece of paper when I recognize this particular one as belonging to a more general class of things.

Many variations on this theme have been proposed since ancient Greece, and most philosophical schools of thought have arrived at one version or another. In modern times, even as the empiricists and rationalists claimed to disagree on all the basic questions, both had to come up with some way for particular experiences to be ordered under more general concepts. The empiricist Hume (1740, p. 69, italics in the original) thus concluded that our specific sensory experiences are ordered under "seven different kinds of philosophical relation, *viz. resemblance, identity, relations of time and place, proportion in quantity or number, degrees in any quality, contrarity, and causation.*" The most famous modern version, however, came dressed in rationalist clothing from the mind of Immanuel Kant. Kant took this distinction to reflect the interaction of two separate faculties of the mind: the faculty of sensibility (whose job is to gather specific sensory "intuitions," as Kant called them) and the faculty of understanding (whose job is to order those intuitions under more general concepts, which Kant called "categories" after Aristotle's own term).

One of the most interesting things about Kant's version of this story is that these conceptual categories we use to order our sensory intuitions are taken by him to reflect something about *us*, not something about the *real world*. While Hume, for instance, believed that we come to order experience under general philosophical relations only by abstracting these (with repeated experiences) from the world, Kant thought just the opposite. Taking the category of substance as an example, Kant would say that, as a category of understanding, substance is a concept used by us in constructing every experience we have of the world. Since every set of sensory intuitions is ordered by us under the category of substance, every experience we have of the world is an experience of substantial objects. But, according to Kant, this only confirms that substance is a concept we always necessarily apply in constructing our experience. It is a feature of ourselves, of the structure of our mind, not the "real world" (whose structure we can never know, since we can only have any experience of it through the application of our categories).

Kant's philosophy thus rests upon a sharp distinction between the *content* of experience (*received* as sensory intuitions by the faculty of sensibility) and the *form* of experience (*produced* by the mandatory application of the categories of understanding). This sharp distinction between form and content reflects an equally sharp distinction between the "a priori" and the "a posteriori" features of experience. For Kant, the categories are strictly *a priori* features of experience: they literally come "before experience," since they are *applied to* each experience. The intuitions of sensibility are, in contrast, *a posteriori*, coming, as it were, "after experience." The whiteness of this paper might be found to be true or false with experience, depending upon the content found in sensibility. Its having substance could never be falsified with experience, since understanding brings a substantial form to all experiences we can ever have.

Indeed, it was based upon the sharp distinction between a priori and a posteriori that Kant (1783, p. 11) divided what he considered to be the proper subject matters of philosophy, psychology, and natural science. Philosophy was to be concerned only with the a priori aspects of experience, while psychology and natural science were allocated the internal and external aspects of the a posteriori, respectively. Thus, while philosophers need to know that some a posteriori content will be available for sensibility to bring to understanding, the specific properties of these contents (colors, motions, temperatures, etc.) are not the philosopher's business.

If we are, as Jaspers directs us, to turn to philosophy in order that we might improve our psychology, then these sharp Kantian distinctions will have to give way.

2. The Breakdown of Some Philosophical Distinctions

Although Kant's a priori status can be maintained for categories if we talk about experience in a very abstract and theoretical way, it becomes much more difficult to maintain in talking about the experience of living, breathing human beings. It is quite possible to retell Kant's story of inter-acting mental faculties in terms of the actual biology of the human brain (which does indeed receive sensory information about the world and then process and order that information in various ways), but this merely changes the language of a priori versus a posteriori into the language of genetic versus environmental influences. If we apply Kant's model of the mind to the actual experience of actual people, we could, in other words, still maintain that certain categories are necessarily applied in constructing any possible experience because these structures are somehow "hardwired" into the system, somehow determined by our genetic code.

This idea is not so far-fetched as it may at first appear. We might imagine, for instance, that evolution has put tremendous pressure on the shape of the brain to reflect the actual structure of the world with fidelity. In one version of this line of reasoning, certain particularly constant features of the world, such as substance, time, space, causation, and so forth, might eventually have written themselves into the structure of our brain. Then, any particular sensory data received by the senses would be analyzed using these concepts, and the system would work much as Kant said it did. Here, the genetic determination of these concepts would correspond to the a priori status Kant claimed for his categories. They would, in effect, tell us more about *us* than about the real world, except that in this version, we rely on the pressures of natural selection to guarantee that these concepts we bring to our experience have been shaped over the millenia by the actual features of that world.

To see why this version of the story is most unlikely, consider the following experiment. We begin with two identical twins born today, both of whose brains have therefore been shaped by evolution in exactly the same way. One twin is raised here on our planet and the other is transported to a different galaxy where things are otherwise similar except that objects disappear and reappear capriciously: sometimes the table breaks up into lots of little tables and then recombines into the original table, like mercury droplets dispersing and coalescing.

If we believe that the concept of substance has been hardwired into their brains by evolution on a planet like ours which manifests the perma-nence of objects, we must conclude that our transported twin will go through life constantly being surprised by the impermanence of objects. This seems most unlikely, and for two reasons. The first is that we already know enough about evolutionary neurobiology to guess that evolution adopted a strategy much more powerful than that of shaping the brain to the structure of the world. This alternative solution was a strategy of maximal *plasticity* to what each individual finds in the world, rather than maximal fidelity to the way things were over millenia gone by (see Wiesel 1982, Sarnat and Netsky 1981).

This notion that each of us develops concepts for certain stable features of the world during the early years of our lives is supported by a good deal of psychological and neurobiological theory. Piaget's (1936, 1937) landmark studies of concept development in children emphasize that we not only assimilate the world using concepts we have, but that our concepts in turn accommodate themselves to the actual structure of the world in a series of stages during early life. In the neurobiological version, Edelman (1978, 1987) has suggested a mechanism by which patterns of neurons coding for constant features of the environment will become stabilized over the early years of life, perhaps again in a series of stages like those observed by Piaget (and all parents, teachers, pediatricians...).

But the second reason to doubt that our transported twin would go through life constantly surprised by the impermanence of objects is even more convincing than our current theories of psychology, neuroscience, and evolution. This is the simple fact that we have actual experience with people raised in the conditions of that other galaxy. After all, the main "objects" in a child's life are not tables and chairs, but mothers and fathers. And sometimes mothers and fathers spend a good bit of time capriciously disappearing and reappearing in cases where they are mentally ill, alcoholic, or otherwise in need of repeated hospitalization, for example. The striking fact about people raised in such an environment appears to be precisely their lack of application of the concept of permanent objects throughout their adult life (Mahler 1965, Spitz 1965, Klein 1959, Bowlby 1969, 1973).

The philosophical implications of these findings should be clear. (For a detailed discussion, see Hundert 1989.) Although it is true that as adults we bring certain concepts to experience a priori, these concepts have themselves been shaped by the a posteriori world—and not only by the forces of evolution, but by the rediscovery and reinvention of these concepts by every infant and child interacting with the world. Thus does the a posteriori infiltrate its way into our categories, contaminating our "pure" Kantian a priori concepts with the contingencies of the real world in which we live.

This blurring of the distinction between a priori and a posteriori is paralleled by the blurring of all related philosophical distinctions. We can no longer maintain a sharp contrast between the form and the content of experience, as Kant did with his separate mental faculties, because we see now how the actual contents of experience act upon the child to shape those form–determining concepts which will be brought to experience throughout life. Indeed, even the distinction between analytic and synthetic starts to blur as we begin to view science as the "search for things worth naming" (Lewis 1923) and realize that experience has abandoned those words (phlogiston, epicycles) that were discovered not to correspond to any natural cleavage found in the world. Analytic statements may be true by definition, but the substantive ("synthetic") information found in these definitional relations have been crafted by many hands over many years.

If the a priori status Kant claimed for his categories has been muddied by the dirty waters of actual experience, with what conception of these categories are we left? An understanding of what has been gained by this infiltration of the real world into our concepts will take us a long way toward a new conceptualization of psychotic experience.

3. The Structure of Sanity

Several important results follow from this blurring of the a priori and a posteriori features of experience. For starters, it *makes valid knowledge possible*. So long as Kant insisted upon the strict a priority of his categories, our experience of the world was determined mainly by these features of ourselves, and so Kant had to postulate an entire reduplicated world of things–in–themselves, in contrast to things–as–we–know–them. With a new understanding of how the actual world shapes these concepts through our interactions with that world over the early years of life, we can discard Kant's superfluous reduplicated world, discovering that the real world is intimate enough with our concepts to make valid knowledge of it possible. This is no small gain, but our goal here is to see how these ideas can contribute to our understanding of psychopathology, not philosophy.

To understand this more complex view of the categories of experience is to change completely our attitudes toward psychopathology. If categories do indeed develop in each of us over the early years of life, then that development can suffer problems in much the same way other developing competencies can become impaired. Two general classes of problems might be distinguished: one in which the mechanisms for generating categories (through interaction with the world) becomes defective, and another in which the early world of the infant does not manifest the "constancies" needed for normal category development, as described above. Either way, our view of categories has become much more fluid than Kant's rigid image of the mind as a steel filing cabinet, and the possibilities for variety in experience become much greater.

Indeed, when psychiatric investigators such as Jaspers (1923), Minkowski (1933), and Binswanger (1946) first began to explore the categorical phenomenology of patients, they were startled by the diversity of the inner experiences of people who otherwise looked pretty much the same from the outside. These explorations soon led to a categorical analysis of a variety of psychotic states, whereby, "the phenomenologist attempts to reconstruct the inner world of his patients through an analysis of their manner of experiencing time, space, causality, materiality [substance], and other 'categories' (in the philosophical sense of the word)" (Ellenberger 1958, p. 101).

Before we examine what these existential explorers found in the categorical structure of psychotic patients' experiences, we should be clear about the implications of even looking to this type of structure for "pathology." Kant believed that his categories of understanding were "necessary conditions of any possible experience." The suggestion here is that his rather sterile categories were in fact not necessary in any real sense, but rather were one set of *sufficient* conditions for one particular sort of experience: the sort of experience we call *sanity*. And if we consider the categories to be a window on the structure of sanity, then surely they define a boundary condition for what has often been called insanity.

This was the reasoning of John William Miller (1983, pp. 9, 135–6), who understood clearly the relationship between normal and pathological mental functioning:

"It is health that defines illness, not illness health... The reason psychiatric conflict is of prime importance is that it is the occasion for the discovery of structures. It reveals how one is put together... Kant showed how to maintain nature, but not how to lose it... This loss occurs as madness, not as error."

4. The Structure of Madness

If sane experience is indeed made possible by a categorical structure supported by the world itself, how then are we to understand the structure of madness? Several lines of evidence now point to a new unifying understanding of psychotic experience as that experience produced by mental faculties whose categories manifest structural defects. Since the concept whose structure has been most studied is the concept of time, let me first illustrate what is meant by a structural defect in a category.

The structure of time can normally be represented by a two–directional number line, with the past represented by the numbers off to the left, the future represented by the numbers off to the right, and whatever number is in the middle (as the numbers continue to move from future to past) is currently the present. We might say that a past, present, and future axis constitute the normal structure of this category of experience.

To illustrate the distortion of a category in the experience of a psychiatric patient, let us begin with Havens' (1973, pp. 139–40) advice and look to one of the most carefully analyzed cases of psychotic depression that we find in the literature. This was Minkowski's male patient who had the fixed delusion every day that the next day he would be tortured and executed. While no one would deny that this man's category of time is severely structurally distorted (in completely lacking a future axis), it is perhaps more usual to think of his depression as leading to his delusion and his delusion as giving rise to this distortion in the form of his temporal experience. But listen to Minkowski's (1933, pp. 186–7) own analysis of this question:

"Isn't the disorder pertaining to the future a perfectly natural consequence of the delusional idea of imminent torture? This is the crux of the problem. Could we not assume, on the contrary, that the disorder in our attitude concerning the future is of a more general order and that the delusion of which we spoke is only one of its manifestations? Probably someone will say that basically this is the outlook of a person who has been condemned to death and that our patient reacted this way because of his delusion that he and his family were condemned to death. I doubt it. I have never seen a person who has been condemned to death. I willingly admit that the description we have given corresponds to the idea that we have of the experience of someone who has been condemned to death. But don't we draw this idea from ourselves? Don't we have it because, at moments, we are all condemned to death—at precisely those moments when our personal *elan* weakens and the door to the future is shut in our face? Can't we assume that the patient's attitude is determined by a more lasting weakening of that same impulse? The complex idea of time and of life disintegrates, and the patient regresses to a lower level that is potentially in all of us. Thus the delusion is not completely a product of the imagination. It becomes grafted onto a phenomenon which is a part of our life and comes into play when the life–synthesis begins to weaken. The particular form of the delusion, the idea of execution, is in fact only the attempt of that part of the mind which remains intact to establish a logical connection between the various sections of a crumbling edifice."

So Minkowski concludes that the delusion does not give rise to the temporal distortion, but rather *vice versa*. Indeed, he suggests that the delusion can best be understood as a secondary or *reparative* effort in the face of a breakdown in the temporal synthesis of the patient's experience— a structural breakdown that actually defines his psychosis.

As Havens (1973, p. 140) reminds us, this model of "primary break-down" with "secondary symptoms" should be familiar from the other schools of psychiatric thought. The psychoanalytic model appeals to primary ego deficits giving rise to secondary symptoms whose content may vary. The cognitive–behavioral model appeals to primary deficits in the patient's mental set giving rise to secondary "depressogenic cognitions" whose content also may vary. And, of course, the biological model appeals to primary breakdowns in neurobiological functioning giving rise to secondary symptoms whose contents vary (and thereby become less impor-tant, as when the content of a drug–induced visual hallucination will typi-cally be ignored for diagnostic purposes).

This question of whether the structural breakdown in the category of time is primary or secondary is clinically crucial, because by "secondary" we may, as stated, refer to a *reparative* effort of the *healthier* part of the patient's brain. I can think of many chronic psychotic patients who believe that they are being punished for sins in a past life or are being tortured for having caused some disaster or another. I am convinced that for many of these patients, suicide (or sometimes murder) is the only *rational* con-clusion that could be reached in the real world, but that the brain evolved nothing if not an instinct for survival—even if the real world must be sacrificed instead. Elvin Semrad (1973, p. 5) once said that "psychosis is ... the sacrifice of reality to preserve life." When we miss the fact that the "delusion" can be a reparative effort of the healthier part of the patient, I wonder how many suicides we precipitate when our well–intentioned therapies finally convince these patients that it is not true that they are being punished for a past life, and so deprive them of the meaning they have created for their lives?

Since Minkowski, many other investigators have continued to study the structure of time in mental disorders, from Lewis' (1932) inroads into the differences between neurotic and psychotic temporal experience to Melges' (1982) grand analysis of *Time and the Inner Future*. What has continued to emerge from these studies is an appreciation that the actual *structure* of the category of time seems to be affected (e.g., asymmetric blocks to the past or future, complete temporal disintegration, etc.) in just those cases where we would ordinarily diagnose psychosis. In contrast, neurotic conditions seem to leave the *structure* of time intact, but involve, for example, simply an over–focusing on past or future.

It seems to make sense that if I over–focus on the past, I may become ruminative and guilt–ridden; but, if I actually lose the future entirely I become psychotically depressed. It is likewise tempting to think about the complete absence of responsibility that so characterizes the poor judgment of manic patients as reflecting a similar loss of the past. But time is only one of many categories, and by shifting back away from this one example we should now be able to conceptualize a larger model for understanding the characteristic shapes taken by experience in each of the various forms of major mental illness.

5. A New Model For the Classification and Understanding of the Major Psychoses

When Kant adapted Aristotle's notion of "categories" as those general concepts that structure our experience of reality, he had in mind a purely philosophical enterprise. His were construed as purely transcendental categories, applied by the transcendental "I" (the *Ich*, subsequently adapted by Freud for his equally synthetic ego) in the construction of experience. When we in turn adapt Kant's own theory to model the actual way we humans construct reality, we begin to see these categories as much more than transcendental a priori concepts. Instead they become the mental structures we actually apply in constructing our experience. As real entities with presumed developmental histories and a neurobiological basis, we can now look to structural defects in such categories as we explore psychotic experience.

It is only appropriate that we should begin thinking about the psychoses in terms of category disorders at this time when ego psychology and object relations theory are focusing on psychoses as disorders of the "I" or ego. As Spitzer (this volume) points out, most of what DSM–III–R would consider delusional can be lumped together under the German term *Ichstörungen*, literally translated "I–disorders," but referring to the *experiencing I,* not the "personality." Since Kant meant by this *experiencing I* precisely that faculty of ordering the contents of sensation under the categories, a disorder of that experiencing I can only mean a disorder of one or more categories—a disorder of the form of experience.

But which categories are implicated in which disorders? It is not my intention to produce here a detailed accounting of, say, affective psychoses as distortions in the category of time (as discussed above), borderline psychoses as distortions in the category of object, schizophrenic psychoses as distortions in the category of causation, etc. My intention here is simply to show why the search for such a detailed accounting might be useful and to warn interested parties about certain pitfalls.

One pitfall is to think that each category can exist independently from the others. Kant himself realized that the categories are completely interdependent even as he recognized each as necessary for our human experience. Indeed, Hegel (1807) believed that by searching our categories for their inherent inadequacies as independent concepts, we could push our knowledge to the limits of the real.

The point here is that, since our categories are themselves abstractions from the unified whole of experience, it is not possible even in principle to distort the structure of one category without distorting others. Arieti (1962 p. 463) thus proposed the term "awholism" to describe the phenomenology of schizophrenic experience. This connectedness of our categories has important implications for work in this area, because if, for example, schizophrenic experience becomes conceptualized as a disorder of causation, then time (which is connected to causation very intimately) will also be affected. Melges' (1982, pp. 133–46) experimental studies of acute psychosis induced by high doses of hashish may thus give us more evidence for this general model than it actually gives him within his more limited model of temporal distortions. He notes (p. 133) that the "progression of psychotic symptoms ... beginning with a mystical awareness and followed by lack of control over one's thinking, fragmentation of identity, and finally feelings of control by outside forces, is quite common during the course of acute psychosis." This picture may well describe the breakdown of our usual category of causation better than any other category, along with, of course, the loss of "ego boundaries" that would necessarily accompany the structural breakdown of any category.

Indeed, another pitfall to watch out for is an assumption like "for every twisted thought, a twisted category" (mirroring the biologist's equally problematic "for every twisted thought, a twisted molecule"). Life is not so simple, as may be demonstrated by the symptom of paranoia. Paranoia is associated with almost every psychotic condition: depressives, manics, and schizophrenics alike tend to become paranoid as they lose touch with reality. With our new view of psychosis, it makes sense that paranoia should become a kind of "final common pathway" in the process of psychosis. No matter which category is becoming structurally distorted, the accompanying threat to ego–boundaries (the inseparable *Ichstörungen* of Kant's original connection between the "I" and its categories) can always lead to a paranoid reaction. One need not have an over–focus on the future (Melges 1982, p. 51) to become paranoid. As the world's normal structure begins to tear along any of its seams, attempts to maintain a self–boundary are almost bound to produce paranoid manifestations. Thus, Minkowski's patient did not come to believe he would drop dead of a heart attack tomorrow. He believed "they" would torture and execute him.

The last possible pitfall I would like to warn against for those who might develop this model further is the notion that this is a new idea. So often we miss the opportunity to learn from the past when we become preoccupied with the novelty of our own discoveries. But if psychosis does fundamentally reflect an alternation in the *form* or *structure* of reality (and the usual idea of "impaired reality testing" is actually a secondary phenomenon), then keen observers of psychotic patients will have noted this in their own ways using their own language.

While the existential school of psychiatry has described these phenomena in the language presented here, each of the major schools has in fact made similar observations. In the biological/medical model, Bleuler (1911, pp. 14–15) himself, in coining the term "schizophrenia," considered its hallmark to be an alteration in the *form* of thought (loose associations) and he suggested that this reveals a "vagueness of conceptual boundaries." We can now take this suggestion seriously as we examine the process of this breakdown of categorical structure and give new meaning to the generic term "formal thought disorders." A similar conclusion is also reached within the psychoanalytic model by Modell. After distinguishing Freud's topographical model of the mind (conscious/preconscious/unconscious) from Freud's structural model of the mind (ego/id/superego), Modell (1968, p. 134, italics added) distinguishes "psychotic states" from normal neurotic states by the presence of "topographic regression *with significant structural alteration*" (neurotic states involving topographic regression without such structural changes). And, indeed, the same conclusion has also been reached by Muscari (1981) in a purely philosophical analysis of "the structure of mental disorder."

I mentioned above one of the fundamental clinical questions raised by this view of psychosis: whether or not certain delusions are not symptoms of psychosis at all, but are reparative efforts to make sense of a psychotic world (where psychotic now refers to the underlying structural disorder). I would like to conclude with another clinical implication, namely, the renewed ability this model gives us for understanding the "loss of control" experienced by psychotic patients. This is a very common and most distressing feature of psychotic disorders, and we can help our patients regain control over their lives only when we appreciate how this control is lost. Kant was impressed by the deeper significance of its being *my* synthesis which unites my sensory intuitions under the categories of understanding. When our patients' worlds begin to crumble, surely this must be our first priority. Only with a true understanding of how we can help them reconstruct their reality can we help them regain control of their lives.

Summary

Philosophers have long known that human experience only becomes possible when particular instances of things become ordered under more general concepts or categories. In this essay, these categories are discussed not as philosophical entities, but as actual structures with developmental histories and a neurobiological basis. In shaping the form of our normal experience, intact categories may be understood as supporting the structure of sanity. When the various categories become distorted, certain "formal thought disorders" become identifiable. This essay proposes a new understanding and classification of the major psychoses as category disorders, and reviews a number of clinical and conceptual advantages offered by this model.

References

Arieti S: The microgeny of thought and perception. Arch. Gen. Psychiatry 6: 76–90, 1962.

Binswanger L: The existential analysis school of thought (1946). Transl. Angel E, in: May R, Angel E, Ellenberger MF (eds): Existence: A New Dimension in Psychiatry and Psychology, pp. 191–213, Basic Books, New York, 1958.

Bleuler E: Dementia Praecox or the Group of Schizophrenias, transl. Zinkin J (1950). International Universities Press, New York, 1911.

Bowlby J: Attachment and Loss, Vol. 1: Attachment. Basic Books, New York, 1969.

Bowlby J: Attachment and Loss, Vol. 2: Separation: Anxiety and Anger. Basic Books, New York, 1973.

Edelman GM: Group selection and phasic reetrant signaling: a theory of higher brain function. In: Edelman GM and Mountcastle VB (eds): The Mindful Brain, pp. 51–100. The MIT Press, Cambridge MA, 1978.

Edelman GM: Neural Darwinism: The Theory of Neuronal Group Selection. Basic Books, New York, 1987.

Ellenberger MF: A clinical introduction to psychiatric phenomenology and existential analysis. in: May R, Angel E, Ellenberger MF (eds): Existence: A New Dimension in Psychiatry and Psychology, pp. 92–125. New York: Basic Books, 1958.

Havens L: Approaches to the Mind: Movement of Psychiatric Schools from Sects Toward Science, repr. (1987). Harvard University Press, Cambridge MA, 1973.

Hegel GWF: The Phenomenology of Spirit (1807), transl. Miller AV with analysis of the text by Findlay JN, Oxford University Press, Oxford, 1977.

Hume D: A Treatise of Human Nature (1740), repr. Oxford University Press, Oxford, 1978.

Hundert EM: Philosophy, Psychiatry, and Neuroscience: Three Approaches to the Mind. Oxford University Press, Oxford, 1989.

Jaspers K: General Psychopathology (1923), transl. Hoenig J and Hamilton MW, Manchester University Press, Manchester, 1963.

Kant I: Prolegomena to Any Future Metaphysics (1783), transl. Carus P and rev. Ellington JW, Hackett Publishing Company, Indianapolis, 1977.

Klein M: Our adult world and its roots in infancy (1959), repr. in: Envy and Gratitude and Other Works by Melanie Klein 1946–1963, pp. 247–63, Hogarth Press, London, 1975.

Lewis A: The experience of time in mental disorder. Proc. R. Soc. Med. 25: 611–620, 1932.

Lewis CI: A pragmatic conception of the a priori (1923), repr in: Feigl H and Sellars W (eds): Readings in Philosophical Analysis, pp. 286–94, Appleton–Century–Crofts, New York, 1949.

Mahler MS On the significance of the normal separation–individuation phase with reference to research in symbiotic child psychosis, repr. in: The Selected Papers of Margaret S. Mahler, M.D., Vol. 2, pp. 49–57. Jason Aronson, New York, 1979.

Melges FT: Time and the Inner Future: A Temporal Approach to Psychiatric Disorders. John Wiley & Sons, New York, 1982.

Miller JW: In Defense of the Psychological. Norton, New York, 1983.

Minkowski E: Lived Time: Phenomenological and Psychopathological Studies (1933), transl. Metzel N, Northwestern University Press, Evanston, Ill, 1970.

Modell AH: Object Love and Reality. International Universities Press, New York, 1968.

Muscari PG: The structure of mental disorder. Phil. of ScNLi. 48: 553–72, 1981.

Piaget J: The Origins of Intelligence in Children (1936), transl. Cook M, Routledge & Kegan Paul, Ltd. London, 1952.

Piaget J: The Construction of Reality in the Child (1937), transl. Cook M, Routledge & Kegan Paul, London, 1954.

Sarnat HB, Netsky MG: Evolution of the Nervous System. Oxford University Press, New York, 1981.

Semrad E: The clinical approach to the psychoses: heuristic formulation of regressive states. Unpublished transcript of the Academic Conference Presentation of September 14, 1973, McLean Hospital, Belmont MA, 1973.

Spitz RA: The First Year of Life. International Universities Press, New York, 1965.

Spitzer M: Kant on schizophrenia. This volume.

Wiesel TN: The postnatal development of the visual cortex and the influence of environment. Nobel lecture repr. in Bioscience Reports 2: 351–77, 1982.

Rationality
and Self

The Irrelevance of Rationality to Adaptive Behavior

Brendan A. Maher

1. Introduction

In this paper I propose to examine some of the issues that arise when psychopathologists apply concepts such as "rationality", "reality testing", "contact with reality" and the like to the description of allegedly pathological states in psychiatric patients. A conference that brings philosophers and psychopathologists together appears to be a particularly appropriate locus for such discussion, the more so as psychopathologists generally tend to ignore philosophical aspects of their discipline, preferring instead to take for granted the assumptions that underlie their work. That they do so is a testimony not to a kind of cavalier indifference to philosophical matters in principle, but rather to a conviction that accumulated practical experience in the clinic provides a sufficiently reliable basis for professional action. This naturally brings with it the conviction that speculative examination of premises does not hold real promise of improving the practical clinical techniques that they employ.

There is substantial validity in this position; hence the main burden of proof of the concrete value of philosophical analysis tends to fall on the shoulders of the the philosopher critic. I am a psychopathologist by trade, not a philosopher; nonetheless it seems clear to me that careful scrutiny of philosophical aspects of psychopathology is an activity not only desirable in its own right, but also possessing some potential for changing the way we think about the concrete clinical phenomena that form the subject of our work. I hope to justify this assertion through an analysis of some specific clinical phenomena and of the way that we think about them.

I turn first to the concept of "contact with reality"—a concept that is central to most discussions of the nature of serious psychotic disturbances.

2. The Concept of Reality Contact

We may begin with some reflections on the terms reality and contact. Implied in these terms is the assumption that there is a reality that exists independently of the patient's perception of it; that this reality can be contacted through the senses, and the adequacy of this contact can be assessed by other people—notably the observing psychopathologist. The tacit model that guides this way of looking at the problem comes from the study of the sensory processes themselves. Thus the individual with impaired vision who misreads the lower case letters on the Snellen chart is mistaken in his reading, the test of his error being provided by the demonstrable discrepancy between his response and the character printed on the chart, supported by the fact that the provision of corrective lenses now brings his response into congruence with the chart. In this specific matter, his contact with reality has been restored.

I do not mean to underestimate the complexity of even this seemingly simple instance, but rather to provide a bench mark against which the extended and more complex use of the concept of reality contact by psychopathologists may be examined. But to return to the example from vision. We assume that the correct identification of the printed character is possible because the patient has a visually experienced representation of the character that is closely isomorphic with the physical structure of the character itself. That is to say that if the printed character on the chart happens to be the letter A in Times Roman font, 18 point size, the patient is not experiencing a visual representation of the letter A in 24 point Gothic, even though both would produce the same response—the spoken "A". The visual processing of the input from the chart is assumed to follow a set of rules which, no matter what transformations occur en route to the visual cortex, produces an end–state in consciousness that corresponds in some detail to the patterning of the physical attributes of the stimulus itself.

Now psychologists have known for well over a century that this is not really the case. Fechner, Weber and the many psychophysicists who followed them, demonstrated long ago that the sensory and perceptual systems are relatively insensitive to small changes in the physical attributes of stimuli (such as the intensity of lights, the amplitude of sounds, the intensity of pressures, etc.). We can measure these changes with suitable instruments at levels of magnitude too low for the human visual or auditory systems to detect. We also know from experiments now a almost half a century old, that the insensitivity of the visual system to small changes can be demonstrated not only by the reports of human observer–subjects but also by direct inspection of retinal activity. Perhaps it is not too long a leap to conclude that selection pressures on the evolving visual system did not convey any marginal survival advantage to the perfect continuous isomorphism of stimulus characteristics and perceptual characteristics.

But we have learned since then that visual perception produces representations of physical reality that sometimes involve active augmentation and diminution of the relative magnitudes of parts of the physical stimulus. Thus boundaries formed by the stepwise juxtaposition of dark and light surfaces of an object produce greater discrepancies in the intensity of neural activity on either side of the boundary than is true of the intensity of the physical gradient measured at the stimulus itself. In brief, the system appears to operate in ways that exaggerate the boundaries of things. Here we can speculate that the system has evolved in this way because the rapid correct discrimination of separate objects in the environment conveys a survival advantage. We might note in passing that this would be, of course, an advantage which, in the dialectic of predator and prey, sets up selection pressure in favor of the development in prey of a camouflage of colors and patterns that blur sharp boundaries between itself and the environment, diminishing the gradients that the predator's visual system is wired to exaggerate. In this volume Professor Emrich has presented examples of the perception of convexity and concavity drawn from the work of Ramachandran, Nakayama and others, suggestive of the conclusion that this kind of perception is heavily influenced by the experienced environmental regularity with which natural illumination tends to come from above rather than below. These effects can be diminished by experience with specific objects, but the powerful nature of visual demonstrations convinces us that the human nervous system has been subject to selection pressure towards the development of high–speed perceptual processes influenced by environmental *probabilities* about stimuli rather than by careful isomorphic representation of them in consciousness.

The introduction of evolutionary concepts into this discussion is intended to set the scene for an examination of the question of human thinking, and the slippery concept of rationality. To develop this theme, I will present some assertions. They are:

a) Natural selection operates upon physical structure and/or upon action, and not upon thinking itself. Organisms fail to survive to reproduce themselves because they run too slowly, are physically weak (a matter of the physics and physiology of their musculature or other bodily structures), have hyporesponsive or hyperresponsive visceral systems, are too brightly colored, etc. Should an organism survive to the age of reproduction, its reproductive success will depend upon additional features some of which will include the capacity to protect and provide for offspring.[1] Illogical thinking is not selected against unless it leads to maladaptive behavior. Maladaptive behavior is always selected against regardless of the conformity to rule of the thinking that led to it. The burglar who commits the fallacy that goes: "Policemen wear blue uniforms; that man coming down the street is wearing a blue uniform; therefore he is a policeman and I should get away" will get will spend fewer years in prison that the one who thinks only according to the formal rules of syllogistic deduction, and whose

---

1 Some of the selective processes that contribute to evolutionary change are abrupt in form, such as in the case of famine, war or other natural catastrophes. However, it is clear that the most continuous form of selection arises through inter- and intraspecies competition for resources and mates, a competition in which the competitors with the best payoff ratio of energy expenditure to resource acquisition tend to come out ahead of those whose behavioral strategies produce less favorable ratios. As the best ratios are determined by behavior that optimizes empirical accuracy, rather than behavior that conforms to logical rules, there is constant selection pressure for the former and against the latter. Although the availability of resources and mates to modern man may make the necessities of competition less acute than in earlier times in evolutionary history, the continuance of optimization principles in thinking conveys no adaptive disadvantage, and hence persists.

behavior is thus influenced by the possibility that the man might a fireman, a naval officer, an airline pilot or any other of the host of people who wear blue uniforms.

Neither penalty nor gain accrues directly from the form of thinking as such; they accrue only to activities. To put the matter simply, patterns of thinking are shaped by the environmental consequences of the behavior that they mediate and not by features of their internal formal relations.

b) Survival of an organism depends upon escape from dangers that might destroy it, and upon the maintenance of a positive increment of energy in the balance between its efforts to obtain energy from the environment and its expenditure of energy in those efforts. *A positive balance need not accrue to every activity provided that it does so on the average over a series of activities. The sea–hawk does not have to catch a fish each time it dives into the water as long as its pattern of searching and diving leads it to catch an adequate number over a series of dives.* This principle is now referred to by behavioral biologists as *the principle of optimization.* As I shall mention later, it was enunciated several decades ago by the linguist George Zipf. (Thus, for example, the building in which we are now meeting, the heating and air–conditioning systems are activated by a computer programmed to do so mainly according to the season of the year. Thus the heat may be on in an unusually hot day in October, and the air–conditioning on in an unusually cold day in May,—but as the energy costs and time delay caused by repeated switching from one system to another are high, and the costs of daily decision making by humans is also high, the relegation of the task of a computer programmed to optimize over the year makes functional sense.)

c) Time spent is an energy cost, as it always involves energy expenditure even when the organism is not especially active.

d) Conscious cognitive activity, such as thinking, attending, perceiving, etc. costs energy and time. Energy and time is saved when activities are controlled at lower, more automatic levels in the nervous system.

e) Adaptive efficiency requires that the organism be minimally consciously preoccupied with monitoring ongoing regularities in its environment or in its own behavior. Conscious attention cannot be effectively divided simultaneously between several activities or environmental events. The automation of the control of activity leaves the field of conscious attention open for the detection of dangers and opportunities, and hence the system has evolved so as to relegate to automatic control as much as is possible. (We know that nervous system activity habituates to repetitive stimulation, a phenomenon that offers a model for the principle contained in this assertion).

f) In order to adapt to regularities in the environment, the individual must be sensitive to patterned sequences that will predictably be followed by other specific elements. Thus the animal that detects the sound which is possibly that of a predator survives better (even if mistaken) if it begins its escape immediately than does the animal which, like a good logician, waits around to check the appearance and scent before deciding that it really is a predator. By the same token the animal that notices a stimulus that does not have the initial characteristics of prey and then spends no further time or effort attending to it may occasionally miss a meal but will, on the average, come out ahead in the energy budget.

Probabilities may assume negative values. Under some conditions the occurrence of an event makes the occurrence of another event less probable than it would be had the first event not occurred at all. Patterned sequences are so important that the organism will persist in seeking for them until one is found, even if it fits only partially with the observable data. Thus, the significant question for the psychopathologist is not simply why does this person seem to hold inconsistent beliefs,—rather it is "what is the consistency that underlies these beliefs".

g) While organisms process events in terms of the probabilities attached them, the motor system can not match responses to probabilities in parallel fashion. If it is eighty per cent likely that a predator is approaching we cannot produce an "eighty per cent " avoidance response; we can produce either an avoidance response or no avoidance response. In human thinking we see this principle formalized in the concept of statistical significance through the convention that leads us to accept a finding as reliable that has only a 1/20 probability of being unreliable. Cognition can conceptualize a wide range of probabilities, but action is less flexible. Hence, action often presents the appearance of having arisen from non-probabilistic thinking. The behavior of a person who never eats in restaurants because he thinks that there is a significant probability that the food might be prepared unhygienically, cannot be distinguished from a person who never eats in restaurants because he is certain that this is the case. One has the premise "Some restaurant kitchens are dirty", while the other has the premise "All restaurant kitchens are dirty". The inferential step retroactively from action to premise is laden therefore with the possibility of error.

From these various considerations emerge some implications for the study of rationality in thinking. In order to consider these implications we should turn first to consider current psychological models of human behavior.

3. Models of Human Behavior

Psychologists and philosophers often write as though there are two kinds of people. One consists of ordinary people living their lives in a real world,—in short, the people we meet everyday, people like ourselves and whose behavior it is our task to understand. The other consists of a set of hypothetical human beings created in the minds of psychologists, and with whom real people tend to compare quite unfavorably. The prototypical hypothetical person is a formal rational person, begotten by social cognitive psychology out of old–fashioned economics.

Real people, on the other hand, are distressingly often less intelligent and perceptive than are these ideal rational creatures. Real people's cognitions reveal an inadequate understanding of statistical principles, biases in their judgments of others, ethnocentricity in attitude, a failure to realize that religion has been replaced by science as a basis for the conduct of life, misattribution of effects to causes, distortion of reality so as to reduce dissonance, failure to recognize that altruism is selfishness, that terms such as freedom and dignity are gross self–deceptions, they are "mindless" when they should be "mindful"—the list goes on.

Astonishingly enough, these real people manage to survive in a world in which one would think that natural selection would have solved their population problem aeons ago. They stand in sharp contrast to the psychologist's rational person, a creature whose cognitions are unfailingly congruent with stimulus input, who lives in constant awareness of the effects of sample size, observer bias, experimenter influence, etc. who is perpetually and mindfully on the alert for the very best solution to each immediate problem presented by the environment, who perceives and interprets simulated non–verbal cues with facility, and whose interpersonal relations are marked by a mature understanding of all of the factors that might influence anything that anybody ever says or does in relation to somebody else. A striking exception to this unflattering contrast between real people and rational people is provided by psychologists themselves, whose reports imply that they survive the comparison with their own creations quite nicely, although years of informal observation of the rationality of the decisions that psychologists make in their own lives, and in the conduct of their professional concerns, leaves room for some doubt about this.

To put some flesh on the bare bones of the provocative assertion that psychologists have failed to distinguish between the real world and the looking–glass world of laboratory artifact, an anecdote may help. Some years ago the writer happened to be a member of a search committee seeking to make a junior faculty appointment in a university psychology department. One candidate presented an account of a research project in which, amongst other things, a group of subjects had been taught the principle of regression to the mean. Later, they had been given a pencil–and–paper multiple–choice test to see how well they could apply this knowledge to concrete situations. Included in the test were many items of a kind of which one went something like this. "John Doe is a salesman who travels all over the country. He enjoys good food, and whenever he happens across a restaurant in which he has a particularly fine meal he recommends it to his friends in that town. To his disappointment he finds that those of his friends who take his advice generally tell him that when they went to the restaurant they had a rather mediocre meal, not at all as good as he had led them to expect."

The respondent is then asked to choose the most likely reason for this, as follows:

"This is because (a) the chef had an off day, (b) his friends have different tastes in food from his, (c) they had gone to the wrong restaurant , (d) very good meals are statistically infrequent exceptions to the mean, and tend to fail to recur because of regression to the mean."

Apparently, many of the subjects of this research did not pick (d) and hence "failrd" this item; nor did they do very well on the test as a whole. Once again real people had failed to live up to the standards of the hypothetical ideal created by the experiment, and worse still, had failed to do even after having been trained to understand what the correct answers were. During the colloquium in which this research, was presented one questioner asked whether or not the creation of the above mentioned item had been guided by prior empirical evidence that good meals in restaurants actually are most often examples of chance combinations of favorable factors. The speaker dismissed the question as irrelevant to the important theoretical point that had guided the research, which seemed to be that people make judgments about things in a much less sophisticated way than psychologists think that they should, and that they do so even when the psychologists have shown them the right way to do it.

One member of the search committee, who supported this response, and was favorably disposed to the strategy of this research, then remarked to the members of the committee who were to go to dinner with the candidate, "I suggest that we go to Blank's Restaurant. The food there is always excellent." That is where we went, and the food was good. Nobody seemed to be unduly concerned about the discrepancy between the real world in which we all lived, (in which good restaurants are good and bad restaurants are bad) and the hypothetical world of the researcher in which the candidate's subjects had failed so dismally to make the correct response. What the subjects had done, of course, was to respond to what they—and the search committee—knew to be true about the real world, which is that there are good restaurants and bad restaurants; the Guide Michelin has done quite well for itself and its publishers by assessing and reporting this difference quite reliably for decades. In order to survive, people's choices must be adaptive, which means that they must be guided by the real variables that control outcomes, not by the application of logical or statistical rules stated in abstract form.

We have little difficulty in applying our understanding of environmental probabilities to the behavior of animals, but often demonstrate a parallel failure to do the same thing with human behavior. It consists essentially of a failure to take seriously those determinants of organismic behavior that came into prominence with Darwin and others who came after. In the case of Darwin at least, there has been a revival of interest in the adaptive aspects of behavior evident in the work of animal behaviorists but little on the part of psychopathologists.. Perhaps we can go some part of the way to rectifying this state of affairs by remembering the seemingly forgotten work of George Zipf, and trying in some measure to revive it.

George Zipf presented a theory of human behavior in two major works (Zipf 1935,1948). For our purposes, his *Human Behavior and the Principle of Least Effort: An Introduction to Human Ecology* (Zipf 1948) provides the most complete summary of his theoretical proposals together with the arguments that he used to sustain them. By way of introduction it is helpful to note that Zipf was primarily a mathematical linguist, but had made substantial efforts to integrate the quantitative aspects of language usage into a comprehensive theory of human behavior.

Zipf's central thesis was that behavior develops in ways that routinize the solution of recurring problems and the performance of recurring tasks, so that the average amount of work expended in their performance is minimized. In the calculation of work expenditure he included the effort spent in developing solutions in the first place. What Zipf referred to as mentation, i.e. the cognitive processes involved in working out an optimal average solution to recurring problems, is a cost. It is included with other costs such as the motor energy employed in performing the solution to the task, the resources used in implementing the solution and so forth. All of this is laid out in his Principle of Least Effort. He put it this way.

"In simple terms, the Principle of Least Effort means, for example, that a person in solving his immediate problems will view these against the background of his probable future problems, as estimated by himself. Moreover, he will strive to solve his problems in such a way as to minimize the total work that he must expend in solving both his immediate problems and his probable future problems. That in turn means that the person will strive to minimize the probable average rate of his work–expenditure (over time). And in so doing he will be minimizing his effort..." (Zipf 1948, p.1).

In actual application, the principle is more complex than this brief quotation suggests. Because behavior in one situation affects the possible solutions available in another, the probable average of work expenditure has to take into account not only the impact of a given solution upon the problem to which it is directed, but also its impact upon the solutions that might be feasible for other problems.

The effect of the operation of this principle is that on a given occasion, the solution that we see somebody apply to a specific instance of a problem may appear to us unintelligent in relation to the concrete details of that problem, until we know the base rate for the occurrence of this problem for the individual concerned. Another way of putting this is that the effort spent in producing the best solution to each instance of a problem may not be worth the increment of gain; hence to spend such effort is maladaptive. If we wish to assess the intelligent deployment of effort, we must assess the effectiveness of the given problem solution on repeated occasions, not just because repeated samples have higher reliability, but because the adequacy of the *average* solution cannot be assessed from a *single* case.

Zipf cited the development of the Morse Code for telegraphy as a good example of the least effort principle in practice. Letters of the alphabet with the highest frequency of use in English were assigned the shortest transmission signal. Thus E is a single short ".", A is ".–",T is a single "–", while infrequently used letters such as Q and X are "—.–", and "–..–" respectively. Although some messages that have an atypically high frequency of Q,X,Y and other low frequency letters, create significant costs in time and effort to transmit, over many messages the code ensures that the average transmission cost will be optimally minimal.

Zipf proposed that what had been developed systematically in the case of the Morse code, develops naturally and inevitably in the human being on the basis of experience. Hence his observation that the frequency of the use of a word in a language is inversely related to its length, and that when a previously low frequency word comes into wide use, it is promptly shortened, as when "television" owned by few people, became "TV" or ("Telly" in the U.K.) when owned by many.

Because carefully thought through decision making is a needless expense when applied each time to repeated recurrences of a common problem, it is natural that decision rules develop at the folk level. These are, of course, the real function of proverbs. Thus the metaphorical meanings of "Take care of the pence and the pounds will take care of themselves", or of "Who sups with the Devil must have a long spoon" are not valid in every case, but perhaps often enough to provide a decision guide that will prove optimally efficient over the long haul. Children are taught in this way, and thus acquire optimal–average solutions without having to evolve them exclusively through costly experience.

Demonstrations that human beings fail to follow "correct" rules of inference suffer from the fact that the investigators expect that their subjects will provide the best possible solution to the specific single problem that is presented. What is lacking however is the analysis of the subject's behavior in terms of what would be the optimal solution to the class of problems averaged out over a variety of common situations.

A good example of this can be found in investigations reported by Tversky and Kahneman, as cited in a recent paper by Herrnstein and Mazur (1987). People were presented with an hypothetical problem, worded as follows:

"Imagine that you are about to purchase a jacket for $125 and a calculator for $15. The calculator salesman informs you that the calculator is on sale for $10 at the other branch of the store, located twenty minutes drive away. Would you make the trip to the other store?" They reported that sixty–eight percent of their subjects said that they would drive to the other store. A second group of subjects was presented with another version of the same problem, except that now the jacket costs $15 and the calculator $125, with the latter being available for $120 on sale at the branch store. Now only twenty–nine per cent of the respondents state that they would make the drive. Given that the actual savings in these hypothetical situations was the same, i.e. $5.00, and the total bill for the same goods would be the same at $140. why would not rational people make the same choice in both cases? We will pass over the fact that the entire problem was verbal and that the investigators did not actually observe what people would do.

We will also pass over the possibility that the person who seriously goes into a store to buy a $15 jacket and a $125 calculator may be a little different from the person who goes in to buy a $15 calculator and a $125 jacket. What is important is that the investigators solved the problem of the "irrationality" of their subjects by concluding that their responses are determined by the way the question was framed, namely by the thirty–three percentage discount that $5 bears to $15 in one case and the four percentage that it bears to $125 in the other.

From the vantage of the Principle of Least Effort none of this is new or surprising. On the average, an individual will save resources by going with the percentages over many cases of savings opportunities, rather than working out the absolute dollar cost in each case. The higher the percentage discount, the rarer the opportunity is likely to be. Going for the rare benefit may be foolish on occasion (as in this case) but wise on the average over many cases. The irrationality of the subjects can only be gauged by looking at the empirical consequences of applying the percentage criterion over many cases of actual sales discounts, i.e. over a *class* of problems rather than specific single instances.

As pointed out above, Zipf emphasized that the mentation that is required to work out solutions to problems is itself a cost, and could be substantial. Complex cognitive activity costs. It must be amortized over the anticipation of the frequent recurrence of the problem to which it has provided a solution.

The Principle of Least Effort clearly antedated and encompassed the phenomena now included in contemporary formulations of optimized rationality. It provided a rationale for studies of foraging behavior, culturally generated evolutionary changes in language, the basic rationality of economy of effort (including mental effort), the natural preference for actuarial decision rules when these have sufficient predictive accuracy,—all of these well before their reappearance in modern forms.

Why, we might ask, do many psychologists fail to appreciate the functional efficiency of least–effort solutions, and fail to understand why these are hard to detect in the laboratory? The answers to these questions are undoubtedly complex, but some possibilities come to mind. The first of these is the nature of the scientific enterprise in general, and in which psychologists are personally engaged. Scientific work, by and large, consists of trying to solve as comprehensively as possible problems as yet unsolved. When a problem has been more or less solved, or at least solved as well as seems possible with the methods and data available, the task of the scientist is completed. He or she can now move on to another problem or can decide to devote more time and thought to developing ways in which the previous solution might be bettered. In neither event can the task be handled by the simple application of an existing solution—this being the rôle of the technician, to whom the application of validated procedures to the solution of routine problems has been assigned.

Because the solution of a scientific problem does not have a direct impact upon the personal life of the scientist who is trying to solve it, it is possible for the scientist to live with an unsolved problem more or less indefinitely. A lifetime may be spent on trying to answer a scientific question; during the search the scientist may systematically fit the available data to various possible models and conclude that no satisfactory model has yet been devised. The interim answer "I don't know why such–and–such a phenomenon occurs" is acceptable to the scientist qua scientist. On the other hand, the scientist at home may be quite unable to give the same answer when faced with, let us say, mysterious comings and goings of a spouse. The explanation of this is personally urgent, and some explanation is better than no explanation.

Most people in the world are not employed in finding unsolved problems to solve; they are mainly engaged in other things, one of which is the development of behavioral practices that save effort and time in dealing with normal tasks of life. Their lives are generally quite unlike those of scientists. New problems are nuisances, or even threats, and their solution is necessary if one is to get on with other matters, the other matters being the real business of living. Real people quite reasonably apply time–tested solutions to such repeated problems as they encounter, unless the effort demanded in applying these solutions is great enough to justify the investment of effort in finding a new solution. Then, briefly, they become scientists. Except for these occasions their daily working life is not like that of the professional scientist; the work of the latter is the exception, that of the former is the rule. Ignoring this, psychologist–scientists are prone to the error of assuming that their subjects should be like them and finding that they are not, they write about them in patronizing tones, and contemplate training programs that might improve them.

4. Rationality and Psychopathology

Delusions present the clearest example of a psychopathology that brings to bear the test of rationality as a measure of the normalcy of the patient's statements of belief. The present writer has offered a model for the development of delusional beliefs (Maher 1972, 1974, 1988; Maher and Ross 1983); in this paper we shall examine the application of the conception of irrational adaptiveness to these phenomena.

One of the most important clues to the confusion that this brings with it is to be found in the definitional problems surrounding the term "delusion" itself. While exact definitions vary from place to place and time to time, they all consist of two components. One is that a delusion is a false belief, and the other that this false belief is held in the face of evidence sufficient to disprove it. As holding false beliefs under such circumstances appears to be irrational, their existence in any individual is seen as *prima facie* evidence of pathological irrationality.

One of the obvious problems that arise from this definition is that when a belief that is false from an empirical–scientific standpoint is held by a large enough number of people, it is no longer defined as delusional. Thus many religious beliefs are held in the face of substantial counter-evidence, but are not defined as delusional. This gives rise to a rather more profound epistemological issue: By what criterion, other than lack of popularity, are beliefs to be tested for truth or falsity? Some delusions do contain assertions about the nature of the sensory experience of the patient, as for example beliefs that the body has changed its physical shape, and these delusions may be held in spite of the counter–evidence provided by a mirror. However, such delusional statements are about perceptions: As such they may be discrepant with the perceptions of other observers, but are not literally false beliefs. Instead, they are best regarded as plausible beliefs derived from disordered perception, and it is in the realm of sensation and perception that the pathology may lie, rather than in the cognitive processes that underlie the development of the stated belief.

However, many delusions do not consist of simple statements about physical aspects of the environment; they consist of statements of inference about an environment, the physical aspects of which are perceived in the same way as they are by normal persons. The abnormal component consists of the *interpretation* of the environment that is made by the patient. Now it is often the case in science that the same set of data permit several alternative interpretations, and that no one of these may account for all of the data. In this sense, an interpretation can only be classified as "false" if there is a piece of evidence available that is fundamentally incompatible with it; it is not rendered necessarily false merely by evidence that reduces its plausibility.

Interpretations are adaptive insofar as they lead to action that promotes survival. Under normal circumstances the adaptive efficiency of an interpretation depends upon the assessment of probabilities duly weighted with regard to the probable consequences of taking actions unwittingly based upon false negatives or false positives. An interpretation based upon minimal evidence but that nonetheless leads to adaptive action is in this important sense more "rational" than an interpretation demanded by some formal rules of inference that leads to less adaptive action.

This kind of consideration gives rise to a dilemma. The dilemma is well illustrated in a study by Huq et al. (1988). Patients exhibiting delusional thinking and comparison groups without delusions were given the task of assessing the probable source of a sequence of colored marbles handed out one by one. The marbles came from one of two sources and patients had been given advance information about the proportion of colors in each source. With each successive marble, the probability of making a correct identification naturally increases as it is made in the face of an increasingly larger sample. Deluded patients drew their inferences on the basis of smaller sample sequences than did the control subjects, but their inferences were no less correct than those of the controls.

The dilemma consists of the fact that the deluded patients drew conclusions on the basis of what, according to the formal rules of statistical inference, were inadequate samples—and this appears to be a maladaptive strategy. On the other hand, they reached the correct conclusion sooner than non–deluded patients, and this appears to be an adaptively superior strategy.

Psychopathologists need to address the issue of the possible adaptiveness of seemingly maladaptive behavior through a careful analysis of the relationship of concepts of formal reasoning to the clinical phenomena of psychopathology. In so doing, we must avoid the simple assumption that rules of inference, formal adherence to statistical principles and the like, define "normalcy" regardless of their efficacy in dealing with real–world environments.

Summary

The argument of this paper is that the cognitive activity of human beings is determined by the survival consequences of the behavior to which it gives rise. Cognitive activity is an energy cost and hence normal thinking is oriented to the economy achieved by producing optimal average solutions to recurring problems of a given class rather than best–fit solutions to each individual case. Concepts of irrationality in psychopathology that do not take this into account, preferring instead to define irrationality against a standard of conformity to the rules of formal deductive reasoning fail to provide a framework for understanding the pathology that underlies delusions, or the processes that determine the various kinds of "normal" irrationality of everyday life.

References

Herrnstein RJ, Mazur JE: Making up our minds. The Sciences: 27, 40–47, 1987.
Huq SF, Garety PA, Hemsley DR: Probabilistic judgements in deluded and non–deluded subjects Quart J Exper Psychol 40A: 801–812, 1988.
Maher BA: Delusional thinking and cognitive disorder. In: Nisbet RN, London, H (eds): Cognitive alteration of feeling states. Aldine Press, Chicago, 1972.
Maher BA: Delusional thinking and perceptual disorder. Journal of Individual Psychology 30: 98–113, 1974.
Maher BA, Ross JS: Delusions. In: Adams H, Sutker P (eds): Comprehensive handbook of psychopathology. Plenum, New York, 1983.
Maher BA: Anomalous experiences and delusional thinking. In: Oltmanns TH, Maher BA (eds): Delusional beliefs: Interdisciplinary perspectives. Wiley–Interscience, New York, 1988.
Zipf GK: The psychobiology of language. Houghton–Mifflin, Boston, 1935.
Zipf GK: Human behavior and the principle of least effort, Addison–Wesley, Cambridge MA, 1949.

Limits of Irrationality

Frank Döring

1. Introduction

For the last two and a half millennia or so, most philosophers have devoted at least part of their careers to the study of rationality. They have wondered, for example, how "reason" can override the "passions" in rational conduct, how thought can proceed in accordance with rational laws, what the first principles of reason are (if there are any), whether they can be justified, and if so, how. Only few philosophers, however, have bothered to ask how *irra*-tional thinking and acting is possible. One of the first, Aristotle, touched off a still unfinished debate about the weakness of the will (*akrasia*). He noticed a curious problem that has bedeviled theories of rationality from their very beginnings, the problem that these theories tend to overshoot the mark. They tend to demonstrate, not only how a person *can* act rationally, but also that, given that she can so act, she cannot *but* act rationally. Theories of rationality tend to have notorious problems in explaining how irrational conduct is possible.

In this paper, I will investigate whether such a problem exists for one theory of rationality which has enjoyed great currency in philosophy over the past three decades. The theory has suitably been labelled the *interpretive view of the mind*;[1] it is associated primarily with the names of Quine, Davidson, and Dennett. The interpretive view certainly appears to make the occurrence of irrational behavior very hard, perhaps impossible, to understand. I will argue that appearances are deceptive, and that in fact irrational behavior is compatible with the interpretive view (which is not to say that the view offers a natural explanation of such behavior). My aim will be to dispel one worry about the interpretive view, not, however, to commend it.

2. The Interpretive View of the Mind

The interpretive view of the mind has three main ingredients. The first is the claim that the contents of mental states are determined by the relations

---

1 Mark Johnston, *Self-Deception and the Nature of Mind*. Speaking of *the* interpretive view is, of course, a crude simplification which serves purely expository purposes. I do not want to suggest that there are no important differences between Quine's, Davidson's, and Dennett's position.

the states bear to other mental states. Davidson, for instance, writes: "we make sense of particular beliefs only as they cohere with other beliefs [...] and the rest [. The] content of a propositional attitude derives from its place in a pattern."[2]

The second ingredient is that in order for mental states to be *rationally* connected with one another their contents have to be related by rules of logic or similar principles. One of the more prominent proposals for one such connection is the following: if a person believes both that p and that *If p then q*, then it is rational for him to believe that q because q follows logically from p and *If p then q*. The rationality of mental states and of the transitions between them is thought to consist in relations of deductive (or other) entailment between their propositional contents. (I will return to the question of what is meant by "consists in.")

The third ingredient of the interpretive view is the claim that the kind of coherence pattern that determines the contents of mental states is a pattern of rational links: rational inference, rational change in desire, rational action are what endows intentional states with content. I call this the *presumption of rationality*. The three parts of the view, taken together, say that mental states have no definite content unless they exhibit relations of rationality to their fellow states, where rational relations are relations of entailment.

This result flies in the face of many an example of folly we observe in daily life. If the interpretive view is right we should not be able to detect these examples. To look out for irrational quirks in an agent should be a self-undermining pursuit because there can be no clear evidence for such quirks. This is the problem which the interpretive view poses for the very possibility of ascribing irrationality: *All evidence for the irrationality of a person's beliefs (desires, actions) is, by the same token, evidence against the ascription of the very contents with respect to which the person appears to be irrational. Therefore there are never sufficient grounds to judge a person's beliefs (desires, actions) irrational.*

I call this the *problem of complementary evidence*. An alleged case of irrationality can always be redescribed in such a way as to make the irrationality disappear: the person may be taken to entertain different contents, or no contents at all. What is more, the alternative description is at least as well supported by the evidence as is the allegation of irrationality. So ascriptions of irrationality are never warranted by the evidence.

If the interpretive view of the mind is correct, and if more scrutiny bears out the result only sketched so far, then there are no ascriptions of blatantly irrational beliefs. Can this possibly be true? Should we not rather infer (rationally!), from the absurdity of this consequence, that there must be something seriously flawed with the interpretive view? Had we not better pay heed to the old warning that "there is nothing so absurd which

---

2 *Mental Events*, p. 221.

some philosophers have not maintained?"[3] I shall now review some of the reasons in support of the sketched result. My conclusion will be that they are indeed too weak to support it.

3. The Argument for Rationality

Most of the discussion among analytic philosophers since the sixties about the determination of mental contents has been conducted in terms of the methodology of two idealized scientific enterprises: field linguistics and cognitive ethology. The interpretive view emerged as the upshot of these exercises in imaginary methodology. The field linguist of the sixties faced the task of translating a radically foreign idiom into his own language, based upon no other evidence than the overt linguistic performances of his informants, plus information about physical features of the environment.[4] The cognitive ethologist of the seventies and eighties attempts to devise a psychological theory which predicts and explains agents' behavior in terms of mental states and their interactions.[5] He has shunned the methodological restraint of his predecessor and helps himself to a generous serving of assumptions about the internal workings of his subjects. Both, the linguist and the ethologist, are concerned with making sense of other people. The one worries primarily about linguistic behavior, the other about behavior more generally. The shift from field linguistics to cognitive ethology as the prototype discipline occupied with reading people's minds largely coincides with the dismissal of behaviorism in psychology and the adoption of the "cognitive" approach. Dennett's cognitive ethologist is very much Quine's old field linguist dressed after the fashion of the new approach.[6] Since the main difference between the two lies in the outmoded behaviorist predilection of the linguist I will simply ignore him in what follows and focus my attention on the ethologist.

The cognitive ethologist seeks to ascribe intentional states to agents in order to explain their behavior as actions whose reasons consist in the ascribed states. The first thing to be noted about the ascription of intentional states is that it is a "holistic" enterprise: we do not ascribe beliefs, for example, on a one by one basis but rather in complex clusters.[7] A person cannot be said to believe just that it is raining outside and nothing else. It would be entirely mysterious *what* she is supposed to believe if she did not

---

3 Thomas Reid, *Essays in the Intellectual Powers of Man*, p. 115. As an aside, Reid himself is a rather questionable authority on the topic of irrationality or "lunacy" because he was primarily interested in it as a characteristic of his philosophical opponents.
4 The *locus classicus* for the approach is Quine's *Word and Object*.
5 This approach has been championed by Dennett in a series of articles (e.g. *Intentional Systems*, repr. in Dennett 1979) and in his book *The Intentional Stance*.
6 If we think, as Schiffer suggested, of determining the contents of a person's beliefs as interpreting the "Mentalese" inscriptions in a box in the person's head labeled "beliefs," then we see immediately a close parallel to the task of translating utterances in a foreign idiom. The parallel is drawn out in a very illuminating way in Stich's *The Fragmentation of Reason*, ch. 2.
7 This point has been stressed especially by Davidson. See, e.g., his 'Mental Events'.

also possess some notion of the differences between outside and inside, rain as opposed to no rain, the belief that she is inside, not exposed to the rain, and so on. There is a linguistic parallel: a person cannot be said to mean by her words "It is raining" that it is raining if this is all she can say. She may, of course, use the words like a gesture in order to express her thoughts, but then the meaning of the gesture is not a function of the meaning of the words because the words do not have meanings.

The second observation is that there is more to those other beliefs than their mere existence. They have to be *connected* in a systematic way to the belief that it is raining outside in order for this belief to be the belief it is. They have to *interact* in the appropriate way. For instance, the belief that it is *not* raining outside must exclude, and be excluded by, the belief that it is raining outside. Without this mutual exclusion the contents of the beliefs cannot be what we first thought they were. More generally, the point here is that the contents of belief cannot be severed from the inferential patterns into which the beliefs enter. The contents *are*, in some sense, the inferential patterns.[8] This is tenet one of the interpretive view.

Third, the patterns mentioned are rational: it is rational, for instance, not to believe both a proposition and its negation at the same time, rational in at least the minimal sense that doing the opposite would be unacceptable by rational standards.[9] The interpretive view holds that this is true in general: the patterns which determine content are patterns of rational inference. How is this claim supported?

4. Rationality Conditions

It is useful to introduce a piece of methodological fiction in order to tackle the question as to how content determination and rationality are connected. Imagine that the propositional contents of beliefs are represented in a person's mind in a "language of thought" (*Mentalese*) whose sentences are syntactically structured in the way sentences of a public language are structured.[10] The meaning of the Mentalese sentences is then a function of the meanings of their syntactic components.

Suppose that we had just begun to characterize the contents of a person's intentional states. Among the patterns exhibited by her beliefs we observe that beliefs of the form p and $*p$ never occur together. (We gathered these forms from the person's utterances or from the deliverance of a fancy cerebroscope.) When the person's belief set contains a belief of the form p and she then adopts a belief of the form $*p$ she drops the first

---

8 One way to spell this out is what Harman calls "conceptual role semantics" (see Harman 1982).
9 Throughout this paper, I appeal to very basic intuitions about rationality which, I think, every theory of rationality will have to respect. This is not to say that all intuitions deserve to be respected. (How could they?) There has been an extensive debate about the status of intuitions about rationality, much of it in response to Nelson Goodman's *Fact, Fiction, and Forecast*. I cannot enter here into this debate. For a recent exposition and references see Goldman (1986).
10 This proposal is developed in Fodor's *Language of Thought*.

one, and *vice versa*. This pattern will lead us to interpret '*' as negation. Other patterns would lead us to different interpretations or to no interpretation at all. If the pattern included the simultaneous occurrence of beliefs of the form p and $*p$, then '*' would not be a plausible candidate for negation. Again, we would tinker with our interpretation until we would no longer feel compelled to diagnose contradictory beliefs.[11]

The situation with binary truth-functional connectives is similar. Imagine someone who typically infers a belief of the form q from beliefs of the form $p\#q$ and p, and also tends to infer a belief of the form *not-p* from beliefs of the form $p\#q$ and *not-q*. This will lead us, one may suggest, to interpret '\#' as a conditional operator whose meaning is that of the logical symbol '⊃' or the English *If–then*. Other inferential dispositions would lead us to detect other connectives. And a similar approach might give us insight into the non-logical areas of the person's Mentalese vocabulary.

This is indeed the kind of pattern one finds in the literature.[12] Yet it is not an adequate picture of what happens in real life and fails to capture what is admissible on even the most demanding standards of rationality. Take the following example. You perhaps believed at some point that if you swore excessively you would go straight to hell. You may also have had good reason to believe that your swearing was excessive. The simple pattern then tells you to adopt the belief that you will go to hell. But luckily you did not accept this consequence. Rationality alone could not force this conclusion upon you. You were quite right to hesitate to infer the consequent from a conditional belief and the belief in its antecedent. Obviously, one of the things one can do, and should do on occasion, is to reject the conditional or the antecedent. This is what you did in the swearing case. You simply rejected the idea that your swearing should get you into hell. You could have also done a number of other things, of course.

The reason why the simple pattern has so much initial appeal is, I conjecture, that it resembles very closely the argument form in logic which is often considered the intuitively most evident form: *modus ponens*. Logic has traditionally been regarded the canonical consultant in matters inferential. So it is tempting to think that proper reasoning has to accord with it. But the resemblance between inference patterns and argument forms is treacherous. As Gilbert Harman is fond of pointing out, logic does not tell you what to believe, it only tells you which consequences follow from which premises.[13] This may be useful to know when you try to find out what to believe, but it does by no means determine what you ought to believe. Not only does logic not decree which inferences ought to be be

---

11 In *A Puzzle About Belief* Kripke gives an example where our best intuitions about belief ascriptions seem to urge us to ascribe inconsistent beliefs to a person whose reasoning is impeccable by ordinary standards. I am not sure what moral to draw from the case, but at least two points seem to be fairly clear: a) One reason why the case is so puzzling is that there is a strong resistance against ascribing inconsistent beliefs to an apparently sane person; b) there is a strong temptation to say that something went wrong with the characterization of the contents of the person's belief. Both points support the idea that interpretation seeks to construe a person's beliefs as consistent.

12 For a refined version see Cherniak (1986), ch. 2.

13 Harman (1986), ch.2.

drawn, it does not even allow for certain inferences which are clearly admissible by rational standards. Logical entailment is neither necessary nor sufficient for rational inference. This is so for the following reasons.

First, from an inconsistent set of premises any conclusion whatsoever follows by the rules of logic (*ex contradictione quodlibet*). But it is not rational to infer any belief *ad libitum* from some inconsistency in your beliefs. It is contentious whether one can believe an explicit contradiction. But there is unanimous agreement, among friends and foes of the interpretive view alike, that it is possible to have implicitly contradictory beliefs, beliefs which entail an explicit contradiction. In fact, such implicit contradictions are probably quite common. Where they occur they entail every proposition you please, but they certainly don't make every inference rational. So logical entailment cannot be sufficient for rational inferability.

Secondly, logical entailment cannot be necessary for rational inferability either, or else one could never make rational changes to a consistent set of beliefs. When we change our minds as a result of careful reasoning we infer the contradictory of a previously held belief: the belief we arrive at via rational inference is logically inconsistent with what we believed before. If p is a newly accepted proposition and B is the initial set of beliefs, then a change in mind means that $p+B$ is inconsistent. Yet if p was inferred from B via logical implication, then B must already have been inconsistent (because a conclusion is inconsistent with a set of premises only if the set of premises is itself inconsistent). Therefore, if you take nothing but logic as your counsel in matters inferential you will be allowed a change in belief (as opposed to an extension) only if your initial set of beliefs is inconsistent. But this is absurd! It must be possible to rationally change one's beliefs starting from a consistent set. So logical entailment cannot be necessary for rational inference.

Thirdly, even in a situation where nothing speaks against accepting a logical consequence of what you believe, the mere fact that the consequence follows logically does not in itself provide you with a reason for believing it. Take for example Church's undecidability theorem (or your own favorite theorem of metalogic). The theorem follows logically from every belief of yours, but this does not mean that you may adduce whatever you like as a reason for believing it. Again, entailment is not sufficient for rational inference.

There probably is a role for logical entailment in a theory of rational inference, but it is much less central than the philosophical tradition thought. Logic can tell you when your beliefs are inconsistent. Since you are interested in having true beliefs, and since you know that not all the members of an inconsistent set of beliefs can be true, you have reason to safeguard yourself against inconsistencies. (This reason is not itself a logical reason; from a purely logical point of view there is nothing worrisome about an inconsistent set of beliefs.) Logic may assist you in exploring your options and thus finding a road to consistency. But there are other ways to do this.[14] I do not see that there is anything more to logic in rational inference than this auxiliary role.

So we need a guide in inference other than logic. Whatever logic has to tell us is neither necessary nor sufficient for rational inference. As a consequence, the second ingredient of the interpretive view has to be reformulated: We have to say that it is not relations of deductive (or other) entailment that make for the rationality of the connection between mental states but rather some other, yet unknown, kind of relation.

We saw that the simple inferential pattern which looks like *modus ponens* is too simple to determine the interpretation of '#.' What, then, would be an appropriate pattern? Let our subject start out with the belief *A#B*, together with a belief in any of *A, not-A, B,* or *not-B,* where '*A*' and '*B*' are abbreviations of propositions. We can then pose the question in the following general form: Are there, amongst all the sets of beliefs that the subject might end up with, given her initial beliefs, patterns that uniquely identify the different binary connectives in her thought?

There are a great many different belief states the person may enter, given the stipulated initial conditions, since her confidence in any of the initial beliefs may vary. The number of states would be entirely unmanageable for us interpreters if we allowed people to have *degrees of belief* which can assume any value between certainty and total disbelief.[15] Let us, therefore, make the idealizing assumption that there are exactly three different doxastic[16] attitudes a person can have *vis à vis* any proposition: she can accept it, reject it, or be indifferent. Rejecting a proposition is the same as accepting its negation, and *vice versa*. Because of this duality we only have to consider, for every proposition *p*, either it or its negation, but not both.

So in our example there are, so far, three different propositions about which the person has to make up her mind: *A, B,* and *A#B*. In addition, she can come to accept any truth-functional compound of *A* and *B*. There are cases where this would be quite acceptable, or even advisable. At some point you might have been shrewd enough to infer, for instance, that either your swearing was excessive, or that excessive swearing would send you to hell, but not both. There are $2^{2^n}-2$ significant distinct (non-equivalent) truth functions of *n* propositions which are pairwise negations of one another.[17] For the two propositions *A* and *B* there are therefore 14 such truth functions, three of which are *A, B,* and *A#B* (assuming that *A#B* is neither necessarily false nor tautological). Since each of them is the

---

14 For example, if belief states were models of the world they would automatically be consistent in all the respects in which they are models.

15 One may wonder why I do not employ, at this point, a Bayesian theory of subjective probability, a theory about the management of degrees of belief. The reason is that people are very poor Bayesians in that their inferences generally do not conform to the probability calculus. This limits the application of Bayesianism as a descriptive tool so severely that it cannot be used for precise predictions of a person's inferential behavior. I leave it to the reader to puzzle out whether Bayesians could instead make *rough* predictions about people's changing degrees of belief which could be used in interpretation.

16 From *doxa*, the Greek word for belief.

17 See next note.

negation of one of the others, and since we have stipulated that accepting a proposition is the same as rejecting its negation, we subtract half of the 14 propositions from the number of different propositions towards which our subject will have a doxastic attitude. This leaves us with 7 propositions. Generally, the number of different doxastic states *vis à vis* n propositions is 3^n (because there are 3 possible doxastic attitudes towards each individual proposition). For our example, we thus have 2,187 different states.[18] (The number will be greater by several orders of magnitude if we allow for the possibility that '#' is not a truth-functional connective, or that there are other truth-functional connectives to build new compounds.)

Bad news for interpretation, it may seem. How shall we pick any sensible pattern out of such a gigantic pool? We might try several measures to trim down the pool to more manageable dimensions. For example, we could disregard states in which the putatively accepted propositions form an inconsistent set. We imposed a consistency constraint once already in

---

18 One may suggest the following simplification. Let us assume that the resulting belief state is closed under conjunction, that is, if the person believes p and believes q, then she believes $p\&q$. This assumption is fairly safe because during deliberation about which inferences to draw one needs to "put two and two together" anyway. (However, as a general condition on belief, even rational belief, the assumption is too strong.) $p\#q$ is, presumably, a truth function of p and q. Therefore, the content of the person's resulting belief state can be given by a truth function of p and q, regardless of the person's attitude towards each of the members of the set $\{p\#q, \text{not-}p\#q, p, \text{not-}p, q, \text{not-}q\}$ individually. The number of distinct truth functions of a set of atomic propositions is an exponential function of the number of atomic propositions: For n distinct atomic propositions there are 2^{2^n})) distinct truth functions, 2^{2^n}))–2 if we subtract the uninformative tautology and necessary falsehood. (Each proposition has one of two truth values so that there are 2^n distinct combinations of truth values of n propositions, which in turn yield 2^{2^n})) distinct truth functions of these combinations). The following table of truth functions of p and q illustrates the combinatorial result:

p	q	T	F	a	b	c	d	e	f	g	h	i	j	k	l	m	n
1	1	1	0	1	1	1	0	1	0	0	0	1	1	1	0	0	0
1	0	1	0	1	1	0	1	0	1	0	0	1	0	0	1	1	0
0	1	1	0	1	0	1	1	0	0	1	0	0	1	0	1	0	1
0	0	1	0	0	1	1	1	0	0	0	1	0	0	1	0	1	1

Since $i = p, j = q, n = \neg p, m = \neg q$, the set of distinct truth functions of p and q is precisely the set we need to consider in order to cover all but one possible combinations of acceptance, rejection, and agnosticism *vis a vis* truth functions of the atomic propositions and *vis à vis* each of the atomic propositions by itself (and, more generally, *vis à vis* truth functions of all subsets of the set of propositions under discussion). For example, accepting i means accepting p and remaining agnostic about q. We thus don't have to consider the case for or against p alone if we consider all truth functions of p and q. The one case not yet covered is: agnosticism *vis à vis* all the atomic propositions. If we rule out the necessary truth and the necessary falsehood and add general agnosticism we are left with 15 truth functions and hence belief states to consider for the purpose of interpreting '#', instead of 2,187.

The objection I have against this construction is that it does not preserve all the information contained in a belief state. Suppose, for instance, that '#' means '⊃', and that the person ends up believing $A\supset B$ and rejects both A and B. On the semantic construction just sketched this would be the same as accepting h, because h is logically equivalent to $(A\supset B \,\&\, \text{not-}A \,\&\, \text{not-}B)$. But if we know that the person believes the conditional we can predict that, under suitable circumstances, she would infer B if she came to believe A (assuming that she forgot to drop $A\supset B$ when she dropped not-A from her beliefs). No such claim can be based on the person's believing h. What can be gleaned from this example is quite a general insight. The proposed simplification attempts to give the content of a belief state in terms of truth conditions in the actual world. It turns out that these conditions don't exhaust the content of the state. In particular, they omit information about counterfactual situations. An adequate account of content has to take counterfactual conditions into account. This morale is of course familiar to philosophers of language (see, e.g., Kripke's *Naming and Necessity*).

order to determine what beliefs our fictitious subject deems to be contradictories of one another. Here, the constraint would be stronger because it would rule out not only overt contradictions but any inconsistency. This would tell us something about what the connective '#' *cannot* mean. If the subject infers sets of propositions that are inconsistent on the assumption that the connective '#' means X, then the interpretation of '#' as X must be dropped. For example, if the subject winds up believing the set {$A\#B$, A, *not-B*}, then '#' cannot be the material conditional because the set {$A{\supset}B$, A, *not-B*} is inconsistent. Instead, '#' could mean *vel* (inclusive *or*), *aut* (exclusive *or*), or something else. (We must obviously rely here on prior correct identification of the symbol for negation in the subject's Mentalese.) Although the consistency requirement rules out a great number of states the resulting number will still be very large.[19] Yet this is not the issue.

Trying to simply reduce the number of possible belief states to be considered is really beside the point. What we are after are patterns of inference which determine the meanings of certain Mentalese symbols. These patterns do neither magically emerge out of the pool of possible states, nor are they determined by mere regularities in our subject's inferential behavior. Regularities in inferential behavior could, for all we know at this point, occur for any number of reasons which have nothing at all to do with the meanings of Mentalese symbols. We need to impose further constraints on how belief states may interact in order to single out sensible patterns. These constraints will have to be substantive assumptions about the internal workings of our subject's mind. It will come as no surprise that they will be conditions of rationality. What we need in order to forge a link between patterns of inference and meanings is a theory of rationality.

So, this is in outline how, on the interpretive view of the mind, the presumption of rationality constrains interpretation. We determine what pattern of inference would be rational, given some interpretation of '#', together with whatever else we claim to know about the person's beliefs, desires, etc., and then find out whether her performance accords with this pattern. To the extent that it does the interpretation is justified.[20] Taking the rest of the person's mind into account and imposing rationality in effect greatly reduces the number of acceptable belief states she may enter in any given situation. Ideally, it reduces the number to whatever the number of rational options is, *i.e.* one, according to some people's intuitions about rationality.

---

19 Remember, from the previous footnote, that there are many sets of propositions which are logically equivalent but doxastically distinct. So there are many more distinct doxastic states *vis à vis* truth functions of A and B than there are distinct truth functions of A and B.

20 Stich (forthcoming) argues that the notion of rationality interpretation appeals to is hopelessly mixed up with all sorts of idiosyncratic prejudices and therefore ought not to be taken seriously. He thinks that we unjustifiably project our provincial notions onto the world while we had better try to purge ourselves from them. Since I am not concerned here with the justification of the notion of rationality that enters into interpretation I will not contest his view.

We do not know, in general, which inference is rational under which conditions. As I said earlier, logic rules out inconsistent sets of beliefs but does not tell us which (consistent) set we should infer on a given occasion. The solution to this problem would require a detailed account of rationality which ranks all the many different possible doxastic states our subject may enter in terms of how acceptable or recommendable they are. I believe that the great number of possible states will make the development of such a theory a much harder task than it would be if the patterns to be expected were as simple as *modus ponens*.

If we had the theory we could make some headway in the *Gedankenexperiment* about reading another person's mind. We started with the question, Are there patterns that uniquely identify the different binary connectives in a person's thinking? In one sense, the answer is *yes*. A theory of rationality would tell us, for every binary connective, what the rational patterns of inference are in which it can occur. So we would know which connectives an ideally rational person employs (a person of whom we know not only what she did infer in the past but also what she would infer in many different counterfactual situations). In another sense, the question is still open. We do not yet know in general what conditions have to obtain in order for statements of the form 'A means X by '#'' to be true. In other words, we do not yet know under what conditions ascribing an interpretation to a person is warranted if the person is not ideally rational. For instance, we have not decided how many of the inference types in the pattern for a particular connective must occur in a person's performance in order to warrant the claim that she really thinks in terms of this connective.[21] Nor have we decided what to say in cases where a person's performance is not entirely included within any of the patterns countenanced by the theory of rationality.

A theory of rationality alone is not a theory of interpretation; more has to be said about how exactly rationality constraints figure in interpretation.[22] The conditions are at work somehow, so much we have seen. But

---

21 Sometimes there will be alternatives that are not ruled out by the person's performance. For example, the subject may never have occasion to infer a set of propositions like {A#B, A, B} that would distinguish between exclusive and inclusive *or* by ruling out *aut*. The nonoccurrence of this set does not show, of course, that '#' is the exclusive *or*.

22 One may harbor the following doubt about the existence of a theory of interpretation. People sometimes make mistakes. A theory of interpretation would thus have to draw a line between "good" and "bad" inferences, between performance which counts as relevant data and performance which doesn't. The trouble is that this distinction can only be drawn on the basis of some prior interpretive assumptions. For example, an inference to a belief set of the form {A#B, A, not-B} is to be dismissed as irrelevant only if it is inconsistent with a certain conjectured interpretation of '#' (e.g. as material conditional). Now, there is obviously a circle here. Without presupposing some interpretation the data relevant for interpretation cannot be distinguished from mere "noise," but without prior selection of the relevant data no interpretation can be supported. A theory of interpretation would have to tell us, independently of the data selection, which interpretive assumptions to make, or tell us how to select the relevant data, independently of interpretive assumptions. But since neither can be had there cannot be a theory of interpretation.

Such reasoning would be a bit rash, I think. Circles often look worse than they actually are. The demanded mutual independence of data selection and initial interpretive assumptions is not sacrosanct. If there were a way to correct initial choices the theory of interpretation might fare quite well with mutual dependence. The circle would pose no insoluble problem if there were an effective

do they always have to be fulfilled? Do they always have to be fully met? Can there be occasional deviations from them? I will now argue that in normal cases the constraints pull in different directions.[23] It follows that they cannot be all maximally satisfied; better satisfaction of one constraint will always be at the cost of worse satisfaction of another. It is this gap between maximal and achievable satisfaction, I think, that allows for the existence of irrational belief.

5. Multiple Constraint Satisfaction

Imagine that we investigate a subject's mental arithmetic. We are already confident about how to interpret her Mentalese numerals, the *equals*-sign, some of the function symbols like '+', '−', and a few other things. Now we want to test the conjecture that by '∗' she means multiplication.[24] As our data we have her calculations in which '∗' occurs, let's say:

$$2*3=3+3$$
$$1*1=1$$
$$4*2=8$$
$$5*2=7.$$

The last calculation somehow does not fit well with our conjecture. Something strange is going on, but it is not obvious what it is. It is not simply that the data are inconsistent with our conjecture. Rather, the data, together with the conjecture, imply that the subject is doing something wrong. There are several ways in which the subject may have gone wrong, and there is of course also the possibility that our conjecture is false. We can test some of the possibilities. We can test, for example, whether '5∗2=7' was a mere slip that we should disregard for the purpose of interpretation. Suppose we find out that it wasn't, that the subject stubbornly holds on to

procedure which, regardless of our initial choice of interpretive assumptions and relevant data, would always converge in the same final interpretation. (Lewis (1983) sketches three iterative procedures for the revision of initial assumptions.) It would be premature at this point to make any conjectures about the existence of such a procedure. I do not think, however, that this vitiates what I will say about how rationality constrains interpretation.

Grandy puts forward a "Principle of Humanity" which seems to be a piece of pragmatic advice for escaping the circle, rather than a theoretical solution to the problem. Grandy writes: "The combination of reported desires and beliefs (even supplemented by facts inferred from nonverbal behavior) do not suffice to determine the expected behavior. Instead we must have some model of the agent that we use to assist us in making a prediction. [...] we consider ourselves in order to arrive at the prediction: we consider what we should do if we had the relevant beliefs and desires. [...] So we have, as a pragmatic constraint on translation, the condition that the imputed pattern of relations among beliefs, desires, and the world be as similar to our own as possible. This principle I call the *principle of humanity*." (Grandy 1973, 442-3). It seems to me that the principle does not replace considerations of rationality, nor is it in place just because no amount of performance data determines a unique interpretation. It is appealed to because there is no other practical way to draw the line between relevant and irrelevant performance data in a non-ideal world.

23 This point is not new; you find it already in Quine (1960).

24 For any given data, there are always infinitely many different hypotheses which are equally compatible with it. I am not concerned here with the general issue of how to choose among them.

it. (If you find this too implausible, modify the example: imagine Chinese numerals instead of Arabic ones; or imagine that the subject asserts 'There are only finitely many prime numbers', instead of '5∗2=7'.) If '5∗2=7' was no slip we would have to consider three more or less plausible alternative hypotheses:

(a) '∗' means multiplication, and the subject lacks the intelligence to recognize the inconsistency in his beliefs.

(b) '∗' means multiplication, the subject notices the inconsistency, but fails to remove it.

(c) '∗' means something other than multiplication, for example, multiplication for all arguments except 5 and 2, for which it means addition. (This non-standard interpretation is likely to have far-reaching consequences for the interpretation of most of the person's assertions.)

With some luck, we will be able to conduct experiments which may convince us of one or the other of these hypotheses; or we may think up other alternatives. No matter which hypothesis we will ultimately adopt, it will commit us to claims about the subject that we will not make light-heartedly. We will have to admit that the subject violates certain conditions, conditions of rationality and others, which cannot be renounced altogether if interpretation is to succeed. To ascribe these violations is to acknowledge that not all constraints on interpretation can be fully satisfied.

What are these constraints? I mention just a few: Every interpretation has to construe its subject as largely consistent, as being reasonably skilled in detecting implications, as being able to draw inferences and resolve inconsistencies, as having largely true beliefs (which comes to: having roughly the same beliefs we have), and as having the beliefs that this kind of subject should have according to our best psychological theory.[25] Each of (a)–(c) balances these constraints in a different way: (a) avoids ascribing overtly inconsistent beliefs at the cost of construing the subject as incompetent; (b) construes the subject as somewhat more competent but not intelligent enough (or unwilling) to remove the inconsistency; (c) ascribes true but psychologically implausible beliefs. By following out the consequences of the hypotheses, we may find that one is clearly superior to the others in the way it does the balancing, but we will not find that one satisfies all the constraints.

This, I believe, is true quite generally. People's inferential behavior is never such that an interpretation can fully satisfy all the constraints. If we think that nevertheless interpretation sometimes (or often, or most of the time) succeeds we have to concede that less than full satisfaction is all that's needed. But this means that the relations which, according to the interpretive view, determine the contents of belief do not have to live up to ideal rationality. On the scale between inferential chaos and ideal rationality there is some vague threshold below which content ascription does not make sense. But above the threshold, I want to suggest, there is

---

25 There are many proposals for rationality constraints in the literature, often under the name of "principles of charity" (Quine); see for example Lewis (1983) and Cherniak (1986).

enough room for failures to recognize implications or to weed out inconsistencies, for jumping to conclusions and the like, in short, for irrational belief.

The argument I offer here for thinking that there is sufficient space for irrational belief above the threshold consists in the following pair of plausibility considerations. First, there can be no doubt that in many, many cases people appear to hold irrational beliefs. It *could* be the case that this impression is wrong and that what's in their minds instead are fewer but rational beliefs, plus a muddle of non-representational gibberish. But this hypothesis is unappealing because it makes unavailable explanations of behavior in terms of those irrational beliefs. It is less appealing, for example, to accept as a brute fact that John jumped off the tree than it is to explain it by his irrational belief that he could fly. (I will shortly say a little more about the relation between contents and actions.) Some explanations of actions which appeal to irrational beliefs are simply better than their alternatives. This is good reason for thinking that the belief states they posit exist. Secondly, it is hard to see how there could be an *a priori* argument to the effect that certain constraint violations, the ones that occur in cases of irrational belief, undermine interpretation. Attempting to construct such an argument would be like trying to decide *a priori* what the threshold should be for the number of hairs on a person's head below which the person is bald. Taken together, the two considerations suggest that there are diagnosable irrational beliefs, and that this fact is compatible with the interpretive view.

At the outset I presented the *problem of complementary evidence: All evidence for the irrationality of a person's beliefs (desires, actions) is, by the same token, evidence against the ascription of the very contents with respect to which the person appears to be irrational. Therefore there are never sufficient grounds to judge a person's beliefs (desires, actions) irrational.* It should be apparent now that the problem is overstated. It is true that a person's deviation from the course of rationality makes it more difficult to balance properly the constraints on interpretation. If a person entertains what looks like irrational beliefs we have to take greater pains than usual to find out what it is that she believes. But it does not follow that in no such case a satisfactory balance of constraints can be achieved. It does not follow, in other words, that the grounds to judge a person's intentional states irrational are never sufficient.

6. The Bigger Picture

So far, I illustrated the thesis that rational relations between beliefs determine content by rather artificial examples. Let me now try to outline a slightly more realistic picture. In the examples we had, as the sole determinants of content, inferential relations to other belief states. For the case of truth functional connectives this is plausible; it would indeed be hard to see what if not inferential relations should determine content. The situation is different with the more "material" contents of people's minds. When you believe, say, that there is a tiger in front of you, it is much less clear in what way mere relations to other beliefs and thoughts should determine what your belief is about. To be sure, some relations must be there, and they are governed by rationality constraints. But at least equally important are counterfactual relations to objects in your environment which are not relations of rational inference.[26] For example, you would not, under normal conditions, believe that the thing over there is a tiger if it were not a tiger or a very faithful tiger replica. And, generally, when you act on the belief that there is a tiger in front of you your actions must be appropriate to the presence of a tiger rather than, say, a squirrel. Neither inferential relations alone nor mere counterfactual relations between your intentional states and the environment make for determinate contents of your mind. Neither kind of relation is sufficient without the other.

Thus the fact that a certain mental state of yours is typically caused by the presence of a tiger in your visual field, and typically (*i.e.* out there in the wild) elicits evasive motor behavior, is not sufficient in itself to establish the claim that the state is the belief that there is a tiger in front of you. Nor is this fact sufficient when it is backed by a gloss about *ceteribus paribus* conditions: that your vision is unimpaired, that your eyes are open, that illumination is fine, etc. Rather, for the state to be a belief about a tiger it has to be linked to your other beliefs and desires in a rational way. You should flee, for instance, only if, in addition to your present perceptual belief, you think that tigers are very dangerous and do not have any current desire to be eaten by one. You should flee precisely because that is the rational thing to do given your present beliefs and desires. On the other hand, reason relations alone do not determine content either. Without causal connections which hook up your mind to the world your mental states would be like the formulae of an uninterpreted calculus: compatible with an indefinite number of different interpretations.

Dependencies between conjectured intentional states, behavior, and states of the environment furnish the cognitive ethologist with a great many clues about the contents of their informants' minds.[27] This is, I think, why we can detect clear-cut cases of irrationality, for example those reported from mental patients suffering delusions. The contents of patients' delusions can be quite transparent to the psychiatrist. There are enough occasions on which the patients behave "normally" enough to convince us that their perceptual beliefs are largely as they would be expected from a normal person. This means that there is a rational core in the patients' behavior that is sufficiently robust to warrant interpretation. But it does not mean that the patients *always* have to be that way. A patient may

---

26 I simply state this without arguing for "wide" as opposed to "narrow" psychology. I am convinced that some form of wide psychology is the only viable option.
27 This is not to contradict Quine's skeptical thesis about the "indeterminacy of translation," the thesis that no amount of data can uniquely determine an interpretation or translation (cf. Quine 1960).

have, for example, the ability to form beliefs *about spies* despite the fact that he thinks that the man living upstairs is a spy only on the grounds that he wears a dark coat. We do not say, in this case, that perhaps his belief is not really that this person is a spy and that by 'spy' he means something like *man wearing a dark coat*. We do not say this because, from other observations, we have reason to believe that the patient still can distinguish between the concept of a spy and the concept of a man in a dark coat. In particular, if he did not believe the man was a spy over and above his wearing a dark coat he would not be as anxious as he is. We would start doubting that his belief is about spies if he did not show any of the reactions that one would expect from a person who believes that the man is really a spy. We would have to rethink our interpretation if the patient agreed with it, realized that he ought not to hold on to his beliefs, yet failed to even attempt a rational reconciliation. In textbook cases of delusions proper there is nothing as salient as this attempt at reconciliation.

Relations between (conjectured) intentional states and the environment provide clues for interpretation over and above those provided by inferential behavior. These clues can be exploited in order to strike an acceptable balance between the rationality (and other) constraints. When we grant that the patient's belief is about spies, for instance, we are are looser on the side of truthfulness for the sake of more coherence. In this way, quite drastic violations of some constraints seem possible as long as they are counterbalanced by close adherence to others.[28]

Summary

This paper explores the question of how rationality assumptions constrain interpretation. In order to interpret a person's utterances (and non-linguistic behavior) as expressions of belief one has to assume that the expressed beliefs are rational. Therefore, it may seem that there cannot be interpretable expressions of irrational belief. It is argued that this impression is wrong. Although there are limits to how irrational a person's beliefs can be without undercutting interpretation it is not the case that beliefs have to be fully rational in order to be interpretable. The rationality constraints on interpretation leave enough room for moderate irrationality.

References

Cherniak C: Minimal Rationality. MIT Press, Cambridge MA, 1986.
Clouser DK., Bernard G: Rationality and Medicine: An Explanation. Journal of Medicine and Philosophy 11: 185–205, 1986.
Clouser DK., Bernard .G: Rationality and Medicine: Introduction to the Theme. Journal of Medicine and Philosophy 11: 119–21, 1986.

---

28 I am indebted to Gilbert Harman, Richard Holton, Rae Langton, Dan Sperber, Natalie Stoljar, and Jonathan Vogel for helpful comments on an earlier draft of this paper.

Davidson D: Radical Interpretation. Dialectica 27: 313–328, 1973.
Davidson D: Mental Events. In: D. Davidson: Essays on Actions and Events, Clarendon Press, Oxford, pp. 207–227, 1980.
Davidson D: Paradoxes of Irrationality. In: R.A. Wollheim and J. Hopkins (eds.) Philosophical Essays on Freud. Cambridge Univ. Press, Cambridge, pp. 289–305, 1982.
Davidson D: Rational Animals. Dialectica 36: 318–27, 1982b.
Davidson Donald: Incoherence and Irrationality. Dialectica 39.4: 345–354, 1985.
Dennett DC: Brainstorms. Bradford, Cambridge MA, 1979.
Dennett DC: The Intentional Stance. MIT Press, Cambridge MA, 1985.
Fodor JA: The Language of Thought. Harvard Univ. Press, Cambridge MA, 1975.
Foley R: Is It Possible to Have Contradictory Beliefs? Midwest Studies in Philosophy X: 328–355, 1986.
Føllesdal D: The Status of Rationality Assumptions in Interpretation and in the Explanation of Action. Dialectica 36.4: 301–316, 1982.
Goldman AI: Epistemology and Cognition. Harvard Univ. Press, Cambridge MA, 1986.
Grandy R: Reference, Meaning, and Belief. The Journal of Philosophy 70: 439–452, 1973.
Harman G: Conceptual Role Semantics. Notre Dame Journal of Formal Logic 23: 242–256, 1982.
Harman G: Change in View: Principles of Reasoning. MIT Press, Cambridge MA, 1986.
Johnston M: Self-Deception and the Nature of Mind. In: McLaughlin PB and Rorty AO (eds) Perspectives on Self-Deception, Univ. of California Press, Berkeley, pp. 63–91, 1988.
Kripke SA: A Puzzle About Belief. In: Margalit A (ed): Meaning and Use. Reidel, Dordrecht, pp. 239–283, 1979.
Kripke SA: Naming and Necessity. Harvard Univ. Press, Cambridge MA, 1980.
Lewis DK: Radical Interpretation. In: Lewis DK: Philosophical Papers, Vol. I, Oxford University Press, New York, Oxford, pp.108–118, 1983.
Maher BA, Oltmanns TF (eds): Delusional Beliefs. Wiley, New York, Chichester, Brisbane, Toronto, Singapore, 1988.
Martin M: Defining Irrational Action in Medical and Psychiatric Contexts. The Journal of Medicine and Philosophy 11: 179–184, 1986.
Quine WVO: Word and Object, MIT Press, Cambridge MA, 1960.
Reid T: Essays in the Intellectual Powers of Man (1785). MIT Press, Cambridge MA, 1969.
Stalnaker R: Inquiry. Bradford, Cambridge MA, 1984.
Stich S, Nisbett R: Justification and the Psychology of Human Reasoning. Philosophy of Science 47: 188–202, 1980.
Stich S: Could Man be an Irrational Animal? Synthese 64: 115–135, 1985.
Stich S: The Fragmentation of Reason.(forthcoming).

Technical Problems with Teleological Explanation in Psychopathology: Sigmund Freud as a Case in Point

Joseph F. Rychlak

1. Introduction

It is generally recognized that modern personality theory dates from the closing decades of the nineteenth century when Sigmund Freud advanced his theories of psychopathology, which were then extended to normals. On first consideration, this seems an odd direction to take—moving from the abnormal to the normal behavioral pattern. But there is something irreducibly human albeit "unnatural" about a disordered mind. Neurotics do not listen to reason, yet they have their reasons. Psychotics believe in the most preposterous things, living out a phantasy realm that is stretched beyond recognition by those of us who populate the everyday, "natural" environment.

When we work with the abnormal person we are brought into the pathological process in a most direct fashion. Not only are we as psychotherapists wound into the neurotic's transferences and the psychotic's delusions, but our own assumptions and valued beliefs regarding what is "normal" and what is "abnormal" in behavior come under scrutiny. Physical scientists have learned in the modern era that they are "participators" in their research findings (Zukav 1979, p. 29). What they discover empirically is influenced by their introductory assumptions in a way that was never appreciated by the Newtonians. Psychotherapists have known of their participative role in the pathological process for over a century. Many have been in therapy themselves even as they were trained for their role as therapist.

There is another matter that arises in the realm of psychopathology in a most telling fashion; the distinct possibility of human agency. The arbitrary logic, the unattainable end being sought, the patent refusal to acknowledge reality, all combine to suggest that the human person is in some way creating or at least significantly contributing to the pathological condition from which he or she suffers. It is this teleological aspect of psychopathology that the present paper addresses. There are decided problems confronting the teleologist in the description of human behavior—normal or abnormal. We would like to present four types of problems faced by the teleologist, using the experience of Sigmund Freud to highlight the points under analysis. We begin with a consideration of the perspective from which theoretical explanations are framed, apply this perspective issue to the use of final causation, move to a definition of predicational versus mediational modeling, and then contrast the oppositional and appositional generation of alternatives in reasoning. The paper ends with a recommendation to correct the current gap in technical usage by employing a concept of telosponsivity in behavioral description.

2. Theoretical Perspective: Extraspection Versus Introspection

The first problem faced by the teleologist has to do with the perspective, the "slant" or point of view from which his or her theory is written. This perspective begins in the very task that a theoretician sets out to accomplish. The importance of theoretical perspective has been empirically demonstrated in a series of experiments by Jones and Nisbett (1971). The purpose of this research series was to find out what the actors and/or observers felt were the relevant causes of the behavior carried out by the actors in a number of situations. The actors claimed that it was the logically relevant factors in the circumstances facing them that caused them to behave as they did, whereas the observers of these same actors were prone to attribute the cause of the latter's behavior to presumed habits or personality traits that directed the actor no matter what the logic of the current situation dictated. In other words, the observers made no real effort to look at things from the point of view of an actor—unless they became actors themselves! That is, when the observer of an action was given a videotape of the actor's view of things, the circumstances confronting the actor were then given weight as a cause of the actor's behavior. And, even more interestingly, when actors took the perspective of observers they too tended to view extra– personal factors as the primary causes of behavior in the situation.

We might now refer to the perspective taken by the observers as *extraspective*, as looking outward at "that" or "it" behaving "over there" (Rychlak 1981, p. 27). As Jones and Nisbett found, the resultant theoretical explanation is likely to be written in third–person fashion. The person qua reasoner and assessor of the current circumstances is downplayed in this account, which is framed entirely from the convenience of the observer who assigns the action to an "it," that is, a *trait* or *habit* that moves the actor along regardless of the latter's understanding of the situational circumstances. The perspective taken by the actor can be called *introspective* (ibid.), in that it is framed by looking with the item (person) under description. In this case, the actor's understanding of the situational circumstances is all important. The resultant theoretical account takes on a first–person rendering in which terms like "I" or "Me" are relevant—quite often subsumed by the term "Self."

If there is one thing that is distinctive about Freudian psychopathological explanations it is that they encompass primarily the introspective perspective. There are probably two reasons for this emphasis. First of all, Freud had a genius for grasping the viewpoint (motives, etc.) of others. But secondly, and probably more importantly, he relied upon his personal dreams and self–analysis to formulate and provide the evidence for his theories. Indeed, the more we learn about Freud the more we find that his core conceptions, from dream symbolism to symptom formation, and beyond, are rooted in his introspective understanding of his personal dynamics.

There is one notable example of Freud attempting to write a completely extraspective theory of behavior in the tradition of the medical models of his education. Goaded by his colleague and confidant, Wilhelm Fliess, he sets out in September of 1895 to write what he was to call the *Project for a Scientific Psychology*. The opening lines of the *Project* are extremely interesting:

"The intention [of the *Project*] is to furnish a psychology that shall be a natural science: that is, to represent psychical processes as quantitatively determinate states of specifiable material particles, thus making those processes perspicuous and free from contradiction. Two principal ideas are involved: [1] What distinguishes activity from rest to be regarded as Q, subject to the general laws of motion. (2) The neurones are to be taken as the material particles" (Freud 1966a/1895, p. 295).

Freud never completed the *Project*, although his collected works number 23 volumes. In fact, by October 29th of 1895, some two months after plunging into this "natural science" effort, Freud could say in a letter to Fliess: "I no longer understand the state of mind in which I hatched the psychology [Project], cannot conceive how I could have inflicted it on you" (Freud 1985, p. 152). Actually, as other letters in their correspondence make clear (ibid., pp. 159, 326), it was Fliess who continually pressed Freud for extraspective formulations of the neuroses, written in the style of medical accounts. Fliess had a kind of biological clock theory of his own, in which both men and women were said to be under the influence of 23 or 28 day physiological cycles. Psychopathology occurred when the rhythmic cyles were thrown out of kilter, and the introspective dynamics of the person concerned were irrelevant to the dysrhythmia.

Fliess was the complete, extraspective observer who did not take the actor's outlook into consideration. Freud was always in empathy with the actor. This empathy made it inevitable that he would be drawn into a teleological account of behavior. As we noted, he invariably understood or came to understand why people behaved as they did, the reasons for the sake of which they behaved, including those reasons that they refused to admit (consciously) to themselves. But how could one possibly hope to describe things in this fashion? Freud had no technical terminology on which to draw at this point. What we find him doing is constantly slipping back and forth between introspective and extraspective formulations of behavior in psychoanalysis. The most notorious example of the latter formulation is his libido theory. Libido is an analogy to physical energy, but totally psychic in meaning so that we find it being used instrumentally by a number of psychic identities (Id, Ego, Super–ego), each of whom can in turn be understood from the introspective perspective. The psychic identities are the agents, and it is in the maneuvering and compromising between these identities that we find the uniquely Freudian style of explanation.

3. Final Causation in Human Description

In shifting perspective from observer to actor, with the resultant shift in causal attribution, we necessarily get involved in the historical debate over the propriety of using final–cause description in science. That is, in framing our understanding of an actor's behavior from his or her (introspective) perspective, we begin to speak of the reasons why one action is carried out rather than another. And reasons are most readily subsumed by what Aristotle called a final cause. The word Aristotle used for what we translate as "cause" was αιτια, which has the meaning of *responsibility*. So, causes get at what is responsible for anything existing in nature, or any action that is carried out by animate or inanimate processes. There are four types of causes to consider: material, efficient, formal, and final.

Aristotle (1952a) defined the *material cause* as the constituent matter "out of which a thing comes to be and which persists...e.g., the bronze of the statue, the silver of the bowl..." (p. 271). We shall refer to the material cause as both matter and substance, but in strict Aristotelian philosophy the meaning of substance is more than this (i. e., the individual thing, constituted out of matter and form; secondly, form as so–called secondary substance; see Aristotle, 1952b, p. 644). The *efficient cause* was said to be "the primary source of change or coming to rest" (Aristotle 1952a, p. 271). Efficient causes name the impetus in events, the instrumental push, thrust, flow, cueing, or triggering of motions in nature, and the actor, in so far as he or she starts an action, a process.

The *formal cause* is the "definition of the essence, and the classes which include this (e.g., the relation 2:1 and number in general are the cause of the octave)..." (Aristotle 1952c, p. 533). By "essence" Aristotle had in mind the overall "synthesis of the whole" that an item of cognition takes on in its meaning (ibid.). Thus, formal causation gets at the pattern, shape, outline, or recognizable organization that occurs in the material substances of nature as well as in the (efficient–cause) motions of passing events. Formal cause makes an individual such a one as it is, makes a thing what it is. It should be noted that some Aristotelian scholars dismiss the importance of shape per se in formal causation, placing their emphasis on form as that into which something is classified or made (e.g., Adler 1978, p. 38; see also Robinson 1989, p. 39). However, since the formal cause (εἶδοσ) makes an individual such a one as it is, indeed, makes an individual what it is, it *then* is the form into which something is classified. It is therefore nonsense to say "the formal cause of N. is wrong", but possible and often sound indeed to say "the classification of N. is wrong". In short, we shall employ formal causation as a pattern/shape concept.

The fourth cause to be employed in accounting for anything is the *final cause* or "the sense of [an] end or 'that for the sake of which' a thing is done, e.g. health is the cause of walking about" (Aristotle 1952a, p. 271). Theories employing final causation are *teleologies*, including explanations relying upon purpose, intention, or the "reason" why things exist or actions take place. There is an implicit tie between the formal and final cause (Aristotle 1952d, p. 255). The formal cause is always embedded in the final cause. For example, a formal cause can be considered as the patterned strategy "for the sake of which" the person behaves. A paranoid delusion is an intricate pattern of manipulation in reaction to an imagined persecution. As such, it can be thought of as the "that" (formal cause) "for the sake of which" (final cause) the paranoid is strategizing. A teleologist might construe psychopathology in this manner. Unfortunately, due to certain historical precedents, an explanation of this type would be considered non–scientific in the strictest circles.

That is, the suitability of final–cause description was brought into serious question and then rejected by the scientists of the seventeenth century. A major reason for this rejection stemmed from Galileo's historic clash with the churchmen of the Inquisition. By a fairly complicated process of thought in later antiquity the geocentric world–picture of Hellenism had been interpreted in terms of a deity teleology, i.e., as the divine intention of the Creator. For the churchmen in question the central position of the earth seemed therefore sanctioned by the Biblical account, turned into a coherent theory of the heavens; Galileo, however, was proposing a heliocentric explanation of the heavens. His house arrest and recantation heralded the beginning of the end for final–cause description in science, which must ever rely upon empirical evidence and not religio–teleological dogma. But there was another, more technical reason for questioning the use of final causes in scientific theory: They can be seen to be unnecessary additions to an already understood "natural" object or event.

To clarify this point we must first return to Aristotle and note that he employed final–cause description in both an extraspective and an intro-spective manner. He viewed nature as working toward ends, and therefore was likely to describe physical structures or events in telic fashion, as follows: "...the purpose of the blood in sanguineous animals is to subserve the nutrition of the body....the blood exists for the sake of nutrition, that is, the nutrition of the parts....[and the] bones are a contrivance to give security to the soft parts, to which purpose they are adapted by their hard-ness" (Aristotle 1952e, p. 175). This is an extraspective use of final causa-tion. Aristotle is not taking the "point of view" of the blood, as it winds its way through the body. He is looking "at" the flow of blood, and suggesting that it has a nutritional purpose, as the bones have a structural purpose. But in another context, Aristotle took the introspective perspective in describing the final–cause actions of human beings, as follows: "For consider how the physician or how the builder sets about his work. He starts by forming for himself a definite picture, in the one case perceptive to mind, in the other to sense, of his end—the physician of health, the builder of a house—and this he holds forward as the reason and explanation of each subsequent step that he takes, and of his acting in this or that way as the case may be" (Aristotle 1952e, pp. 161–162).

Note that in this case, Aristotle is indeed taking the "point of view" of the physician and the builder, whom he knows behave "for the sake of" certain reasons or purposes (ends, etc.). Even so, at about the same time in history that Galileo was being pressured to change his views, Sir Francis Bacon was leveling his guns at formal/final–cause description in science. Of course, we must keep in mind that at this historical period "science" was thought of in exclusively physical terms, as involving studies like astronomy, chemistry, magnetism, metallurgy, and so on. There was no "science" of human behavior to consider. Hence, in his assault on Aristotle, Bacon was specifically aiming his charges at the extraspective form of final–causation. What did it add to our knowledge of the physical world, Bacon asked, to say that the bones are "for the sake of" holding up the fleshy parts of the body, or that leaves are "for the sake of" shading fruit on the branches of trees (Bacon 1952a, p. 44)?

Bacon claimed that by rushing to the telic form of explanation Aristotle had actually hampered the progress of empirical science (ibid.). Indeed, he observed as many later critics of final–cause description in psychiatry and psychology have observed, that when one relies on telic description in science he or she is prone to accept explanations closely allied to human nature. This would later be termed anthropomorphizing natural objects and events. This happens because final–cause description is "...clearly more allied to man's own nature...than [to] the system of the universe" (Bacon 1952b, p. 111). Bacon accepted the use of final–cause description in metaphysical analysis.

But the "Baconian criticism" regarding the extraspective formulations of nature is sound. If we can explain the structure or function of something like tree leaves, skeletal bones, planetary motions, or stomach digestion by relying exclusively on material and efficient causation (with possibly a formal–cause patterning added in), what does it contribute to our knowledge to say that any of this exists or occurs "for the sake of" anything? Natural scientists have repeatedly argued that they are involved in the "how" of things (how they are structured, how they function, etc.) and not the "why" of things (the purpose "for the sake of which" they exist or operate as they do).

In 1912, Freud (1958a/1912) replied to a criticism that had been leveled at his work by Rudolf Reitler. In his *Three Essays on Sexuality,*

Freud (1953a/1905) had used the phrase "nature's purpose" in speaking of the role of masturbation in the dynamics of sexual development (p. 188). Reitler had essentially leveled the Baconian criticism, charging that Freud was going beyond the "facts" in using such phraseology, which added nothing to the account. Freud conceded that he was incorrect, that he would remove the offensive phrase in a later edition of the book (which he eventually did), and then added apologetically "I will renounce my attempt at guessing the purpose of Nature and will content myself with describing the facts" (Freud 1958a/1912, p. 247). But what are the facts of human behavior? When we think about people introspectively, it is factual—or it appears factual—that they embrace purposes, reasons, and intentions. And, knowing something about these latter cognitive states clearly *does* add to our understanding of why they behave as they do. In short, it can be argued that although Freud should not be guessing nature's purpose, he has every right as analyst to guess at the purposes of his patients! And, in fact, this is precisely what he did.

References to purposes, reasons, and intentions abound in Freud's theories. In the *Studies on Hysteria* (Breuer and Freud 1955/1893) we read: "...I already knew from the analysis of similar cases that before hysteria can be acquired for the first time one essential condition must be fulfilled: an idea must be *intentionally repressed from consciousness* and excluded from associative modification [italics in original]" (p. 116). At about this same time, in a letter to Fliess dated January 24, 1895 he says "The purpose of paranoia is thus to ward off an idea that is incompatible with the ego, by projecting its substance into the external world" (Freud 1985, p. 109). In The Interpretation of Dreams (Freud 1953b/1901) we find: "It can be shown that all that we can ever get rid of are purposive ideas that are known to us; as soon as we have done this, *unknown*—or, as we inaccurately say, 'unconscious'—purposive ideas take charge and thereafter determine the course of the involuntary ideas [italics in original]" (p. 528). In a 1908 paper, Freud (1959/1908) distinguished between the primary and secondary *purposes* of a person's falling into neurotic illness (pp. 231–232), and so on.

It is our contention that, in his willingness to view human beings from an introspective perspective, Freud gravitated to final–cause description/explanation. This means he was fundamentally teleological in theoretical orientation, although admittedly, as we noted above, he made great efforts to comply with medical colleagues who urged him to frame a more traditional, extraspective, medico–physical theory of psychopathology. In addition, it is our contention that Freud was in his more psychodynamic explanations *exempted* from the Baconian criticism. There are no grounds on which to charge that an understanding of people's reasons, intentions, or purposes is superfluous or irrelevant information. Recent findings on the classical or operant conditioning of human beings, which are totally extraspective formulations of behavior, suggest that knowing something about the subjects' awareness of the circumstances in a conditioning experiment adds immeasurably to our understanding of how such "conditioning" takes place (Brewer 1974). In fact, the evidence supports the view that conditioning is impossible without a subject's awareness of what is to transpire, and a willingness to cooperate with the purpose of the experiment (as understood by the subject)! This takes us to our next point, concerning the model we are to employ in framing a telic account.

4. Predicational Versus Mediational Modeling

In looking "with" people introspectively rather than "at" them extraspectively we are likely to rely upon a predicational model of behavior. By *predication* we mean a process involving *the act of affirming, denying, or qualifying broader patterns of meaning in relation to narrower or targeted patterns of meaning*. In philosophy, this process has been referred to as reasoning from universals to particulars, or from the genus to the species. The ancient Greeks coined the word κατεγορειν, meaning "to predicate," from which devolve terms like categorizing, classifying, or framing knowledge (information, etc.). There is a specific way in which such categorizing takes place. The course of predication is always from the wider "to" the narrower range of meaning under consideration. A predicational model is therefore conceptual, it addresses the creation of knowledge in a top–down sense whereby the broader context of meaning lends itself to a targeted item situated within this context.

When a diagnosis of psychopathology is made—such as "Albert is an obsessive–compulsive neurotic"—a wider range of meaning (obsessive–compulsivity) is being brought to bear on a narrower range of meaning (specifically, Albert). We could readily diagram this logical arrangement through Euler circles, in which case we would have a large circle labeled "obsessive–compulsive neurotics" and placed within it a number of smaller circles, one of which would bear the name "Albert" (i. e., there are other people within this wider expanse of meaning besides Albert). Predication is not simply a syntactic rule. It is a distinctive process which can be shown to create different meanings even as the identical words are used in a sentence but in contrasting predicational relationships. For example, we can say either "A person is like a tree" or "A tree is like a person." Two quite different meanings are conveyed thanks to this subject–predicate rearrangement of identical words. So, predication is not the result of word meaning per se, but of the organized *relationship* of word meanings.

Predication is also what we refer to when we speak of meaningful contexts. For example, the major premise of a syllogism provides a broad context of meaning within which the minor premise and conclusion are situated, each in succession focusing the wider compass of the major premise to a greater and greater extent until it is quite specific (e.g., *All human beings are mortal. This is a human being. Hence, this human being is mortal*). Meaning creation is central to predication. It makes no sense to speak of predication if there is no meaning under processing. Indeed, once the arrangement is made, once the words are aligned with each other, the meaning–extension from wider to narrower is *immediate*. That is, the process under consideration is literally bringing about or *creating* the meaning(s) involved. Nothing outside the predicational process can create such meaning (information, etc.) "for" this process.

This internal creation of meaning is not true of a mediational model. By *mediation* we mean that something which *is taken in or input comes indirectly to play a role in a process that was not initially a part of this process.* The process under description in the mediation model is not conceived as the "immediate" creator of what is to be active within it, but rather as the conveyor of that which it takes in "as given" and proceeds on the basis of. The meanings under processing are always "mediate," since they are never aligned or framed by the process per se, but merely *employed* by this process. One is reminded here of a conveyor belt, moving items along, each of which has been packaged someplace else.

In similar fashion, the meaningful items under conveyance by a mediational process are "accepted whole hog," as given patterns that have been organized even before they are taken into cognition from environmental experience. The mediational process never articulates or forms this meaning. Something like a predication would only occur secondarily within the mediational process, whereby certain rearrangements of the inputs might be effected; or, having emitted certain words in fortuitous ways, certain combinations would be selected for retention by favorable external considerations. Mediation is a bottom–up process, in which what we have called the wider compass of meaning would have been "shaped" from below rather than serving as the "shaper" of targeted items below.

An introspective formulation of human behavior in terms of formal/final causation invites a predicational modeling of such behavior. Extraspective constructs drawing on material/efficient causation fit nicely into a mediational model. As the father of dynamic psychology, Freud was unquestionably a predicational modeler. The whole point of psychodynamics is to see that the person qua conceptualizer arranges the meanings that will occur in cognizance. Freud, who believed that infants reasoned natively according to a *primary process* which was highly colored by predicate assumptions known as phantasy, based many of his psychodynamic explanations on this subjective cognitive process. Phantasy through day–dreaming "abandons dependences on real objects" (Freud 1958b/1911, p. 222).

It is not external reality that forms the meanings of phantasy: It is the point of view, prejudice, bias, wish, and so forth, under affirmation in the predicational process of the individual—who can distort this reality "at will." Phantasy plays a major role in fixation and the subsequent regressions of psychopathology (Freud 1963b/1917). Probably Freud's clearest statement of his predicational modeling was the following, in which he is talking about the self–deception involved in unconscious dynamics. Freud here aligns himself with the thinking of Kant, who was most assuredly a major predicational modelist in the history of philosophy, viewing meanings as formed by the conceptualizing intellect rather than taken in as a pristine totality: "The psycho–analytic assumption of unconscious mental activity appears to us, on the one hand, as a further expansion of the primitive animism which caused us to see copies of our own consciousness all around us, and, on the other hand, as an extension of the corrections undertaken by Kant of our views on external perception. Just as Kant warned us not to overlook the fact that our perceptions are subjectively conditioned and must not be regarded as identical with what is perceived though unknowable, so psycho–analysis warns us not to equate perceptions by means of consciousness with the unconscious mental processes which are their object. Like the physical, the psychical is not necessarily in reality what it appears to us to be" (Freud 1957a/1915, p. 171).

5. Oppositional Versus Appositional Disjunction

There is one more piece to our puzzle of technicalities in the description of behavior for the teleologist. It has to do with why predication works in the "wider to narrower" sense of meaning extension, and also with how it is that alternatives are brought about in this process. Invariably, the wider context framing a targeted item in a predicational process is bounded by *oppositionality*. This is what always makes the predication a "context," for it intrinsically defines what "is" and "is not" the case. In our example of Albert above, we did not discuss the fact that the wider Euler circle labeled "obsessive–compulsive neurotics" had an "outside" area—the surrounding region of the circle (the "non–circle"). In effect, this means there was an oppositional dimension of "inside to outside" the circle involves. Had we decided that Albert was *not* obsessive–compulsive, our logical arrangment would have been to place the smaller circle labeled "Albert" outside of the larger circle labeled "obsessive–compulsive neurotics."

But in so doing, we would be establishing that there is an even wider realm of meaning within which we are cognizing the mental state of our patient. Since we can place Albert on "this" or "that" side of the diagnostic picture, it is necessary for us to "take a position" on the question at hand. This taking of a position is simply another way of referring to predication. Once we take a stand, we have affirmed a protopoint from which our line of thought will unfold. But note: We will always have that sense of the "other" possibility. This reflects what might be termed *oppositional disjunction*. Disjunction refers to the manner in which separations of meanings arise. In logic, it has to do with the forming of alternatives.

What we are suggesting here is that opposite meanings delimit each other—open up thereby a wide context within which other meaningful items can be targeted. Hence, to separate and opt for one end of an oppositional context is to retain a tie to the other end of the meaningful dimension that frames this wider realm. We cannot know what "abnormal" (obsessive–compulsive) behavior entails unless we know what "normal" (non–obsessive–compulsive) behavior entails. These meanings shade into each other even as they remain distinct. It is not incorrect to suggest that "abnormal" literally defines "normal" by contrast (contradiction, contrariety, etc.). In oppositional disjunction, therefore, we have the case of "either x or y, or both" obtaining.

It is quite different in mediational models. Here we have a complete separation of meanings. There are no intrinsic ties of oppositionality to be concerned with. In a typical stimulus–response theory, for example, though the meaning of a stimulus is opposite to that of a response, the way in which these concepts are interpreted is to presume that they are separate and distinct occurrences, hooked–up, connected, or associated together by so–called reinforcements. The same situation obtains today in computer modeling, which is altogether mediational. Computer logic draws from Boolean algebra, where disjunction is interpreted in the binary fashion of "either x or y, but *not both*" (Reese 1980, p. 64). The resultant information theory as the learning theories of old draws no distinction between the pattern of "good–bad" and the patterns of "good–day" or "bad–luck." It is all a matter of lining up separate units in a row—or side by side, across time's passage—and then having them connected together in some way. This results in what might be termed ·appositional disjunction, whereby an alternative meaning is brought into the process and positioned through external influence rather than decided upon intrinsically, as a choice between opposites.

There is a vast difference in the resultant disjunction achieved. Mediating processes never "experience" having to decide between—or, ignore—opposing alternatives no matter what the "past" environment (the reinforcement history, previous inputs, etc.) dictates. This past influence may be varied, but it is always a variety of competing unidirectionalities. A mediating process can employ one such past unidirectionality against another if the former has been input more freqeuntly, or rewarded more often. But as a mere conveyor of such extrinsic influence, the mediating process per se cannot counter its environment. It can only carry out what it has been given to process (usually termed a "shaping"). On the other hand, a predicating process does have intimations to the opposite of its previous experience. Since previous experience is intrinsically dual it necessarily implies the opposite of what it "has been." This countering of past experience in a predicational process can arise for many reasons—for example, out of pure boredom or a belief that the "old way" can be improved upon. Often these intrinsically disjunctive alternatives are stupid errors. On occasion they are "strokes of genius." People do "learn from experience," but sometimes it is opposite to the lesson being taught.

Freud relied upon oppositionality in his theorizing in a most basic manner. In fact, his very *first* theoretical effort—which reached print before the *Studies on Hysteria* (Breuer and Freud 1955/1893)—was founded on a view of mentation in which opposite or antithetical intentions led to symptom formations. A young mother, who did not wish to disturb her baby's sleep told herself to be quiet, only to enact precisely the opposite intention by loudly clacking her tongue (Freud 1966a/1892). Oppositional disjunction is clearly reflected in the fact that Freud pointed to "the strange state of mind in which one knows and does not know a thing at the same time" (Breuer and Freud 1955/1893, p. 117). Ideas with opposite meanings are entertained by the same mind quite nicely, and such "illogical" occurrences as eating one's cake and having it too continually arise in the unconscious—which also readily accepts ideas that consciousnes finds in contradiction of its moral standards (Freud 1953c/1901, p. 61, p. 85).

In his discussion of verbal parapraxes, Freud observes that the most striking kind of "slip" occurs when a person says precisely the opposite of what he or she intended to say, adding the observation that "contraries have a strong conceptual kinship" (Freud 1963a/1916, p. 34). In his discussion of love, he notes that "loving and hating taken together are the opposite of the condition of unconcern or indifference" (Freud 1957b/1915, p. 133). This is not an appositional arrangement, as Freud conveys a fundamental tie of meaning here. Similarly, in his discussion of analytical work, Freud presents us with a kind of "reverse slip" when he quotes a patient who has said of his dream content: "You [i.e., Freud] ask who this person in the dream can be. It's *not* my mother" only to grasp from this the opposite: "We emend this to: 'So it *is* his mother'" (Freud 1961/1925, p. 235, italics in original). The "damned if you do, damned if you don't" reputation of psychoanalysis takes root from such oppositional twists and turns. In one of his final papers, on the interminability of psychoanalytical treatment, Freud actually drew a parallel between his theory and the early Greek philosopher, Empedocles, whose principles of love and strife in continual conflict were said by Freud to be similar to his life and death instincts (Freud 1964/1937, pp. 245–247).

6. Correcting the Technical Problem: Behavior as Telosponsive Rather than Responsive

It would seem that Freud, almost in spite of himself and surely in contradiction to his medical education, refined a series of theoretical constructs that enabled him to capture the telic side of human behavior in an indirect, subtle fashion. Had he been provided with the technical assistance of suitable terminology, he might have accomplished this feat more directly. His medical education and the injunctions of colleagues like Fliess kept him from conveying the intentionality of psychopathology in a clearer manner. There are aspects of psychopathology that simply cannot be captured in traditional, bio–physical terms. For example, to grasp the etiology of mental disturbances we often must take values into consideration. And value judgments are most assuredly teleological formulations. A value represents the "that" (standard) "for the sake of which" people intend or aspire to direct their lives. Group mores or social norms are extensions of such values. This standard may be underwritten by religious beliefs, or reflect a strictly humanistic system of ethics. All extant legal systems rest on the assumption that human beings with a normally functioning mind can render "right or wrong" judgments on the basis of such standards (Rychlak and Rychlak, in press).

Do we advance the field of psychopathology if we continue to insist upon a non–telic rendering of the abnormal behavioral pattern?   The writer believes we do not. Without sacrificing our interest in the biological substrate of behavior it is possible to examine intentionality and value judgments if we construe the person introspectively, use formal–final cause predicational concepts, and be cognizant of the intrinsic oppositionality on which the predicational model rests. By theorizing in this fashion, we provide a firm base for the psychodynamic explanation of behavior. At present, there is no formal way, no technical conception available in psychological description which can subsume this style of explanation without serious distortion. Psychology has repeatedly limited behavioral description to extraspectively conceived "responsivity," framed in an efficient–cause sense and encompassing appositional disjunction through mediational processing. Today, as in Freud's day, even if a psychologist wanted to explain behavior teleologically, there would be no technical terminology on the basis of which this might be accomplished. As suggested above, the input–output concepts of the computer analogue do not solve this technical problem.

In an effort to rectify this situation, the writer has in recent years advocated that we think of human cognition and the behavior based upon it as *telosponsive* in nature (Rychlak 1987). Τελοσ comes from the Greek meaning "goal or end", and *spondere* comes from the Latin meaning "promise to do"; hence, a telosponse is promising or intending to do something for the sake of an end, goal, or reason. We violate convention in mixing Greek and Latin etymological roots in this fashion, but the result so nicely contrasts with the psychologist's traditional meaning of the "response" that we think it is necessary to do so. Telosponsivity as a technical term subsumes all of the points required for a genuine teleology to be captured: introspective perspective, formal–final causation, predication, and opposition.

It must not be thought that people reason according to "one" telosponse at a time. Each grasp of experience, each perception, attitude, or intuition is framed predicationally according to the telosponsive process. Such meaningful predications can overlap in the same person's cognition. And, of course, since the person always has some sense of the meaning in opposition to what is under affirmation, there is plenty of opportunity for internal doubt, conflict, and denial to take place. These states of psychic tension are not usually construed as reflections of the person's agency, but we would argue that they are and that psychopathology invariably becomes ensnarled in the telic aspects of human nature. In fact, the oppositional capacity that humans have to know yet not admit meaningful predications is the source of unconscious behavior. Freud seems to have recognized this completely, for in once discussing human agency in terms of the popular term "free will" he had this to say: "According to our analyses it is not necessary to dispute the right to the feeling of conviction of having a free will. If the distinction between conscious and unconscious motivation is taken into account, our feeling of conviction informs us that conscious motivation does not extend to all our motor decisions....But what is thus left free by the one side receives its motivation from the other side, from the unconscious; and in this way determination in the psychical sphere is still carried out without any gap" (Freud 1960/ 1901, p. 254).

Freud's treatment of psychic determinism here is clearly telic. Whether conscious or unconscious, the mind *intends* it ends, ends that have been *chosen* or *compromised* from among various contraries to begin with. One side of the mind, with a determination to achieve its ends (wishes, cathexes, etc.), is not given credence in the other, opposite realm. Freud occasionally referred to the illusion of free will, but he meant by this the fact that people naively believe that all their decisions are freely made in the realm of consciousness, when in point of fact we enact unconscious (unadmitted) intentions as well. The critic of such psychodynamic explanations is likely to believe that a natural process like the mind is incapable of intending ends that are at cross purposes, and/or that an intention which is not admitted (consciously) is no longer an intention. Freud's clinical experience, and the experience of any modern psychopathologist reveals that conflict and inadmission are routine cognitive states.

By adding the concept of telosponsivity to the technical terminology of the psychopathologist a more accurate representation of human beings in mental difficulty can be achieved. At the very least, we will avoid the confusion that now exists when two theorists use the same concept—behavior, response, etc.—and yet one is not conveying the same meaning as the other. The teleologist must choose his or her theoretical words with great care lest the intentionality of the person under description be swallowed up by the efficient causality of the terminology carelessly employed. There is need today as never before for clarity in our understanding and description of human nature. We can as professionals dispute and test empirically the soundness of a claim that human beings are teleological organisms. But first we must get clearly in mind what is involved in teleology. Hopefully, by using the concept of telosponsivity this clarification will be forthcoming.

Summary

This paper addresses the technical problems facing a teleological theorist in psychopathological explanation. Four problem areas are singled out for consideration, with documentation taken from the writings of Sigmund Freud as a theorist who actually confronted and adapted to these challenges. The technical questions addressed involve the extraspective or introspective slant from which a theory is to be written, the need to employ final causation in that theory, reliance on a predicational or a mediational explanatory model, and the generation of alternatives via appositional or oppositional disjunction. The paper closes with a call for the interpretation of human cognition and behavior as telosponsive rather than responsive. A telosponse is to be understood introspectively, draws its meaning from final causation, is predicational in nature, and relies ultimately on the human being's capacity to reason oppositionally.

References

Adler MJ: Aristotle for everybody: Difficult thought made easy. Bantam Books, New York, 1978.

Aristotle: Physics. In: Hutchins RM (ed.), Great books of the western world (Vol. 8), pp. 257–355, Encyclopedia Britannica, Chicago, 1952a.

Aristotle: On the soul. In: Hutchins RM (ed.), Great books of the western world (Vol. 8), pp. 631–668, Encyclopedia Britannica, Chicago, 1952b.

Aristotle: Metaphysics. In: Hutchins RM (ed.), Great books of the western world (Vol. 8), pp. 499–626, Encyclopedia Britannica, Chicago, 1952c.

Aristotle: On the generation of animals. In: Hutchins RM (ed.), Great books of the western world (Vol. 9), pp. 255–331, Encyclopedia Britannica, Chicago, 1952d.

Aristotle: On the parts of animals. In: Hutchins RM (ed.), Great books of the western world (Vol. 9), pp. 161–229, Encyclopedia Britannica, Chicago, 1952e.

Bacon F: Advancement of learning. In: Hutchins RM (ed.), Great books of the western world (Vol. 30), pp. 1–101, Encyclopedia Britannica, Chicago, 1952a.

Bacon F: Novum organum. In: Hutchins RM (ed.), Great books of the western world (Vol. 30), pp. 105–195, Encyclopedia Britannica, Chicago, 1952b.

Breuer J, Freud S: Studies on hysteria (1893). In: Strachey J (ed), The standard edition of the complete psychological works of Sigmund Freud (Vol. II), Hogarth, London, 1955.

Brewer WF: There is no convincing evidence for operant or classical conditioning in adult humans. In: Weimer WB, Palermo DS (eds), Cognition and the symbolic processes, pp. 1–42, Lawrence Erlbaum, Hillsdale NJ, 1974.

Freud S: Three essays on the theory of sexuality (1905). In: Strachey J (ed), The standard edition of the complete psychological works of Sigmund Freud (Vol. VII), pp. 125–243, Hogarth, London, 1953a.

Freud S: The interpretation of dreams (1901). In: Strachey J (ed), The standard edition of the complete psychological works of Sigmund Freud (Vol. V), Hogarth, London, 1953b.

Freud S: Fragment of an analysis of a case of hysteria (1901). In: Strachey J (ed), The standard edition of the complete psychological works of Sigmund Freud (Vol. VII), pp. 7–122, Hogarth, London, 1953c.

Freud S: The unconscious (1915). In: Strachey J (ed), The standard edition of the complete psychological works of Sigmund Freud (Vol. XIV), pp. 166–171, Hogarth, London, 1957a.

Freud S: Instincts and their vicissitudes (1915). In: Strachey J (ed), The standard edition of the complete psychological works of Sigmund Freud (Vol. XIV), pp. 117–140, Hogarth, London, 1957b.

Freud S: Contributions to a discussion on masturbation (1912). In: Strachey J (ed), The standard edition of the complete psychological works of Sigmund Freud (Vol. XII), pp. 241–254, Hogarth, London, 1958a.

Freud S: Formulations on the two principles of mental functioning (1911). In: Strachey J (ed), The standard edition of the complete psychological works of Sigmund Freud (Vol. XII), pp. 215–226, Hogarth, London, 1958b.

Freud S: Some general remarks on hysterical attacks (1908). In: Strachey J (ed), The standard edition of the complete psychological works of Sigmund Freud (Vol. IX), pp. 229–234, Hogarth, London, 1959.

Freud S: The psychopathology of everyday life (1901). In: Strachey J (ed), The standard edition of the complete psychological works of Sigmund Freud (Vol. VI), Hogarth, London, 1960.

Freud S: Negation (1925). In: Strachey J (ed), The standard edition of the complete psychological works of Sigmund Freud (Vol. XIX), pp. 235–239, Hogarth, London, 1961.

Freud S: Introductory lectures on psychoanalysis (Parts I and II) (1916). In: Strachey J (ed), The standard edition of the complete psychological works of Sigmund Freud (Vol. XV), Hogarth, London, 1963a.

Freud S: Introductory lectures on psychoanalysis (Part III) (1917). In: Strachey J (ed), The standard edition of the complete psychological works of Sigmund Freud (Vol. XVI), Hogarth, London, 1963b.

Freud S: Analysis terminable and interminable (1937). In: Strachey J (ed), The standard edition of the complete psychological works of Sigmund Freud (Vol. XXIII), pp. 211–253, Hogarth, London, 1964.

Freud S: Project for a scientific psychology (1895). In: Strachey J (ed), The standard edition of the complete psychological works of Sigmund Freud (Vol. I), pp. 295–343, Hogarth, London, 1966a.

Freud S: A case of successful treatment by hypnotism (1892). In: Strachey J (ed), The standard edition of the complete psychological works of Sigmund Freud (Vol. I), pp. 117–128, Hogarth, London, 1966b.

Freud S: The complete letters of Sigmund Freud to Wilhelm Fliess, 1886–1904, transl. and ed. Masson, JM, Harvard University Press, Cambridge MA, 1985.

Jones EE, Nisbett RE: The actor and the observer: Divergent perceptions of the causes of behavior. General Learning Press, Morristown NJ, 1971

Reese WL: Dictionary of philosophy and religion. Humanities Press, Atlantic Highlands NJ, 1980.

Robinson DN: Aristotle's psychology. Columbia University Press, New York, 1989.

Rychlak JF: A philosophy of science for personality theory (2nd ed.). Robert E.Krieger Publ. Co., Malabar FL, 1981.

Rychlak JF: The concept of telosponsivity: Answering an unmet need in psychology. In: Baker WJ, Hyland ME, Rappard Hv, Staats AW (eds), Current issues in theoretical psychology, pp. 247–260, Elsevier Science Publ. Co., Amsterdam, 1987.

Rychlak JF, Rychlak RJ: The insanity defense and the question of human agency. New ideas in psychology, in press.

Zukav G: The dancing wu li masters: An overview of the new physics. Bantam Books, New York, 1979.

Self–Consciousness, *I*–Structures, and Physiology

Hector–Neri Castañeda

1. Introduction

Here I continue *Persons, Egos, and I's: Their Sameness Relations* (Castañeda 1988a), presented at the 1988 Freiburg conference on *Psychopathology and Philosophy* (cf. Spitzer et al. 1988). That paper tackles basic ontological and semantic questions: What does one strictly refer to, that is, thinks, by means of the first–person pronoun? What sort of entity that thinking referent is? How does what a person calls "I" relate to that person? To gain a better understanding of these questions we subsumed the problem of first–person reference under the general case of indexical reference. We found that the *I*'s—like the *now*'s, the *here*'s, the *this*'s and *that*'s—are irreducible fleeting subjective individuals, existing only as contents of experiences. They constitute the framework of the experience they belong to. Their ontology is exhaustively epistemological. They exist merely to make present to the experiencing person objective referents with which they are the same in an appropriate representational sense. That this sameness is not literal self–identity is of the utmost importance: the ontology of the fleeting *I*'s can ground neither an empirical theory of a particular embodiment of consciousness nor a metaphysical doctrine about an immortal soul.

The initial focus of the present paper is the reflexivity of self–consciousness. This is a twofold reflexivity: an external, pedestrian one, and an internal, exciting reflexivity, which rests on the former. The internal reflexivity hinges on *I*'s. We develop complementary evidence for the evanescent and subjective nature of the *I*'s. This nature explains their essential ontologico–epistemological role as points of integration and unification of experiential contents. These are organized in the framework constituted by the *I*–strands. Experiences need not be owned by *I*'s, and when they are the *I*–integration presupposes the unity of the owned experience. Thus we reject the Fichtean thesis—still widely held even among philosophers friends of Artificial Intelligence—that all consciousness involves self–consciousness. (Thus we take issue with Kant's view on the role of apperception.) The Fichtean thesis demands a downwards unity of the contents of consciousness from the experienced–experiencing self to the non–self contents. This runs against the facts of experience, and prevents a unitary account of animal consciousness. Indeed even the postulation of an experienced–experiencing self arises from an unjustified conflation of the external with the internal reflexivity. Hence, whereas there is a momentous problem about the *I*'s, there is no problem of a self–referring self.

Even though no theory of a person's body can be derived from the intrinsic nature of the I's, the phenomenological facts of *I*-experiences reveal certain structures of bodily mechanisms that make those experiences feasible. Thus we may distill a "physiological" schema underlying self–consciousness, that is, the minimal form of a network of bodily mechanisms upon which not only consciousness, but self–consciousness emerges. Its guiding assumption is clear: Discriminations in the contents of what is thought or experienced signal differences in the bodily abilities underlying the making of such discriminations. This assumption must be accepted both by Cartesian dualists and by reductionist physicalists. The Cartesian sees those signals as contingently required by the intimate connection between an embodied mind and its body. The reductionist sees them as analytically necessary, given his reductionist program; he might concede that those necessary truths can, even must, be discovered empirically. We can set aside the modal issue in order to attain the shareable truths. However, here we do not pursue the formulation of the schema of the self–conscious body.

No *I* is a naked or isolated individual. On the contrary, every *I* is a focus of connections to different types of entities in the world, even out of the world, and to the world itself. Since *I*'s exist only as, an only while being, thought of, those connections are constitutive while thinkable. They are instantiations of the possible *I*-structures. These determine the nature of the *I*-contents. Patently, the *I*-structures signal general features of a body upon which self–consciousness accrues.

2. Self–Consciousness and Self–Reference

2.1. The Reflexivity of Self–Consciousness

Ultimately we want to understand the manifold of powers whose join activation ensues in episodes of *self*-consciousness. In such episodes ONE is conscious of ONEself qua *oneSELF*. They are doubly reflexive, and reflexive in two ways. There is the external reflexivity of ONE referring to ONEself, as when shaving ONE accidentally cuts ONEself, rather than another. Externally referring to oneself is, like cutting oneself, a matter of *doing* something, rather than of thinking certain content. Like the refexivity involved in cutting oneself, the external reflexivity of reference to oneself can be unintentionally and unwittingly executed. Thus, a forgetful painter may think that the painter of a certain picture is a very good painter without realizing that he himself painted that picture. There is, on the other hand, the internal reflexivity of ONE referring to something, whatever it may be, as *oneSELF*. The internal reflexivity is the peculiar core of *self*–consciousness. It is the reflexivity of a content of thought, namely: what one expresses by thinkingly using sentences containing used tokens of the first–person pronoun '*I*'.

Both forms of reflexivity are necessary for self–consciousness. Indeed, self–consciousness rests so firmly on its external reflexivity that the expression 'x refers to x as himself' sounds out of order if 'refers' is meant in its strict sense. Merely to refer to something is simply to pick it up in thought as a subject of properties and as an object of a propositional attitude, e.g., believing, doubting, supposing. The use of 'x refers to y as herself' suggests that it would be a special instantiation of 'x refers to y as z' for the case in which x *happens* to be the same as y, and 'as herself' instantiates z. The fact is that one cannot just refer to another person as oneself. One can, to be sure, refer to another person and think that she is (the same as) oneself. But then one is referring to oneself as oneSELF. In short, letting '==>' express logical or analytic implication connecting the concepts in question, we have the following principles, or meaning postulates:

(SC.ER) x (merely) refers to *y* as herself ==> x is the same as y.
(SC.Ex) x refers to x as himself ==> x exists

Clearly, the two occurrences of the suffix '–self' have a very different meaning in the matrices 'one refers to ONEself as *one*SELF' and '*x* refers to HIMself as *him*SELF. Yet it is very easy to think that it has exactly the same meaning and role in both occurrences. Undoubtedly, in some sense that cries out for elucidation the two occurrences of '–self' express a sameness of referent. If one then—as is customary—mobilizes a monolithic concept of identity or sameness, one sees the very same self–identical entity as outside as and inside the referring act. Of course, that entity is called *self*. Then one has the difficult problem of explaining how a self can be at the same time both the subject of and the object of one and the same experience. This is a *fictitious* problem. There is no such a self. Here one must tread with care. That problem of the self does not exist. This, however, in no way justifies a Humean conclusion that there is no self in experience. In fact, Hume was also the victim of his conflating the external ONEself with the internal *one*SELF. There is no external self; but there is an internal SELF. The latter is an important philosophical problem. Since the internal SELF is what one refers to by using the first–person pronoun 'I', we should perhaps say more perspicuously that whereas there is *no* problem of the self, there is a serious problem about the *I*'s.

We can, then, concentrate on the internal reflexivity without loss.

Self–consciousness is executed in episodes of thinking about oneself qua oneself. The contents thought in such episodes are expressed in natural language in utterances of sentences containing (at least apparently) singular–referring uses of the first–person pronoun. The internal reflexivity of self–consciousness is the appearing of the thinker to HIMself as him-

SELF, that is, as an *I*. Self–consciousness is *I*–consciousness. Not because we identify *I*–consciousness with the use of the pronoun 'I'; but because the uses of 'I'–sentences reveal the speaker's thinking *I*–contents, and, consequently, his having a brain *I*–representation. A thinking episode is not an event of uttering. It is embodied in—indeed, in some *appropriate* sense of 'sameness', a thinking episode is the same as—an event or process in the thinker's brain, or thinking box, whatever this may be.

Here we do not endorse the reductionist physicalistic thesis that mental events are just second–order causal properties of physical events. We must, however, insist on an insight that underlies physicalism: mental events and mental dispositions are in the world and are part of the causal order. We must accept causal equations of the mental and the physical, and raise the fundamental issue of the nature of the sameness involved in such equations. Here, however, we do not enter into this issue.[1] One thing is clear to me: the sameness in question cannot be conceptual or analytic equivalence, much less literal (self)identity: hence, such equations cannot provide a reduction of the mental, more specifically, of consciousness, to the physical. Yet they may secure the causal dependence entrenched in the hierarchical emergence of mental states and particulars on and off physical states. In fact, consciousness seems to be an irreducible emergent. This is, however, not the occasion to tackle this topic.[2] In any case, reductionist

---

1 For a theory of the sameness family of relations see Castañeda (1974, 1975), both in *Sprache und Erfahrung* (Castañeda, 1982), the former in *Thinking, Language, and Experience* (Castañeda, 1989), and in *Das Denken und die Struktur der Welt* (Jacobi and Pape 1989). On my view the identity between mental and physical states is the sameness called in those papers consubstantiation. On the other hand, the basic sameness between veridical thought content and what makes it veridical hinges on sameness call consociation. Consubstantiation is also the sameness between the morning star and the evening star. Thus I seem to be endorsing a version of the Contingent–Identity Theory. See, for example, Place (1956), Smart (1959), and Lewis (1966). My version of the contingent identity of mental events and processes to physical ones is not reductionist. See Note 2 below. Furthermore, the theory is mounted on a general theory of contingent identity or sameness.

2 Many different types of mental fact constitute serious hurdles and tasks for reductionist programs. Here I mention just one fact seldom noticed. To me it has for the last thirty years seemed to be, not a mere hurdle, but a stumbling block for the reduction of episodes of consciousness to physical events. That fact is normal veridical, partially illusory visual experience. Not to generalize unduly, let me put the fact concretely. I am looking at the sky and see a triangle having as vertices the moon, the North Star, and the chimney on my house. This is a veridical perception of the objects in question. The triangle is not a physical, but an illusory, one. Because of the time needed for light to travel, the position of the moon I see is one it occupied minutes before, whereas the position of the North Star is years older. My visual experience is precisely the visual presentation of what I see, that is, the mere existence of my visual field. My visual experience consists of the visual field containing the triangle just described. It does not occur in my brain (or whatever my thinking box may be). Of course, events in my brain have caused the existence of the presented visual field. My experience, however, occurs before my eyes, spread about in the piece of physical space containing the objects I see. My visual experience is not reductionally equivalent, let alone identical, to events in my brain (or thinking gadget). Because my veridical visual experience is partly illusory, the contents of my visual consciousness are not identical with a sub–domain of physical entities I see. (I say "entities" to include not so much physical objects in their fullness, but only their seen parts or surfaces.) My veridical visual displays occupy visual spaces which at least overlap with physical space. But even if such overlappings exhausted my visual spaces, there would be in visual space non–physical content. The physics and physiology of vision may causally explain why my visual spaces have certain non-physical, illusory contents. Nonetheless, causal explanation is not reduction. To cause is to bring into existence. (This is a basic truth often forgotten in defenses of reductionist causal claims.) Clearly, episodes of thinking, as well as dispositional states of believing, are individuated by their contents. In brief, my episodes of veridical visual consciousness are not reducible to complexes of physical

functionalists are, or should be, firmly concerned with the reflexivity of
self–consciousness. The better we understand what it appears to be, the
more detailed and secure our reductionist programs can be. Likewise, Artificial Intelligence, whether practiced with a reductionist bent of mind or
not, has a vested interest in the reflexivity of self–consciousness. Clearly,
the production of facsimiles of human behavior or of mental states and
activities needs only the causal dependence of the mental on the physical.
Self–consciousness is the apex of mentality.

We are concerned with thinking reference, the reference a thinker
makes to what he thinks, whether he is reflecting by himself or engaged in
a dialogue. What does it consist of?

Let us examine the *as*–moment in the general formula:

(GR)   *X refers to Y as Z.*

This is a requisite background for our study of the moment *as*
oneSELF in self–consciousness.

An act of referring is a real event in the world. It is, therefore, a part of
the causal order. It involves a relation which can have the selfsame entity in
the positions of agent and accusative. Hence, there is a causal relation that
includes an external dovetailing of reference on to its source. This dovetailing is, as we noted above, not only required for self–consciousness, but
implied by the internal reflexivity of the moment *as oneSELF.*

An act of referring is a mental event. As such it has an internal
content. This is what the sub–form 'as Z' of (GR) alludes to. Content Z is
what the thinker thinks of, refers to thinkingly. What does this amount to?

The physical–physiological process of thinking something about Z, say,
that (... Z ...), is undoubtedly thoroughly computational. It may include a
multitude of computations of brain states, terminating in a complex B of
brain events that contains a *representation* of that (... Z ...). That is, either
there is an isomorphism between some systematic parsing of that (... Z ...)
and a parsing of B, or there is a mechanism for constructing such an isomorphism, or there is a general causal function that assigns (... Z ...) to B.
However, for X to think that (... Z ...) the occurrence of that representational event is not enough. That representational event must deliver a *presentation to the thinker* of what he is thinking of. This is of the greatest
importance. The representations of what the thinker refers (or purports to
refer) to as Z when he thinks thought content (... Z ...) may be stored in
different ways in his brain. This storage is not thinking. Those representations may move from storage to occurrence, yet this transition may not suffice. This is so even if the representation were a perfect replica or image of
the object thought of, and the thinking occurrence of the image consisted

---

events, including those within and those without my body. Patently, no theory of the world or of the
mind, or of consciousness, can be satisfactory if it leaves my visual experience out of account. There
is, however, a reductionism I have adopted: the economical view that reduces visual consciousness to
the occurrence of visual content. For more data for and details of these theses see Castañeda (1977).
This paper is an abridgment of Part IV of *Sprache und Erfahrung.*

in its being a faithful replication of the stored image in the thinking box, screen, or whatever, in the brain. Certainly, to embody an act of referring (or purporting to refer), the occurring representation of the referent must occur in the proper location required by the engineering of the brain. It must, further, occur in the proper presentational way: It must yield the molar state of the possessor of that brain being *presented* with Z through being *presented* with (... Z ...). The word 'presentation' is of course in the family of words meaning consciousness as its basic sense. The threat of circularity indicates that, although, of course, certain amounts of unconscious events, states, or objects do *cause* consciousness, no amount of unconscious states or objects can constitute an episode of consciousness,

The purely mental and crucial sense of '[refers to, thinks of] as (*qua*) Z' is governed by this fundamental principle of the embodiment of thinking:

(Th.PR) In the general sense of '(thinkingly) refers to' (and 'thinks of') what the referrer is presented with is the *selfsame* item as what he strictly refers to (thinks of).

2.3. The Chinese–Box Structure of Attributions of Reference

Let us continue our exegesis of the formula (GR): "X refers to Y as Z." In terminology I don't like, the locution 'as Z' expresses a *de dicto* attribution of content to a mental act. Here, as always, though often not attended to, *de dicto* attribution is attribution by *depiction* of the internal, presentational content of such an act. Suppose I declare: "John believes that Leibniz was a lawyer." Evidently, my subordinate clause discloses to the hearer, not John's words—let alone John's brain representations—, but my alleged replica or picture of John's belief content. The picture purports to reveal, first, an isomorphism between certain doxastic representation of his, concerning Leibniz, with a corresponding representation of mine; the picture purports also to reveal the psychological equivalence between the components of our isomorphic representations. Hence, expressions that occur internally, *de dicto,* in attributions of mental state have, on Peirce's term, an *iconic* function.

The formula (GR) *X refers to Y as Z* is of a mixed nature. The component *to Y* is, as we said, external. It is, in one sense of a companion terminology I also dislike, *de re*. The point often made with this expression is that what a substituend of 'Y' denotes exists. This is of course often true. However, it is just a special case of what people think. The underlying function of so-called *de re* expressions, like 'Y' in the formula (GR), is to express, not existence, but *speaker's (intended) reference*. It is the person proffering (GR) who expresses his thinking of what *he* calls Y. The whole formula expresses that the speaker, *not* the person X, identifies what he calls Y with what X calls Z—regardless of whether Y exists or not. Obviously, to express this identification of his the speaker himself also represents Z as Z. Clearly, then, expressions in *de dicto* positions are points of referential *cumulation*.

Accessing another's thought contents requires connecting those contents with the shared world. For this we must think ourselves those contents, whether we believe they are veridical or not. (This is referential cumulativeness.) Thus, the general sense of (GR) can be diagrammed as follows:

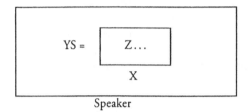

Speaker

where 'S=' denotes the speaker's identification of X's Z with his Y, and each box represents a fragment of the world as conceived by the person mentioned immediately under it.

Statements of the form (GR) are little windows which the speaker opens to her hearers to let them peep into her (conceived) world; these windows reveal internal open windows on the said referrer X's world. To speak (candidly) is thus to perform an act of revelation, of one's–world–window opening.

Internal, *de dicto* expressions are depictions of representations the speaker exhibits as SHARED by him and the person he speaks of. *De re* expressions just vent the speaker's references. *De dicto* indirect speech has a Chinese–box structure, each box revealing the presented representations constituting thinking content—regardless of the existence of what is thought of.

A statement of form 'X refers to Y as Z' discloses to the hearer that the speaker is presented with thinker X as thinker X, with item Y as Y, with item Z as Z. Further, it reveals that the speaker takes Z to be an inter-subjective thinkable. This is simply the cumulative character of the *de dicto* occurrence of Z in 'X refers to Y as Z'. By equating Z with Y the speaker reveals, besides, that Z has an objective status in her world. This status need not be existence. Even if X in fact refers to the speaker's Y as Z, Y may be only an intersubjective thought of item. In short, the externality of the moment *to Y as Z* in (GR) consists of its expressing the speaker's positing the *objective intersubjectivity* of Z as Y. She locates X's referred to item Z in her world, or in the thinkable surroundings of her world. To be sure, the speaker may be in error in equating her Y with Z as thought of by X. It does not matter. The point is that she claims to have penetrated X's mind and have found Z there: Z is shared. Thus, the internality of the moment as Z of (GR) is the subjectivity of Z within X's experience, yet it manifests an accessible *intersubjective subjectivity* of Z. Again, this is the referentially cumulative function of *de dicto* expressions in the Chinese–Box structure.

2.4 The External (de re) Target of Reference and Existence

To understand fully the nature of the acts of referring we must understand (GR) in as general way as thinking reaches. Doubtless, an episode of thinking is typically and primarily oriented toward the physical environment. Typically we think of real objects as having certain properties, and we succeed: the objects we think of exist and have the properties we predicate of them. Occasionally we make mistakes. Sometimes the objects we think do not have the properties we think them to have; sometimes the very objects we assume to exist do not exist. A comprehensive account of experience, thinking, and how language functions, requires acknowledgment that we must sometimes refer (if you wish, purport to refer) to non–existents—as when we conceive failed plans to make certain things, or erroneously postulate certain entities to explain some events. An episode of thinking as a psychological reality is exactly the same whether what one thinks exists or not: the same brain events, the same representational structure. (Just imagine your thinking of a distant existent, which vanishes while you are thinking of it, for instance the star in the example of footnote 1; yet its vanishing does not lame your thinking.) In sum, we must not equate externality of reference with existence.[3]

Thinking is impervious to existence. The sense of 'refers to' and 'thinks of' we need in (GR) lacks an existential commitment to what is thought of. We keep, on the other hand, an existential commitment to X, the referrer. Thus, we subsume the problem of the reflexivity of self–consciousness under a more general problem of thought content.

On the assumption that the speaker makes true statements, what his world windows show is part of the real world. Of course he may be in error; or he may be trying to deceive. The entity Y he locates in his world as being the same as Z as conceived by X may not be real. Clearly, what the speaker calls "Y," his Y, is—like Z in X's alleged act of referring—just a presentation typically (in the default case) pointing to the world. Thus, the item Y is no different in ontological status from the item Z. Both are aspects, faces, *guises* of thought of objects. In the typical episodes of thinking they are posited as real, that is, as existing aspects, faces, guises that compose unitary objects in the real world. If they are real then they have infinitely many properties not thought of in the thinking that the statement reports.

On the assumption that the speaker is telling the truth, we the hearers take it for granted that the aspect, face, *guise* Y put forward by the speaker for consideration is real. That is, we take it for granted that Y has a place in the causal order, and doxastically posit a whole infinite system of existing

---

3 The idea that what one thinks exists and what does not exist cannot have any properties at all is at least traceable to Parmenides's poem. Against him, Plato argued in the Sophist that non–existents are thinkable and can have some properties. Since then this issue has divided philosophers into antagonic camps. For instance, William of Sherwood seemed to have adopted a Parmenidean position, very much like Bertrand Russell's. (See Jacobi 1980, pp. 318ff.) In this century Alexius Meinong and Bertrand Russell argued about the Parmenidean issue. Their focus was Meinong's existing round square. (For references and appraisal of this debate see Castañeda 1985/86. This article contains references to recent discussions of non–existing objects and of fiction.

faces or guises each *existing as being the same as* Y. Under this positing we can equate the speaker's Y with some item H in *our* world and say: "The speaker says of H, to which he refers as Y, that X referred to it [Y] as Z." Thus we become speakers, and assign to Y an intersubjective subjectivity: we and the (previous) speaker think of Y as such. This is the basis for our assigning to Y an objective intersubjectivity through our equating it with H. In its turn, Z gains a deeper intersubjective subjectivity: Z is then a shared item located in the innermost box of a three–membered Chinese Box we have created.

Our H may not be real. We take it to be real, and our (conceived) world is the one we have beliefs about and act on. Metaphysically the basic fact is that we have NO access to an external point of view. All reference is from *our, one's* point of view. (As is well known, here lies the kernel of Kant's Copernican Revolution.)

The speaker's posited sameness between Y and Z need not be recognizable by the person X. It is not the strict self–identity of Y=Y, Z=Z, X=X. As always, the elucidation of sameness is a serious matter.[4] Consequently, we must not prejudge the nature of the sameness involved in referring acts. We remain open to there being several different types of sameness required for the elucidation of storable mental representations, and for their occurrences yielding thinking presentations to a thinker.

2.5 The Internal [*de dicto*] Reflexivity of Self–Consciousness

Now we come to the third prong, 'as (*qua*) *oneSELF*', of our initial formula of *self*–consciousness:

(I*) In an episode of *self*–consciousness
ONE refers to (thinks of) ONEself qua *oneSELF*.

We turn to the meaning of the suffix '–self' in the italicized pronoun '*oneSELF*'. In (I*) this is a relative pronoun having 'ONE', *not* 'ONEself' as its antecedent, whose character it takes. In our schematic formula (I*) the antecedent 'ONE' is a variable; hence, '*oneSELF*' has a variable aspect: its substituends have as antecedents the corresponding substituends of 'ONE'. These substituends of '*oneSELF*' are reflexive pronouns that depict first–person reference: '(he) himself', '(she) herself', 'themselves', 'yourself', 'myself'. Thus, '*oneSELF*' and its substituends are *quasi–indicators*.[5] For example:

(3) The author of "Self–reference and Self–awareness" is thinking [of HIMself] that *he himSELF* wrote *Self–Knowledge and Self–Identity*.

---

4 See the materials mentioned in Note 1.
5 For an extensive study of indexical and quasi–indexical reference see Chapters 1, 4, and 12 of *Thinking, Language, and Experience*, or Chapters II.2, II.5, and II.6 of *Sprache und Erfahrung*.

Here the pronoun '*he himSELF*' refers back to its antecedent 'The author of "Self–reference and Self–awareness"' and depicts this author as referring to HIMself as "I."

Doubtless, the external target of self–reference is ONEself. One always succeed in harpooning ONEself if one thinks of ONEself as *oneSELF*. But what is the presentational representation with which one harpoons ONE-self? Evidently, it is what a use of the first–person pronoun reveals that the speaker is presented with: an *I*. This is a unique, ephemeral, and irreducible representation. The uniqueness and privacy of *I*–reference is established by the fact that nobody can refer to another person in the first–person way. The peculiarity and subjectivity of each *I* is established by the fact that for any third–person individual *i* which is the same as a person X, X may fail to know that he himSELF is (the same as) *i*. The first–person pronoun has a general meaning that determines a framework within which, on each occasion of its use, a speaker confronts a unique and personal representation of the reality he or she is.

In sum, the indexical uses of the first–person pronoun have these central features: (i) they express an ineradicable privacy of the presentational *I*–representations; (ii) because each of these representations is a presentational occurrent it is fleeting, lasting only as long as the presentation (the experience) lasts; (iii) the *I*–presentations, primarily, and the uses of 'I', derivatively, infallibly harpoon an existent beyond the representation, and (iv) they intrude as also infallible the very existence of the presenting representation, that is, the thought of *I* itself. (The other types of indexical singular terms have properties similar to (i)–(iii). The only exception is demonstrative reference to experienced items, which lacks property (iii). Statements of the form "This is F" secure an internal referent, the subject *this*, but do not always harpoon an external target.)

But what exactly is that *I* content one is presented to in episodes of self–consciousness? That it is so peculiar and unique is further brought home by the fact that there is no third–person special characteristic that one has to think that one possesses in order to think of oneself as *I*. Certainly, one *qua* I does not classify oneself as a self, a person, or a thinker—let alone as a human being, female, or whatever is true of all entities capable of *self*-consciousness. To illustrate, a small child at about the age of two can make perfect first–person references fully lacking knowledge involving those categories. In general:

(I*R.9) Where *being F* is not simply *being myself*, or *being thinking*, or *existing*, or their joint logical implicates, all propositions of the form *I am F* are synthetic *a posteriori* in Kant's sense, i.e., non–redundant (non–tautological).

There is just no criterion one can apply to determine whether one is an *I* or not. One simply is an I. This primitive fact is primitively and immediately apprehended by a thinker who is an *I*.

We must fasten to the fact that each *I* is a primitive and ephemeral internal representation of the thinker as the subject of internally occurrent, presentationally convergent experiences. Because of (I*R.9) this representation contains no description or attribution of a property. It is merely the brute unanalyzable presentation of the internal unity of those experiences with their successful harpooning of something in the real world otherwise unknown—whatever it may be. Hence:

> (I**) An *I* is an ephemeral hypostasis that presents a thinker to HIMself as the theater of ongoing mental activity. At bottom an *I* ensues from, and is thus the opaque presentation of, an operational unification of a set of structures that unify the particular contents of a manifold of ongoing experiences. To think an *I* content (... I ...) is to EXECUTE (unconsciously, of course) a unification of presented representations (...) and to be presented with that execution.

The rest of this essay is a preliminary investigation into the unifications underlying an *I*. First we consider the presenting representations constitutive of self–consciousness; then we take a glimpse into the schema of "physiological" processes that make viable those unifications.

3. The Hierarchy of Internal Reflexivity in *Self*–Consciousness

3.1 The Network of Structural Negativities Composing I–Schemata

Once again, an *I* is a hypostatic individual one thinks by means of an indexical internal representation expressible through a token of the first–person pronoun. That individual is a device for successfully thinking of oneself. As such, we have seen, it has no objective properties. Since it reflexively represents the thinker, it is constituted by categorial contrasts that reveal fundamental structural properties of the thinker. Those are the I–structures that mold the contents of *self*-consciousness. They can be gleaned by charting the types of properties and relations characteristic of *I*'s. Each such type is a domain of possibilities open in principle to all *I*'s. Here we will not carry out this cartographical investigation. Our present concern is confined to the internal *I*–structures, bundles of which constitute *I*–schemata. These structures have certain independences; hence, they need not be present all at once. There is, thus, a hierarchy of *I*–schemata. Consequently, the *I*'s can be partially ordered in accordance with the ordering of the *I*–schemata constituting them.

The *I*-schemata provide blueprints for egological development. Under a conception of normality, the *I*-schemata furnish also a master chart against which to check a person for possible *I*-disturbances.

The internal *I*-structures are *I*-strands hinging on contrasts between what one is *qua* oneself and something one is not. Alternatively phrased, an *I*-strand is the polar negation of something intrinsically non–*I*. Because of the polarity, the negation is dichotomous.[6] Thus, an *I*-schema is a complex of *negativities*. To gain a concept of I is to acquire the capacity to pick out immediately *instances* of one or more of those polar negations. This instantiation is of course confronted by thinking of ONEself *qua oneSELF*. Here is a fundamental ingredient in the peculiar reflexivity of *self*-consciousness.

To think of ONEself as *oneSELF* is to think of something *intimated* to be, *felt as it were*, the opposite of each of such and such N's—for the appropriate values of 'N'. I have chosen the words 'intimated' and 'felt' advisedly. We have already seen how to think contents of the form (...I...) is to have a primitive apprehension of the subject one calls "I," not mediated by any identification procedure. That basic truth remains unaltered. Hence, to apprehend oneSELF in the content (...I...) is to apprehend a manifold of polar negations of the different non–I's as one fully unified manifold of *I*-strands. Furthermore, it is to apprehend that manifoldness in a non–conceptual way, as a sensory content. Conceptually one apprehends only the unity. The apprehension of the manifoldness underlying the unitary *I* consists partly of feeling that sensory–like content. Intellectually, such an act of apprehension sets in readiness a hierarchical manifold of propensities to think, especially think believingly, appropriate ranges of propositions. These ranges are demarcated by the felt negativities. The elements of those ranges are determined by the personality of the thinker, the context of the thinking episode, including her surface purposes, and her preceding trains of thought.

Self-consciousness is, thus, erected on a reflexive sensory consciousness. This reflexivity is not reflective (in the sense of reflecting on something); it is of the ONEself type of reflexivity discussed in Part II above. We will see that *self*-consciousness is mounted on other forms of non–reflective consciousness. Also *self*-consciousness occurs on a *doxastic pedestal* composed of propensities to think or to rehearse belief. We elucidate the doxastic pedestal below. The empirical contents of episodes of self–consciousness fall, then, within one or more of the negativities composing the *I*-strands. The most pervasive of these are:

Chief *I*-strands
1. The contrast *I*-this/that
2. The contrast *I*-they [the external objects of the world]
3. The contrast *I*-he/she [this/that (thinker)]
4. The contrast *I*-they [the others]

---

6 For a study of the family of the different types of negation and its contrasts with the family of colors properties, see Castañeda (1988).

5. The contrast *I* [believer/knower]–I [agent]
6. The contrast *I*–he/she [this/that (person: sentient–thinking–and–acting individual)]
7. The contrast *I*–you
8. The contrast *I*–we [partners at a conversation]
9. The contrast *I*–they/we [the members of one's community]

REMARK 1. Here I have been inspired by Ferdinand de Saussure in conceiving a meaning of an expression as a contrast between a usage of the expression and the usages of other related expressions within a family.[7] Each contrast of usage is a semantic strand. To me Saussure's general thesis seems to be correct, but it is particularly suitable for the semantics of the first–person pronoun. Of course here the usages and meanings of words interest us only as avenues for approaching thought contents. The above nine contrasts are contrasts in thought content, in what we find in experience, and what we believe to be in the world.

REMARK 2. I have adopted the hyphen in between the contrasted expressions from Buber. He contrasted "the two meanings" of 'I': *I–It* and *I–Thou*.[8]

REMARK 3. The different *I*–strands listed above divide the full–fledged concept of *I* along different axes. The endpoints of these axes are: (i) what is being experienced vs. what perhaps although not experienced belongs nevertheless to the world at large; (ii) what is internal to the mind vs. what is external; (iii) being vs. not being a person or a mentally endowed individual; (iv) cognizing the world vs. acting on it, which rests on the axis believing vs. intending; (v) being a thinking–acting individual vs. being a member of a community. Undoubtedly other axes must be added for a full account of the *I*–schemata and their strands.

REMARK 4. The nine *I*–strands enumerated above intermingle in many different ways. This yields a spiralic process of steady enrichment of one's concept of *I*. The mingling principles are of different sorts. Some are required by the kind of world we find ourselves in, with its physical, chemical, and biological natures, but also with its social organizations and other cultural products. Some principles of mingling lie deeply seated in the thinker's ontologico–psychological make–up, which manifests itself in the thinker–agent's metaphysical postures. For example, animists mingle the *I*–strands in such a way that everything has its own internal *I*. Solipsists find the total world at large to be merely experiential content of the only accessible *I*. Deists promote the whole of reality to the veridical content of an all–embracing *I*. Pantheists are animist deists. Mystics do all sorts of things; some raise themselves up to the status of partial *I*'s within an all–encompassing one.

---

7 Ferdinand de Saussure *Cours de linguistique generale* e.g. his view of plural as the whole network of contrasts, for instance, 'girl'/'girls', 'potato'/'potatoes', 'ox'/'oxen', etc.
8 Martin Buber, *I and Thou*, 1970.

REMARK 5. The order in which the *I*-strands are listed is logical from the perspective of the experience of thinking. It is not meant to prejudge the philosophical disputes about the possibility, or viability, of solipsistic consciousness. It is not intended to cast any aspersion on, or endorse with its converse, the semantic socialism now fashionable.[9] It is not meant to decide in advance the outcome of controversies (philosophical, pedagogical, or otherwise) about the learning of language or the acquisition of concepts.

REMARK 6. The network of negativities is a network of structures. They have to be filled in with special contents. These are empirical and metaphysical beliefs, or even deep-seated takens-for-granted, at the foundation of the thinker's doxastic pedestal.

3.2 The Hierarchy of Modalities of Consciousness Within Self-Consciousness

The existence of consciousness, hence, also the existence of *self-consciousness*, rests on a complex doxastic pedestal. This is a hierarchy of powers, dispositions, and propensities to think believingly that such-and-such, or disbelievingly of what contradicts what one believes, or skeptically of some other things. That pedestal in its turn pivots causally on, so to speak, an iceberg of unconscious processes. The contents of consciousness are not, however, a uniform monolith somehow above the line separating what is in the light of consciousness and what is submerged in the dark water of the unconscious. Those contents have, rather a hierarchical structure. This is not just a hierarchical logical or epistemic order of those contents; it is also a hierarchy of modalities of mental attitude and of consciousness. The uppermost tiers are propensities to think, which may be also activated, appearing through propositions also present to consciousness; some propensities will manifest themselves in the penumbra of consciousness; others lurk behind perhaps as merely felt in sensory consciousness. Most of the tiers of the pedestal are utterly unconscious. The bottommost ones are metaphysical; yet they are not so much beliefs that can on occasion be brought to consciousness. They are, rather, deep-seated takens-for-granted, built in the hardware of the inferential or computational mechanisms that underlie the embodying of thinking episodes. These cannot (physically, or psychologically) be brought to consciousness. Some of them may be actually unformulable.

Consciousness is suffusive and subsumptive. It is suffusive in that, not only do thought of contents enter consciousness in networks, but the appearing of certain contents mobilize the doxastic hierarchy. This mobilization is, as noted, hierarchical: some propensities to think certain contents are triggered and placed in different degrees of thinking readi-

---

9 See, for example, Ludwig Wittgenstein, *Philosophical Investigations* (1952); Hilary Putnam (1975, 1987), and Burge (1979). For a dissenting argument see Castañeda (1989).

ness. On the other hand, consciousness is subsumptive in that lower forms of consciousness are present in the higher forms, although in an altered nature. In brief:

(Cons*) The unitary structure of consciousness proceeds upwards, but its illumination flows downwards.

In this sense consciousness contains an internal hierarchy of reflexivity. Most important consequences are suggested by (Cons*) about the hierarchical integration of the underlying physiological processes.

Self-consciousness is the highest form of consciousness. It exhibits, therefore, the highest forms of suffusiveness and subsumptiveness. As indicated above, it subsumes all other modalities of consciousness. This is another dimension of the characteristic and peculiar internal reflexivity of self-consciousness.

Now, the subsumptive internal hierarchy of consciousness within self-consciousness includes the following levels:

1. sensory content, conceptually inarticulated
(a) bodily   (b) worldly
2. I–less articulated content pertaining to:
(a) external objects
(b) bodily content
(c) occurring mental acts
3. I–less focal consciousness, the core of which is a complex of perceptual judgments
4. I–owned content articulating the contrast between Self and Object
5. I–owned content articulating intentional agency
6. I–owned content articulating the contrast between Self and others
7. I–owned content articulating an interaction between Self and *you* as well as absent persons.

The maximal degree of self-consciousness has an *I* as its focus and anchor. This fills in the *I*–schema in which all the relevant negativities intersect and have their proper empirical and metaphysical content.

The integration of a manifold of contents as the contents of a unitary self-consciousness proceeds from the lower levels up. That is, we cannot explain the unity of an episode of consciousness in terms of an *I* to whom that episode belongs. This can be established empirically: there are episodes of *I*–less consciousness. It is not just that there is a quiet *I* in the background, which can at any moment come into the open. At this point the positing of an enduring I as the underwriter of the experiences of one and the same person at different times becomes handy. This positing must, however, be grounded on some evidence or reasons. No matter. The consciousness of some lower animals obtains without being owned by any I that can come to the light of self-consciousness.

All consciousness is subsumptive and suffusive. Accordingly, I submit that in gaining full consciousness after a deep sleep we go through all the levels of consciousness as different stages of the process of waking up. As I see things, since each *I* exists only during and within an episode of *self-*consciousness, waking up is really a case of ontogeny recapitulating phylogeny. Anti–recapitulation occurs in cases of falling asleep slowly.

Level 1 is a theoretical posit. We assume that there is a manifold within sensory consciousness, which includes no awareness of objects or events. The primary consciousness is perceptual. We may assume that the sensory manifold is, underneath consciousness, partitioned into masses belonging to the different types of perception.

At *level 2* there is conceptualization of some sort. The minimal sort is what I have called *zero–consciousness*.[10] This is the confrontation of a perceptual field that contains as distinct points some perceptual states of affairs (or propositions) as unanalyzed units, with no logical structure, not even a subject–predicate one. I theorize that this is the kind of consciousness exemplified by animals that respond to differences in color, shape, distance, without any consciousness of objects as such. However, I know so little about animals that I cannot offer a well studied example.

In higher degrees of *level 2* some of the presented states of affairs (propositions) receive some structural analysis. The subject–predicate structure enters the scene. This consciousness is *I*–less and not focal.

A very interesting case of *level–2* consciousness is so–called BLIND–SIGHT. Some persons who have lost part of their cerebral cortex connected to vision illustrate what to many specialists seems to be a paradoxical situation. While declaring that they do not see, such persons are nonetheless able to respond correctly to questions that seem to require clear visual perception. A certain patient named D. B. in the literature is particularly interesting. He had part of his brain removed but had lost only his left visual field. In the experiments items were placed in his visual field. He insisted that he* (himself) did not see anything in his left field. He engaged in "guessing," as he called it. He had a perfect score in thirty "guesses." D. B. sometimes reported having a "feeling" that certain figures he said he* did not see had certain properties, which they in fact had.[11] Similar studies have been carried out with monkeys. Apparently monkeys and men with blind–sight can improve the strength of those "feelings" and also their powers of discrimination of "unseen" objects.

Some philosophers prefer to interpret the cases of blind–sight as cases of no perception at all. To them they are evidence that consciousness is a well–entrenched fiction, which science will eventually vanish.[12] Others see blind–sight as cases of vision, that is, visual consciousness without *self-*consciousness.[13] This is the view I have adopted.

---

10 In *Perception, Belief, and the Structure of Physical Objects and Consciousness.*
11 Weiskrantz et al. (1974), Weiskrantz (1977, 1980).
12 Churchland (1980).
13 Pollock (1988).

As I see it, in blind–sight the integration of the visual contents is, first, incomplete. Then only the fully integrated part of those contents acquires an owning I. The contents of blind–sight remain at *level 2*. Now, the patient learns to link the I–less contents of his left field to those of his I–owned contents of his right field. This produces a partial lopsided integration of his *level–2* contents. There is now an I that owns the new structured experience. This, however, remains mixed because of the partial integration. The contents in D. B.'s left field become accessible to him as if they were seen, but they continue being as if they were not seen *by him*.

Consciousness is subsumptive. Hence, *level 2* is present in the higher levels. Most of what we see surrounds the part of the visual field where we focus, and we see it within consciousness of *level 2*. Sometimes we store such contents in memory in the form of mechanisms for producing visual images. These mechanisms can be turned on by using the memory of the focal contents of the original field, so to say, as handles, or push–buttons. Then the produced image can be inspected by changing the focus. This way one can *ex post facto* promote contents of consciousness from *level 2* to *level 3*. This posthumous promotion is feasible because of the integration of the contents of these two levels within a consciousness of *level 4*. This provides the stage. The promotion itself, executed by a voluntary action, occurs within consciousness of *level 5*.

An external reflexivity with a crude internal pointing operates in consciousness of *level 2*. At this level what appears in a perceptual field is determined in part by the perceptual powers of the perceiver. The contents of the field reflect to HIM what he is, but of course he does not find himself* reflected in them. By hypothesis there is no I that could find anything.

Consciousness of *Level 3* is a modification of consciousness of *level 2*. A central nucleus appears. It brings perspectival organization into the contents of the perceptual field. This perspective is a mixed, albeit blind, external–internal reflexivity. The perspective quietly reflects an orientation of the perceptual contents with respect to the perceiver. This orientation is certainly physical, especially in the case of visual perception. It is also psychological because the nucleus of the perceptual field exists thanks to the perceiver's attention. What is attended to reflects the attender's attention. Yet in the absence of *self*-consciousness the perspective is not apprehended as such.

Perceptual experience is primarily a phenomenon at *level 3*. One faces not merely a uniform perceptual field, but a focal and perspectival one. The perceptual judgments in which a perceptual experience culminates are judgments about the focal contents. These are demonstrative judgments about *this*'s or *that*'s, or *here*'s or *there*'s in the perceptual field in the now of the perceiving. Palpably, all of these items have an implicit reference to a potential, or actual, perceiving *I*.[14] The reference is implicit. As noted, it evinces a blind mixed external–internal reflexivity.

---

14 Castañeda (1987).

At *level 4* an explicit reflexivity enters the stage. As this level has been described, the I here is just a blend of the reflexive sides of the contrasts *I–this/that* and *I–it* [external object of the world]. This I is a crude solipsistic one, which rounds up all the present experiences and unifies them as an I exhausted by them. This I collects and formalizes the internal/external axis.[15]

As characterized here *level 5* is a solipsistic consciousness. On the chart offered, it is the last solipsistic level. As remarked above, the chart is merely a distillation of consciousness of *I*-strands; it says nothing about the causal independence, or dependence, or the chronological order, of the strands. For all we know at this moment, perhaps solipsistic episodes of consciousness occur as the extreme cases within a non–solipsistic experience, or life. Be this as it may, the execution of an act of will presupposes a consciousness in which an intended content of the form *I to do A [here] now* is brought into the causal process. This consciousness must not at the time of execution be concerned with other persons or objects. Its topic and concern are its effective causation. To be sure, other persons may still be involved in action A, as accusatives, beneficiaries, or circumstantial factors. However, action A need not involve any relation to any other: A may be a purely personal action for the exclusive benefit of the agent with no involvement of others. Hence, the consciousness of will, the acme of *level 5*, must always be not non–solipsistic. The *I* of deliberation is broader. The reasons for doing action A may involve all kinds of relationships to all sorts of persons. In principle, however, the deliberating I may believe that there exist no other *I*s or persons. This belief may, of course, be a symptom of mental illness.

Level 5 necessitates a special internal reflexivity. In deliberation the agent seeks to ascertain the range of his/her causal powers. Nonetheless, the search is not an intellectual aiming at a description of those powers. The search is a practical aiming at locating them, however blindly, in order to activate them. Hence, the agent's causal powers need be present in a *level 1* of consciousness.[16] Everything else is supernumerary.

At *level 6* the internality of *self*-reference becomes enhanced. Here a non–solipsistic *I*-strand appears. Yet the *I*s with this I–strand as their social limit are isolated. They observe each other, but do not converse with one another. They can just contemplate their sharing of mental properties.

At *level 7* the internality of the reflexivity of *self*-reference grows by big strides. The full panoply of negativities determine the one instance that is apprehended in its total individuality. To reach this level of consciousness a person must have resources for basking in personal relationships, for enjoying cooperative plans, for experiencing personal conflicts.

Living requires that one raises to higher levels of consciousness when one encounters problems, and has to deliberate and then adopt plans of action. However, when one is engaged in carrying out those plans, one

---

15 See Castañeda (1967).
16 For a discussion of this see *Thinking and Doing* Chapter 10, Section 3.

better not squander one's *self*-consciousness. Yet one need be attentive to the drift of events and be ready to make new decisions when obstacles turn up. Hence, the central level of consciousness for human living is *suffused level 3*, that is, suffused with the higher *I*-strands as potentialities for appropriate response.

3.3 Upwards Integration of Self–Consciousness on Converging *I*'s

Given the subsumptive nature of consciousness, the lower levels of consciousness can exist independently of the higher levels. *A fortiori*:

(C.–SC) NOT all consciousness is *self*-consciousness.

This thesis is the exact contradictory of one of the fundamental presuppositions of Fichte's idealism. The naturalization of consciousness requires not only the anti–Fichtean thesis (C.–SC), but also our whole subsumptive thesis. The ontological dependence of higher forms of consciousness together with their greater epistemic scope is accounted for better, under the thesis of their incorporating the lower forms on which they are grounded and which they illuminate.

From (C.–SC) it follows that:

(UC.–S) The unity of an episode of consciousness is not explicable by virtue of that consciousness belonging to a self, or *I*.

The unity of content of an episode of consciousness has to be understood in its own terms. In fact, the unity of each content of consciousness is presupposed by the unity of experience under an *I*. That is:

(UC+.S) If an episode of consciousness is internally owned by an *I*, then the unity of that consciousness is an element in the constitution of that ownership, hence, it is an internal presupposition of the existence of that *I*.

Yet the Fichtean assumption is still widespread, even in contemporary philosophers decidedly anti–Cartesian.[17]

---

17 See for instance J.G. Fichte, *Science of Knowledge*. On p. 41 we read: "Without self–consciousness there is no consciousness whatever." For contemporary echoes of this, see, for example, Pollock (1988), Chisholm (1981), Shoemaker (1968). Kant seemed to have allowed for some forms of egoless consciousness in his famous slogan: "The *I think* must be able to accompany of my representations." Yet in his transcendental deduction of the categories in his *Critique of Pure Reason* he adopts a Fichtean position. The result is that his conclusion is weaker than it should have been, namely: the categories apply to objects thought of in experiences subordinate to self–consciousness. He needs a stronger conclusion: consciousness of objects, whether subsumed under self–consciousness or not, involves the application of the categories. He did not know about blind sight—discussed above—; nevertheless his remark that if the *I think* does not accompany my representations these would be "nothing to me" is applicable to blind sight. Note, firstly, that for this he must move up from "is able to accompany my representations" to "accompanies my representation." Note, secondly, that my

To elucidate the integration of self–consciousness from below let us consider a slightly revised version of an example discussed in *Persons, Egos, and I's*:

Friedrich's Bee Watching. At a park Friedrich is fully absorbed watching the bird and the bees carrying on their usual affairs. He is then having an *I*–less experience, of the sort of thing Sartre made a big fuss as irreflexive consciousness. He even feels some pressure on his bend knees, and without jumping to an I–owned experience he simply stands up and then sits on the grass. Then he becomes aware of himself. A thought that the experience was pleasant made him think that he himSELF was enjoying it. He continues watching some bees descend on some flowers, pick up some pollen, and then fly away—in full awareness of himself. Then his whole experience is present to him under a diachronic *I*–unity. This unity is in fact a diachronically fusive succession of overlapping *I*'s existing alongside a succession of overlapping specious presents. Friedrich is enjoying several sub–experiences. He is attending to one big yellow jacket. He sees it move from a red flower to a yellow one. This seeing occupies a specious present: "From here to here." There is thus the subject of that seeing. During that interval he hears several drones from different bees. Each hearing has its own subject, an *I* that lasts less than the seeing *I*. Similarly, during the same interval he throws off several ants crawling up his legs. Each one of these seeing and throwing episodes has its own subject, again very short–lived. Also about the middle of Friedrich's seeing his favorite yellow jacket he feels an itching on his head; he scratches. An itching *I*, a scratching *I*, and an itching–and–scratching *I* come into existence and quickly vanish.

The itching–and–scratching *I* overlaps the other two *I*'s. During the first moment of just itching the itching *I* coincides with the itching–and–scratching *I*. Then this *I* is the subject of the integrated experiences of itching and scratching. Likewise, Friedrich's whole experience of seeing the yellow jacket flies from one flower to another pivots on one *I*. This ensues from the integration of the different sub–experiences into one comprehensive reflexive consciousness. That *I* is a unit built up from the subjects of the sub–experiences. The specious present determined by a succession of overlapping of co–consciousness determines in the normal human cases the short–lived *I* of the interval.

Because of the suffusiveness of consciousness, there is in Friedrich's normal case a total *I* of the totally integrated experience. Here the law of fusion that governs the phenomena is this:

---

representations, whether they mean anything to me or not, they must nevertheless involve the application of the categories—as in the case of blind sight. Hence, rather than, as Kant claims, the application of the categories and the unity of consciousness hinging on a transcendental apperception, it is the apperception that pivots on the lower levels of consciousness, which already involve the application of the categories.

(SC.I*) A real I of an episode of self–consciousness at a given time T is the reflexive subject of the maximal co–conscious integration of experiences at T.

REMARK 1. So far nothing precludes that there be one *I* unifying experiences across different persons or bodies. There must be, however, a suitable underlying "physiology" connecting the bodies.

REMARK 2. The sub–experiences of a person at a given time may fail to unify into one subject of experience. In principle, for instance, Friedrich may have been mentally disorganized. Some of the experiences mentioned above may have failed to integrate at all, or may have integrated only partially. These are empirically matters that may appear in many different degrees. Psychiatric practice may have already established many types and families of such failures of *I*–integration.

3.4 Major Integrating Internal Relations

The integrated contents of an experience of self–consciousness involves, internally as framing the experience, a good number of primitive relations. These relations are structural emergents upon the physical–physiological mechanisms upon which consciousness accrues. At the second level a primitive relation of CO–CONSCIOUSNESS links the contents of a simple experience (or sub–experience) as the contents of *one* (sub–)experience. Each experience (or sub–experience) has its own *now–here[there]* spatio-temporal framework. More or less simultaneous experiences normally combine into more comprehensive experiences. This requires an intimate organization of the different synchronous experiential spaces and times. Let's call CO–INTEGRATION the network of structural relations through which a unified total experience is built. Thus, the unity of a person's normal, fully organized total experience at a given time T is wrought out by a system of low–level instantiations of CO–CON-SCIOUSNESS, and by a thorough system of instances of CO–INTE-GRATION. Let's call META–INTEGRATION the relations that struc-ture unowned reflexive experiences. Let's call SUBJECTIONS those structural relations that subordinate an experience to a subject, that is, relations through which an I is posited, or hypostatized.

In the normal case every mechanism runs perfectly and all run in marvelous unison. In the normal case of self–consciousness all the contents of the experience are unified into sub–experiences, and these into a fully unified experience, each sub–experience is experienced as a strand of consciousness that forms part of a unified experience and is owned by an *I*. In such cases the *I* referred to is the maximally integrated and unified *I*— the *I* subsuming all the *I*'s of the unified sub–experiences. Likewise, the *now* of the total experience is the hierarchical cumulation of the *now*'s of the sub–experiences.

In an abnormal case a single mechanism by itself or a combination of such mechanisms fails to work properly. Abnormal cases are data about the distinctness of strands in reality that normally go together. The closer the togetherness in question, the more informative is the abnormality that breaks it. For instance, a person whose mechanisms eliciting the CO–CONSCIOUSNESS, CO–INTEGRATION, and META–INTEGRATION relations work well may yet suffer from disruption of a SUBJECTION mechanism. He may experience a sub–experience as if it were not his.

In the case of blind sight, the "unseen" contents are present and even connected by the appropriate CO–CONSCIOUSNESS relations. These include the relations of VISUAL CO–CONSCIOUSNESS, which prepare the visual manifold for CO–INTEGRATION as a unitary visual field. The visual data of the person suffering from blind sight has a visual field containing the blind data. These are, thus CO–INTEGRATED with the remaining data he sees. The visual field fails, however, to be META–INTEGRATED as an undividedly presented field. This crucial gap in META–INTEGRATION precludes the whole visual from being structured under SUBJECTION to one masterful *I*. Nevertheless, the whole field is there under the surface of consciousness. The patient learns to posit an abstract SUBJECTION of the not META–INTEGRATED data. Because of the deficiency in META–INTEGRATION the posited extended SUBJECTION must remain hypothetical: the postulated extended *I* is not a visual *I*, although by (SC.I*) it comprehends suffusively a concurrent visual *I*.

The preceding list is of types of internally integrating relations. Their respective species must be charted in order to achieve a useful profile of consciousness. Such a profile could be of help to psychiatry. Conversely, psychopathology, by furnishing detailed descriptions of cases in which some integration relation is missing, must contribute the criteria for differentiating such relations from one another.

3.5 Naturalization of Self–Consciousness

The internal hierarchy of an episode of consciousness sits on top of an underlying hierarchy of physical–physiological mechanisms. Mere sensory consciousness is underwritten by, accrue on, complicated networks of physiological mechanisms. At bottom these are simple stimulus–response patterns. They combine into simple thermostatic–like feedback subsystems. These in their turn bundle up in systems containing fine tuning in the adjustment of response to stimulus. In complex cases such fine–tuned adjustment amounts to a physical, blind *monitoring*. This monitoring involves something like representations of degrees of stimuli which cause the corresponding degree of response. This brute reflexivity of such systems underlies the internal reflexivity of episodes of self–consciousness supervening on them.

Clearly, the physical–physiological monitoring of stimulus–response patterns may provide the basis for the emergence of presentations of stimuli, without the emergence of a presentational representation of the monitoring itself. Then there would be consciousness without self–consciousness. Of course, each monitorial subsystem may be enlarged into a system that *records* the monitorial activity. This "recording" is meta–monitorial activity. Then there would be a representation of the subsystem. Something like this recording underlies self–consciousness; of course, such a physical–physiological recording is not identical with self–consciousness, nor is it by itself sufficient to yield self–consciousness.

Patently, a network of monitorial subsystems *cum* self–recording meta–compartments can all operate at unison. Unison operations of that sort provide the physical basis of an *I*-owned experience. Here we can see the basis for each local *I*—as in Friedrich's many *I*'s, e.g., his itching, his scratching, and his itching–scratching I's. Evidently, some of those physical–physiological mechanisms may out of tune, delivering then no *I* at all or a separate, non–integrated *I*. Such are the physical basis of the different types of *I*-disturbances. In any case, survival value accrues to the following psycho–physical connection:

(Ps–Ph.I*) In a well functioning system S endowed with mentality, S's *I* at time T is the fusion of the different *I*'s that emerge from the meta–activities of the distinct monitorial mechanisms underwriting episodes of consciousness at T.

Obviously we must investigate very carefully the bodily structures needed for the realization of the diverse *I*-strands. However, the preceding little glimpse into the appropriate structural properties of a body endowed with self–consciousness is all we can do here.

Summary

This partial study of the nature of self–consciousness focuses on the twofold hierarchical reflexivity of self–consciousness. It can be reasonably described as follows: (R–SC) In episodes of *self*-consciousness ONE is conscious of ONEself *qua oneSELF.*

Fundamental is the *external* reflexivity of ONE referring to ONEself. As such it has nothing to do with consciousness. It the the reflexivity of a reflexive relation: Rxx, whether R is an action or not. One is, for example, as tall as ONEself; a sleepwalker may wound HIMself accidentally and fully unawares by stepping on a shaving blade. Acts of referring are of course the cores of episodes of consciousness. As such they have an internal referent. Nevertehless, self–reference, the backbone of self–consciousness, is built up on the external reference of a thinker's referring to HIMself. Patently, a thinker may think, believingly, that the such–and–such ist this or that, without having any idea that he is in fact the such–and–such in question. In this case: *the such–and–such refers to the such–and–such as the such–and–such*—yet there is no self–reference. What is missing is the *internal* reflexivity of ONE referring to something, whatever it may be, as *oneSELF*. This internal reflexivity is the peculiar core of *self*-consciousness. That self–consciousness rests so firmly on its external reflexivity is brought home by one linguistic fact. The expression 'x refers to x as himself' is redundant. It is part of the logic, or semantics, of the expression 'x refers to y as herself' that this entails that y is the same as x.

We can, then, concentrate on the internal reflexivity of *self*-consciousness without loss. This internal reflexivity, constitutive of the moment *qua* oneSELF, is expressed in natural language by means of singular–referring uses of the first–person pronoun. It is the reflexivity of the appearing of the thinker to HIMself as himSELF, that is, as an *I*. Self–consciousness is *I*-consciousness. Not because we identify *I*-consciousness with the use of the pronoun 'I'; but because the uses of 'I'–sentences reveal the speaker's thinking *I*-contents, and consequently, his having a brain *I*-representation. A thinking episode is not an event of uttering. It is embodied in—indeedd, in some *appropriate* sense of 'sameness', a thinking episode is the same as—an event or process in the thinker's brain, or thinking box, whatever this may be.

The preceding reflection suggests that *I*'s may exist only as internal referents in episodes of self–consciousness. This suggestion is strongly supported by further data. These additional data include an ontologico-epistemological analysis of the so–called *de dicto/de re* contrast in attributions of psychological states to others. In the formula (R–SC), as well as in the general schema 'x refers to y as z, the component 'to y' is *de re*, whereas the component 'as z' is *de dicto*. Internal, *de dicto* expressions are depictions of representations the speaker exhibits as SHARED by him and the person he speaks of. *De re* expressions just vent the speaker's references. *De dicto* indirect speech has a Chinese–box structure, each box revealing the presented representations constituting thinking content—regardless of the physical existence of what is thought of.

A psychological statement that has as its core an attribution of the form 'X refers to Y as Z' discloses to the hearer that the speaker is presented with thinker X as thinker X, with item Y as Y, with item Z as Z. It reveals that the speaker takes Z to be an *intersubjective* thinkable. The *de dicto* occurrence of Z in 'X refers to Y as Z' is thus cumulative and shared. It manifests an accessible *intersubjective subjectivity* of Z. However, intersubjectivity is not always objectivity. By equating Z with Y the speaker reveals, besides, that Z has at least a vicarious objective status in her world. This status need not be existence. Even if X in fact refers to the speaker's Y as Z, Y may be only an intersubjective thought of item. In short, the externality orf the moment *to Y as Z* consists of the speaker's positing the *perhaps vicarious objective intersubjectivity* of Z through Y. The genuine objectivity of Z consists of Z being as such, as Z, an autonomous part of the shared world. Now, when X refers to HIMself [that is, to X] as himSELF, he is presented with what he calls "I"—but this cannot be present in anybody else's experience. Hence, the vicarious objective intersubjectivity of the *I*'s captured by the quasi–indexical mechanism 'he himSELF' or 'oneSELF' does not evolve into their genuine objectivity. The *I*'s are not as such parts of the world; they are only vicariously in the world by means of the persons they are the same as, when such persons enjoy episodes of self– consciousness.

If *I*'s exist only within episodes of self–consciousness, then different episodes have different *I*'s. Since, as noted above, consciousness does not presuppose, or require, self–consciousness, the contents of self–conscious- ness must be built up from the contents of self–less consciousness. These contents must be, hence, integrated prior to the appearance of a subordi- nating self. Further, the self–less contents and their unity impose constraints on the type of *I*–unity they can be subordinated to. Thus, we must distinguish different *I–strands* that characterize the different types of integration of the contents of episodes of self–consciousness. We engage in a very preliminary investigation of the most important *I*–strands, and their combinations into *I*–schemata.

The basic *I*–less contents of consciousness are themselves hierarchical. They are built of the integrated contents of many different sub–experi- ences. Each of these is the content of a potential *I* under which it can be subordinated. The *I* of a comprehensive reflexive consciousness is a unit built up from the subjects of the sub–experiences. The specious present determined by a succession of overlapping of co–consciousness determines in the normal human cases the short–lived *I* of the interval. The integrated contents of an experience of self–consciousness involve, internally, *de dicto* as framing the experience, a good number of primitive relations. These relations are structural emergents upon the underwriting *de re* chemico– physiological, chemico–electronic, whatever, mechanisms upon which consciousness accrues. A prmiitive internal relation of CO–CON- SCIOUSNESS—whatever its underlying neuro–physiological may be— links the contents of a simple experience (or sub–experience) as the contents of *one* (sub–)experience. Each experience (or sub–experience) has its own *now–here* [*there*] spatio–temporal framework. More or less simul- taneous experiences normally combine into more comprehensive experi- ences. This requires an intimate organization of the different synchronous experiential spaces and times. Let's call CO–INTEGRATION the network of structural relations through which a unified total experience is internally built—again, whatever its physiological underpinning may be. Thus, the unity of a person's normal, fully organized total experience at a given time T is wrought out by a system of low–level instantiations of CO– CONSCIOUSNESS, and by a thorough system of instances of CO– INTEGRATION. Let's call META–INTEGRATION the internal rela- tions that structure unowned reflexive experiences. Let's call SUBJEC-

TIONS those internal structural relations that subordinate an experience to a subject, that is, relations through which an I is posited, or hypostatized.

In the normal case every mechanism runs perfectly and all run in marvelous unison. In the normal case of self–consciousness all the contents of the experience are unified into sub–experiences, and these into a fully unified experience, each sub–experience is experienced as a strand of consciousness that forms part of a unified experience and is owned by an *I*. In such cases the *I* referred to is the maximally integrated and unified *I*— the *I* subsuming all the *I*'s of the unified sub–experiences. Likewise, the *now* of the total experience is the hierarchical cumulation of the *now*'s of the sub–experiences.

In an abnormal case a single mechanism by itself or a combination of such mechanisms fails to work properly. Abnormal cases are data about the distinctness of strands in reality that normally go together. The closer the togetherness in question, the more informative is the abnormality that breaks it. For instance, a person whose mechanisms eliciting the CO–CONSCIOUSNESS, CO–INTEGRATION, and META–INTEGRA-TION relations work well may yet suffer from disruption of a SUBJEC-TION mechanism. He may experience a sub–experience as if it were not his. He may, as in the case of *blind sight*, fail to experience a sub–experience as his own altogether.

The ruptures of the internal, *de dicto* structurings is what the psychiatrist investigates directly through the study of the logical connections between the patient's speeches, and between practical speech and behavior.

The internal hierarchy of an episode of consciousness, as remarked, sits on top of, or emerges on, an underlying hierarchy of physical–physiological mechanisms. Mere sensory consciousness is underwritten by, accrue on, complicated networks of physiological mechanisms. At bottom these are simple stimulus–response patterns. They combine into simple thermostatic–like feedback subsystems. These in their turn bundle up in systems containing fine tuning in the adjustment of response to stimulus. In complex cases such fine–tuned adjustment amounts to a physical, blind *monitoring*. This monitoring involves something like representations of degrees of stimuli which cause the corresponding degree of response. This brute reflexivity of such systems underlies the internal reflexivity of episodes of self–consciousness supervening on them.

Clearly, the physical–physiological monitoring of stimulus–response patterns may provide the basis for the emergence of presentations of stimuli, without the emergence of a presentational of the monitoring itself. Then there would be consciousness without self–consciousness. Of course, each monitorial subsystem may be enlarged into a system that *records* the monitorial activity. This "recording" is metamonitorial activity. Then there would be a representation of the subsystem. Something like this recording underlies the self–consciousness; of course, such a physical-physiological recording is not identical with self–consciousness, nor is it by itself sufficient to yield self–consciousness.

Patently, a network of monitorial subsystems *cum* self–recording meta–compartments can all operate at unison. Unison operations of that sort provide the physical basis of an *I*–owned experience. Evidently, some of those physical–physiological mechanisms may be out of tune, delivering no *I* at all or separate, non–integrated *I*. Such are, schematically, the physical basis of the different types of *I*–disturbances.

References

Buber M: I and Thou. transl. Kaufmann W, Charles Scribner's Sons, New York, 1970.

Burge T: Individualism and the Mental. In: French P, Uehling T, Wettstein H (eds): Midwest Studies in Philosophy: Metaphysics 11: 73–121, 1979.

Castañeda HN: Semantic Holism Without Semantic Socialism. In: Midwest Studies in Philosophy. Philosophy of Language II, 14: 101–126, 1990.

Castañeda HN: Consciousness and Behavior, in HN Castañeda (ed): Intentionality, Minds, and Perception, Wayne State University Press, Detroit, pp.121–158, 1967.

Castañeda HN: Identity and Sameness, Philosophia 5:121–150, 1975.

Castañeda HN: Negations, Imperatives, Colors, Indexical Properties, Non–existence, and Russell's Paradox, in: DF Austin (ed): Philosophical Analysis A Defense by Examples, Kluwer Academic Publishers, Dordrecht, Boston, London, 1988.

Castañeda HN: Persons, Egos, and I's: Their Sameness Relations. In: Spitzer M, Uehlein FA, Oepen G (eds): Psychopathology and Philosophy, pp. 210–234, Springer, Berlin, Heidelberg, New York, London, Paris, Tokyo, 1988.

Castañeda HN: Objects, Existence, and Reference: A Prolegomenon to Guise Theory, Grazer Philosophische Studien 25/26: 31–66, 1985/1986. (reprinted in Jacobi and Pape 1989).

Castañeda HN: Perception, Belief, and the Structure of Physical Objects and Consciousness, Synthese 35: 285–351, 1977.

Castañeda HN: Sprache und Erfahrung, transl. H Pape, Suhrkamp, Frankfurt am Mein, 1982.

Castañeda HN: Thinking and the Structure of the World, Philosophia 4: 4–40, 1974.

Castañeda HN: Thinking, Language, and Experience, University of Minnesota Press, Minneapolis, 1989.

Castañeda HN: Self–Consciousness, Demonstrative Reference, and the Self–Ascription View of Believing. In: Tomberlin JE (ed): Philosophical Perspectives: I. Metaphysics. Ridgeview Publishing Co, Atascadero, California, pp. 405–450, 1987.

Chisholm RM: The First Person. University of Minnesota Press, Minneapolis, 1981.

Churchland, PS: A Perspective on Mind–Brain Research, Journal of Philosophy 77: 185–207, 1980.

Fichte JG: Science of Knowledge (1798/1800/1801), transl. Heath P and Lachs J, Appleton–Century–Crofts, New York, 1970.

Jacobi K, Pape H (eds): Das Denken und die Struktur der Welt, De Gruyter, Berlin, 1989.

Jacobi K: Die Modalbegriffe in den logischen Schriften des Wilhelm von Shyreswood E. J. Brill, Leiden–Köln, 1980.

Lewis D: An Argument for the Identity Theory, Journal of Philosophy 63: 17–25, 1966 (reprinted in: Philosophical Papers, Vol. 1, Oxford University Press, Oxford, 1983).

Place UT: Is Consciousness a Brain Process? British Journal of Psychology 47: 44–50, 1956.

Pollock, J: My Brother, the Machine, Nous 22: 173–211, 1988.

Putnam H: Meaning Holism and Epistemic Holism: In: Cramer K, Fulda HF, Horstmann R–P, Pothast U (eds): Theorie der Subjektivität. Suhrkamp, Frankfurt a.M., 1987.

Putnam H: The Meaning of "Meaning". In: Gunderson K (ed): Language, Mind, and Knowledge. University of Minnesota Press, Minneapolis, 1975.

Shoemaker S: Self–reference and Self–awareness, Journal of Philosophy 65: 555–578, 1968.

Smart JJC: Sensations and Brain Processes, Philosophical Review 68 (1959): 141–156, 1959.

Spitzer M, Uehlein FA, Oepen G (eds): Psychopathology and Philosophy, Springer, Berlin, Heidelberg, New York, London, Paris, Tokyo, 1988.

Weiskrantz L, Warrington EK, Sanders MD, Marshall J: Visual capacity in the hemianopic field followed by restricted occipital ablation, Brain 97: 709–728, 1974.

Weiskrantz L: Trying to Bridge Some Neurophysiological Gaps Between Monkey and Man, British Journal of Psychology 68: 431–455, 1977.

Weiskrantz L: Varieties of Residual Experience, Quarterly Journal of Experimental Psychology 32: 365–386, 1980.

Wittgenstein L: Philosophical Investigations, transl. Anscombe EM, Oxford, Blackwell, 1952.

When the Self Becomes Alien to Itself:
Psychopathology and the Self Recursive Loop

Alfred Margulies

"What an abyss of uncertainty, whenever the mind feels overtaken by itself; when it, the seeker, is at the same time the dark region through which it must go seeking..."
M. Proust, *Rememberence of Things Past*, p. 49

I. Empathy with Oneself: The Recursive Spiral of Self

The concept of self is an elusive thing, always one step ahead of attempts to capture it and bring it down to earth. One working definition of self I have used is: "The self can be defined as that psychic structure that comes into being with the enigmatic process of self–reflection—that is, the self as simultaneously both subject and object."[1] How I have struggled with such a definition! It seems not right to have a proposition that includes the same term on both parts of the equation, that is, a definition that in circular fashion uses itself to define itself. Perhaps, perplexed by enigma, I have merely compounded the problem.

But paradox is not something that can be side–stepped in definitions of the self.[2] Circularity goes straight to the heart of the self phenomenon— the self itself is a process that is recursive, iterated, and folds back upon itself. The self of self–awareness is continually coming into being. It is that capacity of mind that constitutes itself in the very act of reflecting on itself. The self becomes itself in its own reflexive action; it is born in paradox and achieves its substance in the uniqueness of its personal, unrepeatable experience.

These musings come from a clinical orientation rather than a philosophical one per se. As a therapist, I daily ponder on the nature of empathy, how it is that one person ever presumes to approximate the inner experience of another. In particular, it has become apparent to me that whatever notions I have about empathy, the very process of attempting to be empathic with another person throws that other into his or her own self reflective spiral. That is, the other will now reflect on his or her self

---

1 Portions of this talk have been adapted from A. Margulies, *The Empathic Imagination*.
2 See Mann (1989) for another approach to the paradoxical features of the self.

through the medium of my presence and my attempt to be empathic. I call this process empathy with oneself through another.

What can that mean though, "empathy with oneself"—to feel into one's own experience? It seems a sleight of hand, a linguistic solution to a mystery, no doubt one of a whole family of such terms whose primary function is to manage paradox, to acknowledge, and then move on from some fundamental, mind–boggling problem that would only take us astray or leave us paralyzed in our tracks. And though such preoccupations are perhaps merely a language problem posed by a western mind demanding an artificial clarity, they are after all problems common to many of us caught up in our reflections about ourselves, reflections broken through the imperfect prism of the language of our culture and our times. Many of my patients suffer in their search for themselves, and for those groping for the truth of self, calling it a language problem will not do.

In this paper I will explore some problems of self–definition resulting from this recursive, circular property of the self examining its own perception of itself. In particular, I will examine the self's confrontation of the alien in itself and how it rejects, incorporates, or finds itself confounded in the face of its own self–pathology.[3]

Let me first illustrate the process of empathy with oneself as a general feature of self and introspection.

1.1 Case Example: The Mirror of Tears

An astute woman is recounting to me the troubling events of her childhood when her father had been insensitive and psychologically abusive. She had been the most sane person in the family, the parentified child. As she relates her story to me she becomes tearful. Though it seems as if it should be obvious, I am confused and ask her what she is experiencing at that moment.

"I suddenly had the thought that this must seem a very sad story *to you*." It is—she is here empathic to me and my experience. She had just imagined *what I, as listener, must have felt in hearing her story*. Interestingly, she was not sad for herself so much, but for me.

She then becomes even sadder, this time for the little girl she had just been talking about, the girl in the distantly recalled memory, the girl she once was. It still is *not herself–now* she is weeping for, but almost a *generic girl*, how any girl would have felt in those circumstances, an empathy for troubled children.

Then, quickly, her perspective shifts once again becoming even more specific to her split off experience: She cries now for *herself–then, as a little girl*. This empathy is curiously projected into the past, capturing who she

---

3 I am here focussing on the organizing concept of "pathology" and the consequences of so naming for the self integrating process. The self may use medical metaphor for the process of empathy with itself, but often it creates an altogether different language for finding meaning. Rather than "illness," the self, for example, may turn to cosmic good or evil to explain the infiltration of the alien.

was then, and sewing together the scraps of that distant time, what her mother, sister, grandmother had been like, her school and so on. It is empathy with her historical self.

Only a brief moment later, she grieves for *herself–now*, as an adult, experiencing her difficult childhood. This is how she feels about herself—but now, in the present, with me, in the moment.

In a rapid succession of events she had experienced a complex and vivid series of emotions, each with a slightly different context and nuance. She began with me and my imagined experience of her story (that is, she empathically imagined how I would empathically imagine her experience as a little girl). The narration itself became a vehicle to recapture her own distanced experience through another: I served mirror–like for her to see herself. She then empathized with what she would feel if she were a little girl going through the experience she had just narrated. That is, she first placed herself through imagination into her own lost experience, as if she were watching a movie about herself. It was only then that she captured it in memory—a memory that is different from any previous memories of the same events because now she has changed and hence the context of the memory in the remembering–self has changed. Lastly, she could place her present self into the experience as the one who had lived these events and was now recalling them. In each instance there is an important shift of perspective from inside the immediate frame to one of being the observer of a larger process. The self–observing–self evolved, shifted, and encompassed more of itself through the medium of the other (me as therapist) and the imagination of enlarging perspectives. I provided a new vantage point through my presence, my wish to understand, and her wish to help me understand what it is like for her now and then.

In my recounting this clinical vignette, the disjointed quality of the experience may seem odd or unusual. I am convinced that it is neither, that this is in fact common in psychotherapy, though I had not been sensitized to the complexity before.

Through a continuous feedback loop of a series of perspective shifts, the self envisions itself, captures itself, and even creates itself in an ongoing, spiralling process. With the process of empathy with oneself, one goes outside of oneself in imagination to find oneself.[4] In this instance, the mirror of the other is the catalyst for change and the medium of self–reflection; the mirroring creates the observing distance that is necessary for recapturing (or capturing) oneself.[5]

---

4 In art and literature we speak of aesthetic distance, the requisite emotional distance to capture experience. Analogously, in historical studies we need a distance in time: It is hard for us to explore ourselves in the present. Our selves need to change first, shift their perspectives—we need to be outside of ourselves, as it were—before we can locate ourselves. Oddly, the very proximity to experience can make it difficult to assimilate.

5 With this example, I am stressing a drive toward growth, insight, and integration mediated through the very separateness of another, rather than the search for wholeness in the needed complementarity of the other (that is, the hunger for the other that aims to complete one's incomplete self through union with an ideal). Words like "mirroring" come to mind. No doubt what I am talking about has to do

2.The Alien Experience Rejected as Pathological

We might at this juncture ask: How does the spiral of self reflection monitor its own processes, rejecting or accepting aspects of itself? What makes my world view my own—that is, me—and when does it seem not-me? What constitutes the feel of a world view? How does one keep it coherent and consistent? What happens when what one discovers in oneself no longer feels like oneself? These questions are intimately bound up with the concepts of character, the relatively fixed essences of a person's style, as well as with such ideas as syntonic and dystonic. The notion of character, though, has an external emphasis, how the person is experienced by others in the interpersonal. By the coherency of world view I mean to emphasize the lived experience of familiarity and reliability. That we are internally divided and inconsistent as well is a fundamental of our work, certainly since Freud. Interestingly, even in its estrangement, uncanniness, or alien aspects a world view may be consistent; we each have our own particular experience of the strange.

I am here reminded of the guideline by Rümke suggesting that a valid diagnosis of schizophrenia rests on the "precox feeling," that is the inner conviction that it is impossible to empathize with the patient (Leon 1989).[6] Though I disagree with much of that statement (anyone who learned about empathy from Elvin Semrad would recoil from the assertion), I do think that experience of the praecox Gefühl points to a fundamental alienness that is in its way impossible for the external observer fully to comprehend. This same experience of alienness and the impossibility of empathy might actually be experienced by the self to itself. The self may experience itself in its recursive processes as foreign and unempathizable; that is to say the self has the precox feeling in the presence of itself, the self is unable to empathize with itself.

2.1 Case Example: The Man with Two Psychoses—Which Madness is My Own?

One patient seen in consultation was impressively psychotic. He was both the devil and God; there was a cosmic conspiracy for his soul; a former girlfriend (dead, I later learned) would someday come back to him as part of the Trinity. He had been admitted to the hospital not because of his psychosis—which had been longstanding and familiar to everyone—but because of a drug reaction which had been dangerous physically and which had added a toxic psychosis on top of his more chronic schizophrenia. He himself, moreover, knew subjectively that his mind was now not right

---

with Kohutian considerations of selfobjects, but it is more: One finds—and loses—oneself through the other.
6 See also Haven's discussion (1973, pp. 124–132) of Jaspers' approach to the alien.

compared to his own baseline! That is, he could easily differentiate one psychosis from another. What does this mean?

It has been noted, depending on the exogenous toxin administered, that patients with schizophrenia will often be able to distinguish one psychosis from another. For example, a chronically schizophrenic drug abuser can tell the addition of LSD, recognizing that he or she is now tripping. The very inability of schizophrenic patients to make such an identification with the addition of amphetamines (that is, the schizophrenic person merely gets more psychotic and without self aware-ness) has been suggestive evidence for endogenous dopamine as an etiologic factor (Griffith et al. 1972; Janowsky et al. 1973). That is, amphetamines exacerbate the underlying schizophrenic psychosis rather than introduce a new one.

My point is that functional psychosis, even in its very fragmentation of experience, is a consistent point of view. This is, after all, one of the rationales of the early pioneering efforts in phenomenology for exploring psychopathologic states of mind—there is a coherency of experience. One *lives within* a psychosis. The broad outlines are relatively limited (and hence we can describe syndromes); the individual coloring is, however, always unique. In the above example, the self reflecting on itself, even though it remains within its psychotic perspective, nevertheless recognizes an alien warp imposed on its perception. Empathy with one's own experi-ence is disrupted. The self distinguished two different kinds of alien experiences, one that was alien–but–familiar (the intrusive, warring cosmic forces) within the context of the self–in–psychosis, and one that was alien-new (and so inconsistent and fragmenting of this particular world view).[7] We might now ask, can an alien process—recognized, objectified and consensually validated as such—be taken into the self spiral, indeed, desired as the longed for self?

3. The Alien Experience Incorporated into the Self

Dostoevsky, meditating on his epileptic seizures:

"The air was filled with a big noise and I tried to move. I felt the heaven was going down upon the earth and that it had engulfed me. I have really touched God. He came into me myself, yes God exists, I cried, and I don't remember anything else. You all, healthy people... can't imagine the happiness which we epileptics feel during the second before our fit. Mahomet, in his Koran, said he had seen Paradise and had gone into it. All these stupid clever men are quite sure that he was a liar and a charla-tan. But no, he did not lie, he really had been in Paradise during an attack of epilepsy; he was a victim of this disease like I was. I don't know if this felicity lasts for seconds,

---

7 With first psychotic breaks, the alien is often experienced profoundly as strange, mystical, religious, or evil. Only over time does the experience become everyday–alien. In parallel the self, stymied in its recursive spiral, becomes affectively dull and accepting.

hours or months, but believe me, for all the joys that life may bring, I would not exchange this one.

During a few moments I feel such a happiness that is impossible to realize at other times, and other people can't imagine it. I feel a complete harmony within myself and in the world, and this feeling is so strong and so sweet that for a few seconds of this enjoyment one would readily exchange ten years of one's life—perhaps even one's whole life.[8]

3.1 Syntonic Brain Damage

What if Dostoevsky had known he had the interictal personality features of temporal lobe epilepsy? I don't mean the fall down on the floor grand mal seizures—these he valued beyond price. Here he could touch God. But in our present day sophistication, we recognize more subtle features of the disorder. We can point to inter–ictal, that is between seizure, aspects of the personality of those suffering from such a brain lesion. These features are well documented: viscosity (or a certain adhesiveness to the personality; a sticky, argumentative quality, a refusal to cede even minor points: everything is serious and weighty), hypergraphia (the compulsion to write, to document, often resulting in lengthy works), hyper–religiosity (often with multiple religious conversions. These are people who care too much about God to leave Him to the professionally religious)... Curiously, these features describe Dostoevsky, and truly Dostoevsky would not have been himself without them.

But, again, what if Dostoevsky had known about this? Would it have concerned him? Would it have mattered to his wife, his editor? What if he had been born to responsible parents in our modern society? What if he had been treated early on? How would this knowledge have been iterated into his evolving self? Would he, rightly from the perspective of history, have valued his quirky interictal pathological character traits as a gift from the gods?

3.2 Case Example: Cortical Damage and the Process of Individuation

A man is admitted to the hospital after mutilating his arm with a knife. The hospital staff is worried that he may be suicidal.

I interview him in the context of teaching medical students and I know little else about him. He is a pleasant, gentle man in his interactions with me, soft spoken, and eager to please. He is fluent and articulate, although there is a certain droning, unmodulated quality that is, despite his dramatic and tragic story, monotonous. The students and I learn that he did not want to kill himself at all, but that under stress he had often turned his frustration and rage onto himself, mutilating his flesh in awful

---

8 From Alajouanine, 1963, p. 212

and visible ways. A t–shirt exposes his arms and the savagery of these self attacks which go back to childhood.

Prior to his own hospitalization he had become involved in a family therapy that focused on his suicidal stepdaughter, his wife, and her ex–husband. The patient had taken much responsibility in this regard, eager to help, and was quickly identified and enlisted as the mediator by daughter's caregivers. Over time this had become burdensome to him and in an effort to explain himself to the clinicians, he had written his own history of severe childhood psychological and sexual abuse. In the process he began to relive his trauma and to feel out of control. It was here that he had hurt himself.

To complicate matters further, about a decade ago he had been severely assaulted by an unknown stranger. The attack had been unprovoked and unusually brutal. The patient's head had been broken like a clay pot, with shards punched into his left temporal area. Moreover the blow itself had been heavy enough to bounce the right side of the brain into the skull in contra–coup fashion. The patient knew the medical lingo and related the story painfully, but with a certain detachment. He had since suffered frustration, humiliation, and sadness over the loss of facility with engineering and mathematical conceptualizations. Moreover, on psychological testing he had become aware of difficulties with pattern copying and manipulation. The assault and its neurological aftermath had drastically altered his life and his potential for certain intellectual endeavors. Though he had grieved, he still felt the pain of losing his previous professional promise.

In our first interview he felt grateful that we had a chance to talk, particularly in clarifying his own tendency to react to frustration with a destructive personal fury. This had been a life–long pattern, much better in recent years, and a response that had deep resonant origins in childhood trauma.

As I talked to him, I felt the terrible waste, the tragedy of this man's life with his intellectual talents literally crushed by a stranger. How extraordinarily difficult that would be: to contemplate your self as having lost part of your brain and inner world. I was impressed, nevertheless, at how intact his intellect had seemed—this was not someone whose pathology would be obvious without the history of his intellectual baseline.

A few weeks later I had an opportunity to talk to him again. The complex family situation was coming under control, and he was feeling better. I was with new students unfamiliar with the patient, and so we talked again about the events of his life. Only this time I noticed something I had not considered before when I had been overwhelmed by the tragedy of his situation and his attempts to cope.

He noted, almost in passing, that he had been more impulsive and self destructive a number of years ago. I asked what he attributed the settling down to. He was unequivocal—the brain damage. Not quite getting it, (and here I apologized in advance: Please forgive me, I do not mean to underestimate the difficulty of your experience) I asked if he were saying that the assault had been helpful in this regard. (And I wondered if this were the functional equivalent of a lobotomy. Again I had missed the point.) To him it was clear: as a result of the brain damage he had turned away from his frenetic life. His interests were quieter, he had found the humanities and writing (And still I wondered, "Was this a sign of temporal lobe epilepsy, that is, hypergraphia?" But there had been no history of overt seizures, unusual olfactory sensations, etc.—I asked.) I persisted in spite of myself to look for the pathology. How could brain damage work to one's advantage? How could he see it as a kind of blessing? Is this his denial, a refusal to look at external reality? No, he was squarely confronting his deficits and was even unusually medically informed. It was I who persisted in looking elsewhere; in a sense, it was I who was denying.

I asked him to explain further what brought about these changes for the better. He was thoughtful and reflective about this, it was after all central to his life and who he thought he was. To begin with, he noticed that he could not think as rapidly as before. This slowing down, a tragedy in the professional sphere, made him more attentive to others—he listened better. In this sense, he had become more empathic, and others found him more receptive. He observed his difficulty in switching from one thought to another, that his mind lacked the fluidity it had once possessed (that is, he had a certain perseveration). But before, he felt, he had been too flighty and impulsive, never settling down to think seriously about anything. Previously he abused drugs and alcohol; now he felt an aversion to any psychoactive agents. In general he had acquired a certain patience for life and was no longer swept away by affective storms.

The brain damage was now being integrated into his self experience, and in the overall weighing of debits and assets, he had come out ahead. The pathology itself, originally a deep source of grief, had become transmuted into the gold of personal strength, profoundly transforming his life. In his empathy for himself, his traumatic, exogenous and awful brain lesion became part of his process of growth and individuation—he felt himself to be a new and better person. He now embraced the alien and created a new self.

It should be noted that, ironically, his old, non–defective self might have been too mercurial to accept traumatic changes to itself. In his empathy for himself, his new self, changed to being more deliberate and thoughtful by the brain damage, was able to incorporate an image of self that was simultaneously defective but now also calmer and wiser. The brain damage, curiously, may have changed the self in such a manner as to accept this very damage. The trauma itself created the conditions for its own acceptance, setting a new context for the self to have empathy with itself traumatically changed.

4. Breaking the Self Spiral: Dilemmas at the Synapse

Empathy with oneself speaks to a synthetic process of mind, a push toward the integration of experience. This, broadly speaking, is a basis of most psychotherapeutic work. But what happens to experience that cannot be integrated by its very nature, when the person is thrust into insoluble dilemmas of self–definition? The very triumph of psychopharmacology presents new philosophical questions, unique to our age and culture. I am here referring to the advent of molecular prostheses, the bionic mind—and the brain/head/self/soul reflecting on its own molecules. Of course, these words are merely metaphors, however powerful they may be in shaping how we think about ourselves and our place in the world. They are not "real" or "true" but are culture bound and have historical antecedents in western thought. But that is my point, the self as a recursive process refracts itself through its own lens of meaning in a spiral of significance, understanding, and discovery.

As clinicians we often operationalize disease concepts in terms of "target symptoms," mental status markers helpful in monitoring the course of an illness. In this fashion, for example, no longer is the prescriber of medications treating mania per se, but its objectifiable, measurable manifestations. Disease then becomes: sleep disturbance, euphoria, grandiosity... each a target along the way to health. Side by side with the clinician, the allied patient joins the watch for the advancing and retreating forces of illness, adjusting medications accordingly. Targets, alliances— martial metaphors seem natural in this war against disease. But an insidious process develops: The self becomes a pitched camp, inspecting and sus- pecting itself in a constant scrutiny of its internal borders. Now the enemy has infiltrated the interior of the psyche itself: I hunt myself down.

Descartes found his epistemological bedrock in "I think..." The ground slips from under us when we question such fundamentals. One horror of psychosis is the loss of ownership of experience (for example, "they" are making my body tingle this way). A "disease of affect," a "thought disorder"—to what can the self anchor itself when the basics of feelings and experience are questioned? The question is not only "Who am I?" but "Is what I feel really me, or is it something that I wouldn't feel if my lithium level were higher?" Does the lithium get rid of some part of me– that's–really–me? It feels that way when it takes away my happiness, my "manic euphoria." But it doesn't feel that way when it gets rid of my depression, which seems not–me, alien. What of my experience do I trust as me? How can I even empathize with myself and what I feel when part of me may not, should not, even belong to me?

The prescribing of psychoactive medications seems particularly rele- vant in that it is so mundane. There is something about "accepted thera- peutic practice" that is both reassuring and unsettling. Knowing that a treatment is widely prescribed gives a certain historical safety in numbers;

things seem worked out, side effects described and dealt with. But what about the subtle side effects for the soul, for the meaning that one attaches to experience altered by exogenous psychic molecules? Problems in finding oneself have always presented in a myriad of forms and situations—but our technological age creates troubling new possibilities and dilemmas for the self empathizing with itself.

Summary

The objectification of personal experience as pathological has a profound impact on the self's attempts to define itself. Given the recursive features of the self, it must constantly assimilate and accommodate to its own conception of itself in a never ending spiral of self definition. Certainly the clinician's own participant observer status contributes to the process of meaning—there is no neutral ground from which to observe and not interfere. Whether the reflective process becomes part of a broader growth toward individuation or whether the recursive spiral becomes paralyzed and stymied is not always so predictable. The metaphor of body and disease, when applied to the mind, becomes drawn up into the evolving self and spills into the very soul.

References

Alajouanine, T: Dostoewski's epilepsy. Brain 86: 209-218, 1963.
Griffith J, Cavanaugh J, Held J, Oates J: Dextroamphetamine: evaluation of psychomimetic properties in man. Arch Gen Psychiatry 26: 97-100, 1972.
Havens LL: Approaches to the Mind, Movement of the Psychiatric Schools from Sects toward Science. Little, Brown and Company, Boston, 1973.
Janowsky D, El–Yousef M, Davis J, Sekerke H: Provocation of schizophrenic symptoms by intravenous administration of methylphenidate. Arch Gen Psychiatry 28: 185-191, 1973.
Leon RL: Psychiatric Interviewing. Elsevier, New York, 1989
Mann D: A simple theory of the self. (Presentation to the Department of Psychiatry, The Cambridge Hospital, Harvard Medical School) 1989.
Margulies A: The Empathic Imagination. Norton, New York, 1989.
Proust M: Rememberence of Things Past, vol. 1, transl. Moncrieff CKC, Kilmartin T, Random House, New York, 1981.

Perception, Thought and Schizophrenia

Verbal Hallucinations and Pre–Conscious Mentality

Julian Jaynes

1. Introduction

There is wide agreement that verbal hallucinations are the most pre–eminent symptom in the psychopathology of schizophrenia, even though the phenomenon does not apparently occur in every case. Some psychiatrists, indeed, think that schizophrenic episodes *always* begin with such hallucinations, but this is very difficult to establish, just as it is very difficult to study hallucinations in schizophrenics at all. Very often a patient will deny hearing voices for any or several of three reasons: either at the command of his hallucination, or because he fears some treatment such as electro–shock, or because he does not want his voices probed into. In this paper, I shall first present some of the data we have found in our studies and then suggest a theoretical framework into which they can be placed.

Our first study, naturally enough, was of hospitalized schizophrenics in a New York psychiatric ward. It was done by my student Michael Rosenberg. A tape recorder was sometimes used but usually not because of its obtrusiveness. Mr. Rosenberg had in his mind a list of questions which was loosely followed. After each interview, he reconstructed what had been said into a paragraph. Here is a typical example:

> VIOLA: The voices appeared somewhat suddenly and gradually got more and more intense. At first there were only angels. These would tell me good things. For instance, "Viola, you're a good person". But then sometimes diabolical voices appeared and would say things like "You're lying". These diabolical voices would tell me that I was bad and should die. They told me that I was going to hell. When these voices spoke, I could see fire and I definitely felt burning on my body from this fire. The angels were often my sisters talking to me. The diabolical voices were the devil talking and he was trying to pull me down into hell, but I resisted.

In answers to questions, the patient said she had been very religious as a child and that her grandmother had had a church in the basement. The voices sounded as if they were coming from behind her. She said they never sounded like her mother, father, or son. She thought they started because she was trying to communicate with "the soul of my son's father." The angels did not like this and the devil tried to take advantage of this opportunity.

I use this as an illustration because it shows certain characteristics common to the hallucinations of hospitalized patients: The suddenness of onset, the deeply religious nature of the experience, the self–contradictory nature of the messages, and their critical emphasis either positive or negative. All these factors are I think very familiar to most of you.

Now the question here is why? Why the religious quality? Why the admonitory nature of the voices?

Let me give some other examples of verbal hallucinations in these hospital patients.

JEREMY (A 25 year old black man who had started taking drugs when he was nine, well groomed, somewhat sedated): I kept on turning around, but there was never any one there... In a 'crack house' a couple of weeks ago, the voices started screaming really loudly and I just flipped. The police came and took me to the hospital. The voices almost always occurred several at a time being both male and female. I didn't ever recognize any of them as being friends or relatives. When I was taking a lot of drugs, the voices would be nice and tell me how good a person I really am inside. However, whenever I stopped taking the drugs, the voices would change very quickly. They became evil and would tell me to do some very bad things. They were always very specific in their commands. For instance, they would tell me "go rob that store", "go mug that lady", ...the voices wouldn't leave me alone until I had done what they had told me to do. I couldn't ever shut the voices down and they just got louder and louder until I couldn't deal with them. Then I would do what they wanted.

It is interesting to note the relationship of the hallucinations to drugs and therefore to brain chemistry. This case also illustrates the sex differences in hallucinations, that males hear more commands to commit some act than do females.

MERCEDES (Hispanic female in her mid twenties, dishevelled, responds only after being offered a cigarette): If the thinking thoughts stop, then I will die. They have taken over my mind and control it, you understand? I am able to communicate with you, but they are telling me things and explaining some information to me. ... They usually come from behind me but I know they're in my mind. They go on all day. They're talking right now. At night they let me sleep, but start talking to me in the morning again. They say all different kinds of things to me. Sometimes nice things, sometimes bad things, sometimes just repeating whatever I say. They tell me about other people, before I even meet them. The voices didn't tell me about you. But now they're talking about you and listening. They won't let me tell you what they're saying.

TOBAS (20 years old, neatly dressed, from the Dominican Republic, about to be moved to a more permanent ward for schizophrenics): I felt the Lord in me. This is when the voices began. At first they were only whispers, but then louder, but still soft. It was Jesus speaking to me. He would tell me what to do and ask me questions. Jesus would speak to me alone and no one else. ... Then I became a backslider. The Devil started talking to me. (He was unable to imitate the voice of The Devil). The Devil told me bad things. He told me to kill myself. The Devil just wouldn't leave me alone because I was a backslider.

ANGEL (An hispanic male in his mid twenties well groomed, quite willing to talk, carrying a spanish comic book): About three weeks ago the voices started and I would look around to see if anyone was there but there never was. At first they were almost funny. There would be a poster advertising a movie and the voices would say "Angel, look at that poster over there saying such and such". I would look and the posters always said what the voices had said they would. After a while though the voices started getting louder and talking more often. ...They would just say really bad things over and over. They would tell that I am a bad person and I'm going to die. When I couldn't take them anymore, I tried blinding myself by looking at the sun, but this didn't work. At around 3:00 in the morning I went to the church to find a preacher, but the church was locked. I started to walk up and down Broadway. The voices just kept talking and talking day and night. I don't know why I went to the church since I had never been very religious, but, I guess, that I thought the preacher might be able to explain where the voices were coming from. When he wasn't there, I just didn't know what to do anymore. After a couple of days the police picked me up and brought me to the hospital. With the medicine, the voices have stopped, but I'm not better yet. (Angel was then afraid to say anything more about the voices "because he could not control these voices and they did not let him control his own mind.")

In general, most of our hospital interviewees were Hispanic. 80% at sometime heard multiple voices. Most of the voices were male and were frightening to 63% of the subjects. 22% of the hospital subjects could not understand some of the time what the voices were saying. Of some pertinence to hypotheses of the relation of schizophrenia to laterality is the finding that 56% of our hospitalized subjects were left handed or ambidextrous.

2. Hallucinations in the "Homeless"

We next turned to a rather haphazard selection of so called "homeless" people in New York City, particularly along Broadway and in the huge Port Authority Bus Station. Interviews were casually begun by Mr. Rosenberg and might continue over coffee or a pizza. The subject of hearing voices was casually introduced into the conversation. In contrast with the hospitalized patients, they seemed not at all anxious in talking about the voices, even eager at times and very cooperative. Also of interest was the phenomenon of hearing multiple voices all speaking at once. Obviously some of these subjects had at one time been hospitalized and some were on medication. The voices were again admonitory and usually religious, often telling the person what to do which in most oft hese subjects is resisted. Here are some examples.

GABRIEL (A poorly dressed 32 year old Puerto Rican man outside the Port Authority): Yeah, I hear voices sometimes. I'll tell you about them if you give me money. O.K., I'll tell you anyway. Man, it's a really scary experience. Really frightening. They can tell you anything. No, I don't ever do any drugs. I don't know whose voices they are. They just talk; sometimes in other languages. Yeah, sometimes Spanish. They are hard to understand. They can say a lot of different things. They can tell you bad things to do; so you just do them. For instance, "hit that man", "spit on her". Sometimes you just say out loud what they told you like "she's ugly". You can't control or stop them. They can go on and off all day long lasting about a minute.

BREHMAN (A 32 year old black man sitting on the ground leaning against a wall on 43rd street and 8th avenue; well groomed for someone whom is living on the streets.): I don't hear any imaginary voices. I hear real voices. I was in a fight last March in Atlanta... When the doctor stitched me up he implanted some kind of monitoring device so that they can keep track of me and communicate with me. Now whenever I'm in the city I see people on the street or anywhere and they can start yelling at me. See, there are a lot of evil people in cities. There are some good people, but the bad ones in the city start yelling at me through this monitoring device. In the country nobody's voice yells at me through the device. ... It can get real bad, especially at night. You see these people could get on the same frequency as you and start yelling at you. They don't leave you alone. Yeah, sometimes they say nice things but almost never. They come at you five, six at a time ... When they yell at me now, I yell back real loud at them and they shut up after a while.

BRUNO (A bearded white man in his thirties living in a hotel for homeless men, met on Broadway at 96th street while sitting on a bench talking to some 'winos'; he seemed open, honest, and happy, and was very excited and anxious to discuss his voices): I hear voices a lot. It's perfectly normal, but you can't tell the doctors or they give you medicine that makes you sick. ... But I just hear the voices and don't do what they say to do. That's normal, right? A couple of minutes ago I was on a bus and the voices told me to get off the bus. They're usually men talking. They can say your thoughts. Sometimes they say "Bruno, you're a good guy", but at the same time there are other louder voices saying "Bruno, you're a real bad person". ... The voices come from in my head. Actually from in my right ear. ... I don't do anything bad they tell me to do. They told me yesterday to "hit an old lady", but I didn't because I knew it was only a voice in my mind.

THE ECHOLAILIC (a 25 year old black man in the Port Authority bus terminal whose hands were shaking perhaps from having been on psychotropic medications for too long; when asked about voices, he responded in short, stuttered speech): I hear voices talking to me a lot. They yell at me and bother me. I don't know who they are or what they say, but they annoy me. They started, I don't know, yesterday? They go on and off a lot. "What's it about? What's it about? What's it about? (At this point, he became echolailic, repeating everything and no longer looked as disturbed as before. Then he suddenly stopped repeating what the interviewer had said and spoke about food and what he might eat later.)

THE STREET MAN (A black man in the corner of the Port Authority, relatively kempt above 35): Voices? I hear all the voices. But they don't tell me nothing I don't already know. You see, I know everything. My thoughts are always ahead of everything. What voices do you want to know about? Cosmologian terrestrian, solarian, universalian...? You see, it's the psychology. Yes, listen, when everything started the earth was made and God did it. I know all that. Jesus knows it. I already know everything even if they're yelling. I know what's wrong and what's right. You see, I'm always trying to catch up with my reality. I don't even try anymore. It's always so far ahead of everything. I can't even keep up with it. ...No one can ever know me or understand me.

MR. JOHNSON (A 42 year old black man in the Bowery with a wooden cross hanging from some beads around his neck): I used to want to be better, but I'm too old to be cured. The problem began because I just was too smart. Jesus would talk to me and he took my brain away because I was too smart. Hitler would tell me nice things sometimes (he used Hitler and Jesus interchangeably). There were other voices too. They would yell at me and tell me to do bad things. They wouldn't leave me alone. I've been having these voices for a long, long time. After a while, you just get use to 'em. I'm a very very religious man, but I don't go to church. I pray to God all the time in my own way... I don't think the voices are ever going to stop. The ones that yell are mainly men.

THOMAS (A 43 year old white man in ragged clothing on the third floor of the bus terminal playing around with a small broken television set and its antenna; he offered to sell it for twenty dollars; when the subject of voices came up, he became very serious, almost paternal.): Listen! Don't you pay any attention to those voices. They're bad. They'll get you into trouble. Just ignore them and after a while they won't bother you as much. I was in the hospital for a long time because of those fucking voices. Those little bastards would just start yelling at you. Listen to me! Start ignoring them now before they get too bad... The voices can talk to you through the television. That's how they first started. It's really frightening because you think the T.V.'s talking to you. I'm not going to sell you this TV if you hear voices. It might scare you too much.[1]

These examples are fairly typical of those homeless people who do hear voices. Although we made no effort to make an estimate of what percent of the people wondering the streets of New York are hallucinating, it seemed that almost half of those approached did so. Most of these street subjects were black. 72% of positive cases at sometime had heard multiple voices. Almost all voices were male. As with hospital subjects, most of them were afraid of their hallucinations and about the same percentage (21%) could not understand what the voices were saying some of the time. But in contrast to the hospital patients, only 21% of the homeless were either left handed or ambidextrous, although that is still more than double the frequency in the general population.

All this material is quite familiar to most of you and would obviously come under the heading of psychopathology. But what follows is more controversial.

3. Hallucinations in Normal Students

We next turned to study verbal hallucinations in a normal population. The subjects were 74 Princeton students taken from the student telephone directory by a strict and careful randomization procedure. Each of the subjects filled out a carefully worded questionnaire in private and anonymously. None of the students so contacted refused to participate. Again, the study was done by Michael Rosenberg (Rosenberg 1988). 27.8% replied "yes" to the statement "I am positive that I have heard a voice at some point when no one had spoken to me." 12.5% clearly recall hearing a dead relatives voice. 3% had heard God's voice, and or a minor level, 78% could still hear a song after it had stopped, and 67% replied "yes" to the statement "I've heard my name being called when no one has called me." The important figure here I think is the first, namely, that roughly 28% of all Princeton University undergraduates have experienced at least one auditory hallucination.

Many of the descriptions they provided of verbal hallucinations were similar to those of psychiatric patients. The voices they heard were parents, relatives, friends, dead relatives, or God. Some had only heard one voice speaking while others had heard more than one voice. Both male and female voices were heard. Some were slow deep voices while others spoke quickly. The great difference is that these hallucinations of normal

---

1 When the interviewer tried to correct Thomas's misunderstanding by saying that he didn't hear voices but was a student at Princeton University doing research with Professor Jaynes, Thomas immediately cut in, "That's just the kind of thing they tell you! I said don't listen to them."

students were of much less intensity and frequency than those of psychiatric patients.

These results are consistent with those found previously by Posey and Losch (1983) in a questionnaire given to 375 college students. I suggest that it is now clearly established that about 1/3 of the normal population hear verbal hallucinations at some time, and that such hallucinations do not therefore indicate pathology as biological psychiatrists have been taught to believe.

4. Hallucinated Playmates in Children

The spectrum of incidence of auditory hallucinations not only has to include normal non–schizophrenic adults but also children. Those who have studied the phenomena of "imaginary playmates" (which should read hallucinated playmates) are convinced that such children hear the 'voices' of their to–us–unseen friends in their conversations with them (Harvey 1918; Pines 1978). In my own research, I have found that about half of women students at a religious college had had such hallucinated playmates, and half of those clearly remembered the pitch and quality of the voices.

One of these women is of special interest. She came from a very poor family in which both parents had to work, leaving the girl in the care of a schizophrenic grandmother who was hallucinating voices in various rooms of the house. The girl developed hallucinated playmates, different ones for different rooms. Her mother, realizing the situation, quit her job, sent the grandmother to a mental hospital, and tried to train the child out of such hallucinations—which was successful in part. But the girl, now grown up, still has her hallucinated playmates who are also grown up like her, and appear in times of stress and try to tell her what to do. Their voices were clearly 'heard' and not imagined. She did not impress me as being psychotic. She was concerned as to whether her hallucinated playmates were innate or learned, I imagine because she was going to be married and was not going to have children if it was possible that they would go through what she has gone through.

And I will report here the case that happened just the other day to a friend of mine. A precocious 3 1/2 year old boy had an hallucinated playmate named Henry. He was visiting his grandfather with his parents. While playing with some toy dinosaurs on the living room coffee table, he suddenly looked startled, jumped up and ran over to a ventilating grill on the floor and cried out into it, "Go back Henry! Don't come any further! You'd get stuck. Go back down to the cellar!" He then returned to his dinosaurs as if nothing had happened. I mention this case as another demonstration that it is not an imagined voice in the conscious sense of imagination but a true hallucination. This small vignette will remind some of you of hallucinating patients in the hospital who are convinced that the voice emanates from some one stuck in the ventilating system.

5. Verbal Hallucinations in a Nonverbal Population

A group that I would like to mention has been discovered only recently (Hamilton 1985). These are cerebral palsied spastic–athetoid nonverbal congenital quadriplegics who have never spoken in their lives. They must be fed, bathed, toileted, and moved by others, and they are often regarded by the nursing staff as "vegetables." Surprisingly, some of them are fully capable of understanding speech at a normal level—even though they have never learned how to speak. Using finger, lip, or eye movements, communication can be established with a known technique, something like the game of "20 questions," in which thepatient can indicate yes or no (see Moore 1972).

When asked privately through this technique about the possibility of hearing voices, most of these patients "gave startled expressions followed by excited 'yes' signals". The voices were usually the same sex as the patient,s ounding like a relative, but identified as God. They spoke as from outside the patient, usually from the upper left (when hearing the voice the patient's eyes shifted to the left as if involuntarily), told the patient what to do and what was right, and made the patient miserable when disobeyed. Usually the voices were helpful, telling the patients to cooperate with any training program that was initiated. The patients felt they could not communicate with the voices. The data were checked for possible Clever Hans effects by having a second questioner who did not know the earlier results. This work has recently been carefully extended, demonstrating that these speechless subjects can present the content of their own phenomenal field accurately and that investigators' interpretations are accurate (Sappington et al. 1988). Unfortunately, CAT scans on these patients were not available.

6. Other Observations

The variety of verbal hallucinations is remarkable. I have in my files unsolicited letters from many correspondents who wish to tell me about their hallucinations. One of the most unusual was from a transsexual who as a boy suffered considerable sexual molestation and then as an adult, after a spell of Scientology, became "overwhelmed" with voices until his sex change operation when they abated. Others had been shipwrecked sailors during the war who conversed with an audible God for hours in the water until they were saved. A woman in her car heard a voice from the left car window telling her to write her funeral, and when she got out paper and pen "the words poured visually into my head." She had never had a similar experience. Another was a deeply religious man who one summer, following an interest in spiritualism, heard at least 20 divine voices extremely similar to the voices heard by Schreber described in his famous autobiography. While he was hospitalized at the demand of his family,he never received medication or therapy or lost his objectivity, and was sorry when the voices went away. If you have a tendency to say this was a chizophrenic episode with spontaneous remission, I wonder what you would say about Emanuel Swedenborg, the brilliant early 19th century scientist who heard voices he identified as everyone from Socrates to Jesus, and whose verbal hallucinations founded the Swedenborgian religion. Or his one time follower William Blake whose poems were heard from believed–in angels all about him. It is to be noted through this material the important relation to belief in those voices and particularly religious belief.

Why are verbal hallucinations so common in such disparate groups, both normal and pathological? Why are hallucinations so often admonitory, 73% commands in men and more often criticisms in women? Why are they often religious in nature? Why do criminal psychotics commonly feel they must obey their voices?

7. Hallucinations in Ancient Civilizations

As a way of trying to answer these questions, let us look back into the earliest history of civilizations for evidence of verbal hallucinations. The earliest text of any size that we can translate with relative assurance is the *Iliad*. I would point out two characteristics. First, verbal as well as visual hallucinations are everywhere in this poem. The voices are, of course, called gods and they manage and control the actions and emotions of this bloody story. The gods or verbal hallucinations begin the Trojan War, determine its strategy and its end.

A second characteristic of the Iliad is that in its older layers there is no introspective consciousness. Nor are there words in the original text for conscious operations, such as think, feel, experience, imagine, remember, regret, etc.[2] The hallucinated voices or gods *were* human volition. The springs of action were not in conscious decision making or introspective musings of what will follow from one specific act versus another. We should always be vigilant in realizing that consciousness is not the same as cognition or perception as common street knowledge assumes, but something added to them, something learned through language and its power of metaphors and analogies.[3]

The older parts of the Iliad, then, display a pre–conscious mentality, one in which verbal hallucinations called gods are absolutely central. This mentality I have called in other work the bicameral mind—a rather inexact metaphor to a bicameral legislature of an upper and lower house. Such bicameral individuals moved through their lives on the basis of habit—just as we do, but when any novel occurrence or situation came along, a choice–

---

2 Modern translations are notorious for naively projecting modern consciousness into the text.

3 I apologize for what must seem contentious and provocative in its brevity. I go into these matters fully in Jaynes 1976a, Chapter I.1, and Jaynes 1988, particularly pages 140–142.

point as we might say, in came an hallucinated voice telling the person what to do, precisely the point at which consciousness in modern times would be choosing our own behavior.

What triggered these hallucinations? I suggest it was even the slight stress of making a decision in a novel circumstance, whereas in ourselves in modern times the stress threshold for such triggering of a verbal hallucination is much higher. The reason they are so prevalent in all cultures today, in the hospital patients and homeless I have talked about, in children and speechless guadriplegics, is because they were once the genetic basis of this ancient mentality, and the genes for this potentiality are with us today. Verbal hallucinations, we think, evolved along with the evolution of language during the late Pleistocene (Jaynes 1976b) as the response part of the brain register of all admonitory information. It's survival value at first was simply to directan individual in various long–term tasks which cued their occurrance. By 9,000 BC, such voices were called what we call gods.[4] The bicameral mind produced a new kind of social control that allowed agricultural civilizations to begin. Historical speculation, yes, but touching data points in archaeological evidence all along the way.

Let me broadly summarize a huge amount of data by several assertions at this point. Civilization, by which we mean human beings living together in large groups, begins in various sites in Mesopotamia, spreads into Anatolia (modernTurkey), westward into Egypt, then into Africa, from Anatolia into Greece and Southern Russia, then India, Thailand, and China, and then independently in a series of civilizations in Mesoamerica and the Andean highlands, and *all* these early civilizations show some kind of evidence of being bicameral or organized by hallucinations called gods (which is the same thing), be it the presence of idols, or depictions in murals, reliefs, or seals, or, where there was a written language, actual descriptions of such interactions between men and their hallucinated gods—not entirely unlike the descriptions of modern hallucinators earlier in this paper.

8. Some Ancient and Modern Parallels

Now let me briefly draw your attention to a few instances of the similarity of some modern phenomena that I have already mentioned and ancient bicameral ones. One is the business of idols. This is an important topic that nopsychologist has studied. Idols are material efigies that provoked and sustained verbal hallucinations in ancient times. They are everywhere in all ancient civilizations. It is as if they make the voices plausible. We can remember here the little boy running to his hallucinated friend under the floor grating wheret he voice seemed to be coming from. Or "Thomas" with his broken television in the Port Authority Bus Station. I have seen on city streets what I regarded as homeless men making imaginary telephone

---

4 This theory is thus one that explains the origin ofgods and therefore religion.

calls at a pay booth, never putting in a coin, and flubbing the fingers over the dial without ever dialing, and then conversing at length with what I assume is a verbal hallucination. In another instance, something which probably some of you have observed, a patient in the hospital was sitting in a chair intently watching a blank television screen, and saying in amazement, "But how does President Reagan know so much about me?" Note the hierarchical underpinings of this. Almost always verbal hallucinations are of somebody above the person in a hierarchical relationship just as it was in bicameral times. It may seem strange to regard a ventilation grating, or a broken television, or a silent telephone as an idol, but such is their function.

A second note I would add concerns hallucinated playmates, in particular the case I have mentioned of the woman whose playmates grew up with her and tried to tell her what to do in times of stress. Hallucinated playmates appear to occur in almost 50% of children, although many are forgotten or suppressed. We can at least imagine that something parallel happened in bicameral times where all children, encouraged and supported with expectancies by the cultural values of the society, developed hallucinated playmates that grew up with them and became their personal god, their *ili* in Mesopotamia and the *ka* in Egypt.

I think it can easily be inferred that human beings with such a mentality of hearing hallucinations had to exist in a special kind of society so that the hallucinations would agree. It would be one rigidly ordered in strict hierarchies with strict expectancies organized into the mind so that the social fabric was preserved. And such was definitely the case. The texts clearly show that bicameral theocracies were all hierarchical, submerged in ritual, with a god, often an idol or robed statue as throughout Mesopotamia at its head from whom hallucinations seemed to come, or else, more rarely, with a human who was divine (that is, heard in hallucination by those just below him in the hierarchy) being head of state as in Egypt. The Iliad with its loose organization of hero–warriors may seem to be an exception, but archaeological evidence from the period of the Trojan War show idols were common, and Linear B describes a strictly hierarchical society. For the evidence of all this, I have to refer you to my earlier work (Jaynes 1976a).

9. The Breakdown of Hallucinations and the Beginning of Consciousness

Such theocrasies with their strict hieracrchies require stability, require children to be brought up with similar expectancies. When there is social unrest, particularly when people are forced to migrate and leave their stability–inducing temples and idols, the voices heard by the individuals of a society no longer agree and the bicameral mind no longer can function. The Exodus and the ensuing turmoil in Canaan was just such an event. The whole of the Hebrew Testament can be read as the slow inevitable breakdown of this hallucinatory mentality and its replacement by wisdom. In Mesopotamia one of the chief causes of the breakdown of the bicameral mind was overpopulation because of its huge success in running agricultural city states. And there too, the second millenium BC towards its end is seeing more and more wars and invasions. Social chaos was most certainly exacerbated by the great eruption of Thera (sometimes called by its Christian name Santorini) that devastates the Near Eastern world and began several centuries of migration and invasion. And the success of writing in relaying the commands of the gods weakened the power of auditory hallucinations. With the social underpinnings of the bicameral mind gone, with people no longer hearing their voices, what could people do?

In this talk I have not had time to go into the nature of consciousness and why it is reasonable to suppose that consciousness is not a biological given evolved in some mystical fashion somewhere back in animal evolution, but is a specificly human ability built upon the basis of the power of language to form metaphors and analogies just at this time. This can most clearly be seen in the earliest Greek literature. Beginning with the Linear B Tablets, going through the Iliad and then the Odyssey, through the lyric and elegiac poets of the next two centuries to Solon in 600 BC provides the clearest description of the breakdown of the bicameral mind and the development of the vocabulary of consciousness of the basis of metaphor. Such words as *thumos, phrenes, kardia, psyche* change from external objective referents to internal mental functions (see Snell 1953; Adkins 1970). And this process is going on elsewhere at the same time. I have gone into this in much more depth elsewhere (Jaynes 1976a). In the Hebrew world, I would ask you to compare the oldest pure book, *Amos*, an almost bicameral man[5], with the most recent, *Ecclesiastes* of about 200 BC.

So in this talk we have started off with several contemporary studies of verbal hallucinations which sometimes may be regarded as psychopathology and sometimes not. Then we looked back into history and found that the ancient literatures show the phenomenon to be practically universal and every day. Schizophrenia then is a partial relapse to the bicameral mind, but only partial, because the person has learned consciousness in childhood, and is desperately trying to hang on to it. I think the evidence warrants the conclusion that the evolutionary origin of the phenomena of verbal hallucinations seen so clearly in schizophrenia is in this ancient preconscious mentality I have called the bicameral mind.

---

5 By "pure" I mean books of the Bible that for the mostpart are not mixtures from various sources as is most of the Old Testament. Prophets such as Amos were transitional persons retaining enough bicamerality to relay the words of gods to others with an authenticity that convinced.

Summary

Verbal hallucinations were studied in a variety of groups. In a sample of hospitalized schizophrenics and a sample of homeless people on the streets of New York City, such voices were often multiple, critical in women, but more often commands in men, and commonly religious. In a carefully randomized sample of normal college students, a questionnaire study revealed that almost a third had "clearly heard a voice when no one had spoken to me". The voices were identified as parents, friends, dead relatives, or God. From a study of "imaginary playmates", it was concluded that verbal hallucinations were occurring here also. And a non–verbal group of congenital quadriplegics, who had never spoken but with whom communication would be established, heard voices they identified as God, such voices being usually helpful.

Parallels were then drawn between modern verbal hallucinations and what is revealed in ancient texts. Ancient civilizations seem to have been governed by such hallucinations called gods, a mentality known as the bicameral mind. It was concluded that the reason verbal hallucinations are found so extensively, in every modern culture, in normal students, schizophrenics, children, and vividly reported in the texts of antiquity is that such hallucinations are an innate propensity, genetically evolved as the basis of an ancient preconscious mentality.

References

Adkins ADH: From the Many to the One. Cornell University Press, Ithaca, 1970.

Hamilton J: Auditory hallucinations in nonverbal quadriplegics. Psychiatry 48: 382–392, 1985.

Harvey NA: Imaginary playmates. State Normal College, Ipsilanti, 1918.

Jaynes J: The Origin of Consciousness in the Breakdown of the Bicameral Mind. Houghton Mifflin, Boston, 1976a. (German translation by Neff K: Der Ursprung des Bewusstseins durch den Zusammenbruch der Bicameralen Psyche, Rowohlt, Reinbeck, 1988).

Jaynes J: The evolution of language in the late Pleistocene. Annals of the New York Academy of Sciences, 280: 312–325, 1976b.

Jaynes J: Consciousness and the voices of the mind. Canadian Psychology 27: 128–186, 1986.

Moore MV: Binary Communication for the severely handicapped. Archives of Physical Medicine and Rehabilitation 53: 532–533, 1972.

Pines M: Invisible playmates. Psychology Today 12: 38–42, 1978.

Posey TB, Losch ME: Auditory hallucinations of hearing voices in 375 normal subjects. Imagination, Cognition, and Personality 2: 99–113, 1983.

Rosenberg ME: Auditory hallucinations in Princeton University Undergraduates. Senior thesis at Princeton University on file in the MuddLibrary, 1988.

Sappington J, Reedy S, Welch R, Hamilton J: Validity of messages from quadriplegic persons with cerebral palsy. American Journal on Mental Retardation 94: 49–52, 1989.

Snell B: The Discovery of Mind. Harvard University Press, Cambridge, 1953.

Schizophrenia and the Quantification of Semantic Phenomena:

How Can Something Mean Something?

Hinderk M. Emrich

1. Introduction

The Putnamian and Quineian part of this paper: how can something "mean" something?, referring to *The Meaning of Meaning* and the *Roots of Reference* may be taken as a dedication to the great philosophical climate of Harvard, and it is also to remind us of Wittgenstein's sentence in his *Blue Book* (1958, p. 15): "For an understanding 'of meaning' you certainly also have to understand the meaning of 'explanation of meaning'." Wittgenstein, in another context, has argued that philosophy is going to try to cure the wounds language produces, when it tries to overcome its own borders; and it is especially due to this problem of intentionality, that cognitive science comes into trouble when its main focus is on philosophy of language. The method I am going to propose here represents an operationalizing and quantifying approach to semantic phenomena and is non-linguistic. It may be regarded, therefore, as an interesting new paradigm bringing together functional neurobiology and philosophy of mind.

2. Three–Component–Interaction in Perception and Its Disturbance in Productive Psychoses

The three–component–model of perception assumes that perception is principally made up of three components: firstly, sensory input ("sensualistic" component); secondly, the internal production of concepts ("conceptualization"–component); and thirdly, control ("zensor"–component). It also assumes that the special interaction between these three components is responsible for the biologically fruitful and efficacious conscious internal representation of the external world during perception, and it is also assumed that the equilibrium between these three components is disturbed during psychosis.

The "conceptualization"–component can also be termed "phantasy-component", "hypotheses–generating–component" or "constructivistic-component". Its representation in the present model takes into account the fact that the processing of data is possible only on the basis of a conceptualization which has to be applied to the set of data, before a successful interpretation is possible. The "zensor" function can also be termed a "correcting" function and may be characterized as partially due to an "erasing"–system and partially to a "suppressing" or "rejecting" –system. From the point of view of a systems–theory of psychosis, schizophrenia appears not as an inherited disorder of metabolism, but as a weakness of a neurobiological "system", i.e. as an interactional disorder of a complex of networks, in which the interaction between different substructures is labile in such a way that under special conditions (e.g. "stress"), a decompensation (functional breakdown) results. In this sense, "vulnerability" to schizophrenia may be interpreted as a consequence of a constitutional deficiency of the brain which results in an inability to stabilize, under specially challenging conditions, the interaction between different substructures of the human brain.

The question arises as to which equilibrium between the three components of perception is "labilized" or disturbed during psychosis. The hypothesis to be established here is that the main disturbance in psychotogenesis is manifested in the equilibrium between the constructivistic component and the zensor function. For example, a weakness of the zensor system controlling auditory function, in relation to the endogenous production component, would explain patients experiencing "hearing voices" in addition to their normal auditory experience, since the correcting system is overwhelmed by an overproduction of the internal hypothesis-generating system: i.e. normal perception is always achieved by an internal process of "betting" (Gregory 1973), in the sense that more or less plausible hypotheses are falsified on the basis of external data sets, in relation to acquired experience, and that this "betting procedure" is disturbed in schizophrenia. According to Gregory, conscious perception is possible only on the basis of "perceptual hypotheses", and in "illusions, generated by ambiguity", "with hypothesis–switching, the data remain the same, but perception changes—so any changes must be 'sensual' and attached to specific hypotheses" ... "Hypotheses affect data, and data affect hypotheses" (Gregory 1973, p. 86). Having this in mind, it appears plausible to assume that schizophrenia results from a disequilibrium between an internal conceptualization processor and an (adaptive) correcting processor, leading to an amplification of internal (partially "nonsense") productions in this illness.

2.1 Binocular Depth Inversion

The phenomenon of depth inversion is documented impressively in the "Haunted Mansion" at Disneyland in California, where visitors see a pair of human faces that appear to rotate precisely as they walk by. In reality, these faces are three–dimensional inside–outside masks, which are perceived incorrectly as normal faces. This illusion of binocular "depth inversion" had been investigated by von Helmholtz and Mach in the 19th century; questions as to its basic mechanisms have been reconsidered by Gregory (1973). It has been demonstrated, especially in experiments by Yellott (1981) that visual experience is the result of "a process in which the brain tests hypotheses about the 3–dimensional shape of objects against the evidence provided by their retinal images". Binocular depth inversion does not occur under all conditions with inside–out 3–dimensional objects, but does so in those instances "with an overwhelmingly improbable real form so that it looks normal only when it is seen inverted in depth" (Yellott 1981, p. 120, cf. also Wolf 1987). Mental preconceptions appear to measure the sensory input in a critical way, creating visual experience, and this interaction is conceptualized by unconscious perceptual learning. From this point of view, visual depth inversion can be regarded as representing an indicator of the "correcting processor", mentioned above.

2.2 Impairment of Binocular Depth Inversion as an Indicator of Psychosis

A three–component–hypothesis of perception has been presented above, giving rise to the idea that the equilibrium between a constructivistic and a correcting processor function is disturbed in psychosis. Thus, the correction of preconceptions is assumed to be impaired in psychosis; and if the processor that is relevant for visual perception is disturbed in the way predicted by the present model, an impaired binocular depth inversion should be observed in psychotic patients. Such experiments have in fact been performed (Emrich 1988), using a stereoscopic projection–device and linearly polarized light: 40 schizophrenic patients (20 productive, and 20 non–productive schizophrenic patients) were investigated in comparison to 20 healthy volunteers. All the normal probands saw the three-dimensional inside–out faces as normal (not hollow) human faces, when the glasses were exchanged (i.e. the information for the right eye was given to the left eye and vice versa), whereas schizophrenics were unable to perform this binocular depth inversion completely; they all observed hollow face parts in these experiments, at least partially. The extent of this effect was dependent on the productivity of the psychosis, i.e. on the extent of the presence of actual hallucinations and delusional experiences.

This finding appears to support the idea that schizophrenic psychoses are not primarily due to a deficiency of a "filter" which protects the brain from an overload of information arising from the outer world, but results from a deficiency of an active correcting processor which interacts with both internal conceptualizations and external sensory data (i.e. the results indicate a deficiency in "correction" of the sensory data (cf. Emrich 1988, 1989).

Though developed independently, this concept has some analogy to Huxley's (1954) interpretation of the mode of action of psychedelic drugs, developed under the influence of Bergson and Broad, which states that these psychotogenic compounds tend to weaken an internal zensoring function, which is relevant for perception.

Also Malenka et al. (1982) observed central error in the correcting behavior of motor control in schizophrenic patients. The view of the basic deficiency in psychosis, elaborated here, appears to be in line with the concepts both of Huxley and of Malenka et al., insofar as it is assumed that internal correcting systems are deficient or in imbalance, in relation to conceptualization during a psychotic state.

3. "Subconscious Voting": The Interactive Structure of Mind

Within the recent past, a new science of mind has evolved, called "cognitive science", and it is assumed that this type of research will contribute substantially to the fundamentals of psychiatry. Within this science, the theory of consciousness is going to play an increasing role, an assertion which has e.g. recently been documented in a book on consciousness, edited by Tony Marcel and Eduardo Bisiach (1988). Consciousness is not a unitary entity, not a single well defined phenomenon, but is described by an array of terms such as "phenomenal awareness", "conscious decision–making", "intention", "emotion", and so forth, as described by Allport (1988). According to these recently developed concepts, "conscious phenomenal awareness" results from a dynamic interaction between several consciousness–producing subsystems, and the result of this interactive process is the conscious experience. The aim of the methodology introduced here is to look into this interaction of subsystems and to show which role a quantification of semantic phenomena plays within this interaction.

According to the three–component–hypothesis of perception, described above, the interactive process is taking place between the components of conceptualization, sensory data, and "zensor unit". Perceptual experiments e.g. with three–dimensional representations of Egyptian cuneiforms show that the degree of aquaintance with an object is critical for the perceptual experience together with other important factors, such as the direction of shadowing, as Ramachandran has shown (1988). Our preconscious system is accustomed to an environmental situation in which the light always comes from above. Another greatly contributing factor in the subconscious construction of depth–perception is the degree of disparity of retinal images. Interactive effects of these factors can be demonstrated in familiar vs. unfamiliar semantically meaningful structures such as e.g. animal masks (see above). As a result of such experiments a systematic variation of three variables is possible whereby we may perform a "titration" of the "semantic pressure" of such objects, since changes of the direction of shadowing, variation of disparity of retinal images, and the semantic content of accustomed objects, lead to different subjective conscious perceptual experiences; this allows for a quantitative insight into the inter-active processes which subconsciously take place and lead to the conscious perception of something which is "meaningful". Preliminary data in this regard have already been acquired.

4. How Something Can Mean Something: Intentional Hypersystems

Questions as to how something may "mean" something are intricately connected with the basics of the mind–body–problem. Max Planck has alluded to this in his sentence: "Science cannot solve the ultimate mystery of Nature. And it is because in the last analysis we ourselves are part of the mystery that we are trying to solve". Harold Rugg (1963), in his book "Imagination", gives an introduction into dualistic phenomenalism with the following sentences: "Man must live in two worlds the external physical world of other men and events and his inner psychophysiological world of sensations, images and ideas, moods and phantasies, wishes and needs". Donald MacKay, in several of his articles, especially in "A Mind's Eye View of the Brain" (1965) discriminates between "mind talk" and "brain talk" and argues: "What impresses me more and more is the element of irreducible mystery that attends our human condition (...) we have to face an irreducible dualism in our nature—not, of necessity, a dualism of 'stuffs', but a dualism of aspect which no mechanistic analysis can exhaust." The question how a system can be "intentional", how must it be organized to have the property of "aboutness" as Searle (1988) terms it, how can it contain the property of "meaning"?, may be analyzed if one considers the argument of Max Planck " ... we are part of the mystery we are trying to solve". In the recently developed theories of constructivism, as formulated by e.g. Watzlawick, von Förster, Luhmann, we are accustomed to argue that "informations are always internal constructs" (Luhmann, 1988). The "phenomenal awareness" we have when we experience perceptions, e.g. inversion–illusions, demonstrated above, is a constructivistic product elaborated by a system on a meta–level (called here "hypersystem"), which has the intrinsic capability to construe on its own two types of programs which can appear in the horizon of consciousness, one objectifying program, under the influence of which we are able to perceive "things", "objects", "systems", and one mentalizing program, which enables us to experience mental states like "qualia", "raw feels", etc. up to the level of thoughts, egos, etc.

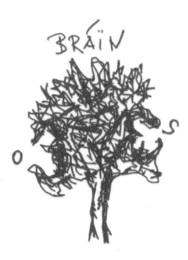

Figure 1: Interpretation see text.

The scheme in figure 1 represents these two types of programs (O: objectivity; S: subjectivity) and purposely has no formal similarity with the structure of the human brain, since it is to demonstrate that what science discovers when it investigates a "system", e.g. the neurobiology of the brain, is a result of the categorical schemes produced by the objectifying programs of the system organized at a meta–level. This "hypersystem" represents the empirical condition for the possibility of having a "mind–talk" as well as a "brain–talk". To signify this, it is termed here "bräïn" (in contrast to the common term of the empirical research object "Brain") and it is assumed—and insofar the end of this paper has associations to Kant as well as to Whitehead—that "bräïn–talk" is the monistic reality behind the phenomenological dichotomy between "mind–talk" and "brain–talk". Donald MacKay (1965) may be interpreted in this sense when he argues: "We have no grounds for postulating two sets of events, one mental, one physical, with tenuous links between. All our evidence so far justifies only treating human agency as a unity, which however does have two undeniably distinct aspects the inside aspect, which is what I feel and know, when I am making a decision, and the outside aspect, which is what the physiologist might see, if he had the means of looking inside my head."

Summary

One of the main topics of the present philosophy of mind is intentionality and the modes of generation of semantics. Quantitative experiments as to a subcomponent analysis in the generation of illusionary perception has the great advantage to be free of language and to be highly operationalized. Interestingly, schizophrenic patients and normal subjects under the condition of a "psychedelic state" experience a "desillusionized" perception in the 3–dimensional depth inversion paradigm. The philosophical implications of these findings in regard of a non–reductionistic monism are discussed.

References

Allport A: What concept of consciousness? In: Marcel AJ, Bisiach E (eds): Consciousness in Contemporary Science. Clarendon Press, Oxford, pp. 159–182, 1988.

Emrich HM: Zur Entwicklung einer Systemtheorie produktiver Psychosen. Nervenarzt 59: 456–464, 1988.

Emrich HM: A three–component–system hypothesis of psychosis. Impairment of binocular depth inversion as an indicator of a functional dysequilibrium. Brit. J. Psychiatry 155 (supp. 5): 37–39, 1989.

Gregory RL: The confounded eye. In: Gregory RL, Gombrich EH (eds). Illusion in Nature and Art. Freeman, Oxford, pp. 49–96, 1973.

Huxley A: The Doors of Perception. Chatto & Windus, London, 1954.

Luhmann N: Neuere Entwicklungen in der Systemtheorie. Merkur 42: 292–300, 1988.

MacKay DM: A mind's eye view of the brain. In: Wiener N, Schad JP (eds): Cybernetics of the Nervous System (Progress in Brain Research, Vol. 17). Elsevier, Amsterdam, pp. 321–332, 1965.

Malenka RC, Angel RW, Hampton B, Berger PA Impaired central error–correcting behavior in schizophrenia. Arch. Gen. Psychiatry 39: 101–107, 1982.

Marcel AJ, Bisiach E (eds): Consciousness in Contemporary Science. Clarendon Press, Oxford, 1988.

Ramachandran VS: Perception of shape from shading. Nature 331: 163–166, 1988.

Rugg H: Imagination. Harper & Row, New York, 1963.

Searle J: Minds and brains without programs. In: Blakemore C, Greenfield S (eds): Mindwaves, Blackwell, Oxford, pp. 209–233, 1988.

Wittgenstein L: The Blue Book. Basil Blackwell, Oxford, 1958.

Wolf R: Der biologische Sinn der Sinnestuschung. Biologie in unserer Zeit 17: 33–49, 1987.

Yellott JIJr: Binocular depth inversion. Sci. Amer. 245: 118–125, 1981.

Why Thinking is Easy

Steven Matthysse

1. The Facility of Thinking

The facility of ordinary thinking is one of the unexplained marvels of psychology. There is no sign that we calculate before we speak, nor that we struggle to form our thoughts correctly. Normal thinking demands no special concentration and takes hardly any time. We do not have to sift through a mixture of logical and illogical or grammatical and ungrammatical thoughts. The mind is free to spend its energy on selecting the effective thought or the appropriate expression from the possibilities offered to it. There is not even any sign that as children we once were clumsy in our thinking, but have practiced the skill to the point where it has become automatic. The child's thoughts occur as abundantly as the adult's, and they spontaneously obey rules of form appropriate to his age. He moves as easily in that realm as we do in our own.

Thought seems to operate as if it had available an intrinsically well behaved raw material. Of course there is effort involved—to maintain focus, to put ideas together in new ways, to convince, impress or amuse— but well–formed elements of thought come to the thinker, prior to any active work on his part, in abundance and with an inherent tendency to combine in ways that are logically appropriate.

In severe psychopathology, this preconditioning of thought is lost. Either nothing at all comes to mind (as may occur in Alzheimer's disease) or the thoughts that do come to mind combine in perverse ways that violate logic and common sense (as in schizophrenia). Through conscious mental effort, thought can be redirected into normal channels, and indeed schizophrenic patients in the early stages try to regain control over their thinking, but usually they fail. Their substitution of conscious mental effort for what is normally an automatic process accounts in part for the slowness and poor performance of schizophrenic patients on nearly all psychological tests.

2. Mechanical versus Formal Laws

I do not think that this disability is a loss of normal "filtering". Normal people do not need to filter out ill–formed thoughts. They choose among good candidates. It may be that schizophrenics "fail to screen their own potential responses for appropriateness" (Chapman et al. 1977, p. 164), but their minds seem to be offered possibilities for ideation that just would not occur to normal people. Consider this excerpt from a dialogue with a schizophrenic woman who was asked to complete the sentence "a fish can live in water because...": "Because it's learned to swim. *What if it couldn't swim?* Not naturally, he couldn't. Why do certain gods have effects on seas like that? What does the earth have such an effect to break their backs? The fishes near home come to the surface and break. *Why?* I think it is due to bodies that people lose. A body becomes adapted to the air. Think thoughts and break the fishes." (Cameron 1938, p. 25) The normal brain does not offer thoughts like these as candidates for ideation. For most people, it is more difficult to think an abnormal thought than a normal one.

I find it hard to believe that any process of unconscious random generation and testing could be efficient enough to account for the facility of normal thinking. Rather the actions of neurons on each other must, in some unknown way, automatically fulfill the laws of thought (Matthysse 1987).

At first such a process is hard to imagine, because the kind of law that characterizes thinking is very different from the kind of law that characterizes processes in the brain. What makes thought lawful is its limitation by what linguists call *rules of competence*. These are rules that well–formed expressions must satisfy, but not rules for producing them (Chomsky 1965, p. 9). Our thought must conform to rules of syntax, semantics, logic and emotional coherence. It must avoid the twenty categories of thought disorder (Johnston and Holzman 1979, pp. 69–70). We cannot yet formulate the rules of competence precisely, but we can instinctively tell thought disorder when we hear it. Like mathematical axioms, the laws of thought are strict in what they exclude but allow great freedom in what they include. They evaluate and criticize but do not determine. They are *juridical.*[1]

The lawfulness of brain–processes, on the other hand, is a lawfulness of *operations*. Neurons act on each other, electrically and chemically. It is the same kind of law that characterizes bodies colliding in space: mechanical, inescapable, acting only at the moment of interaction without regard for consequences.

Throughout nature, however, mechanical laws are found to fulfill formal laws. Light always traverses the space between its origin and its destination in the shortest possible time, although the light beam does not stop to calculate, and it is not in a hurry. In economics the "invisible hand" of Adam Smith (in theory at least) causes the free market to allocate

---

1 Dr. Maher (this volume) stressed that thinking evolved for its survival value in the real world, not for its logical perfection in the world of formal mathematics. Thought is nevertheless lawful in its own way; discovering its empirical laws is one of psychology's greatest challenges.

resources optimally, even though each agent blindly pursues his selfish gain.

Valence in chemistry is another familiar example, which thanks to John Stuart Mill became one of psychology's favorite analogies. "When many impressions or ideas are operating in the mind together, there sometimes takes place a process of a similar kind to chemical combination...The Complex Idea, formed by the blending together of several simpler ones, should...be said to *result from*, or be *generated by*, the simple ideas, not to *consist of* them." (Mill 1881, p. 592). The laws of valence, like the laws of thought, are permissive as well as strict. Dimethyl ether and ethyl alcohol, for example, have the same atomic compostion (C_2H_6O) but different structures (CH_3–O–CH_3 and CH_3–CH_2–OH). Large molecules typically have many isomers.

3. Fast and Slow Processes in Dynamical Systems

Snowflakes are a beautiful example of harmony between mechanical and formal laws. The crystal structure of ice has symmetries—a hexagonal screw axis, mirror planes and glide planes—which constrain the forms snowflakes may take, but still allow endless variety. When supersaturated water vapor from a reservoir at water temperature T_w is allowed to freeze on a fine hair at a colder air temperature T_a, snow crystals form artificially (Nakaya 1954, Fig. 286). The geometrical forms of the crystals depend systematically on T_w and T_a (Nakaya 1954, Fig. 444).

Light beams, the market place, chemical bonding and snowflakes are examples of the fulfillment of formal laws by mechanical laws, but they are so diverse that they leave us without any general principle. There is a more universal way of looking at the relationship between mechanical and formal laws that may help us understand how these concepts apply to the brain.

As the science of mechanics flowered in the 18th and 19th centuries, the notion gradually arose of picturing the states of a physical system as a geometrical space, called a *phase space*, with one coordinate for each degree of freedom. There might be a large number of dimensions; to describe the motion of the solar system one would need 9 x 3 coordinates for the planetary positions, and an additional 9 x 3 for the velocities. The "phase point" moves in a 54–dimensional space. Constructing such a large space is worth the trouble because if you know the system's location in phase space at one time, you can predict its trajectory at all future times.

After a system is allowed to run undisturbed for a long time, its trajectory usually settles down to a small portion of its phase space. It may converge to a single point (a steady state) and stay there, as in a chemical reaction coming to equilibrium. It may converge to a periodic orbit, or *limit cycle*, as in the motion of the planets. It may also converge to a very complex trajectory, called a *strange attractor*. The meteorologist E.N. Lorenz first discovered strange attractors in a simplified model of weather prediction, where the coordinates of the phase space represent temperature gradients and convective air flow (Lichtenberg and Lieberman 1983, Fig. 1.19). After a long time the system converges, but it does not become quiescent. On the contrary, its motion remains turbulent and unpredictable, even though it is restricted to a limited part of the phase space. Any slight perturbation will be amplified indefinitely at later times. Motion of this kind is called "chaotic". If the length of time it takes the phase point to sample its limit cycle or its strange attractor is sufficiently short, the details of its trajectory will average out within the time that it takes for the system to exert any action. In that case, its effective states can be enumerated by the attractors themselves.

In dynamical systems, *multiple* attractors often coexist. If rain falls on the Continental Divide it heads either for the Atlantic or the Pacific ocean. The whole region west of the Continental Divide is the *basin* of the Pacific attractor, and the eastern region, the basin of the Atlantic attractor.

As the number of degrees of freedom of a dynamical system increases, the number of co–existing attracting states can become astronomical. Solid state physics provides striking examples. Consider first an ordinary ferromagnet, where the atoms are arranged regularly on a crystal lattice. Each atom influences its neighbors to orient their spins in the direction of its own. There is a temperature (the "Curie temperature") above which the noise of molecular motion wins out, and alignment of atoms is random. Below the Curie temperature, all atoms become aligned in the same direction. In this case the number of attracting states is small, just one for each direction in which the overall magnetic vector may lie. There are also anti-ferromagnetic substances, such as manganese oxide, in which neighboring atoms tend to orient opposite to each other. Below the Curie temperature anti–ferromagnetic substances become as uniform as ferromagnets, except that instead of all atoms pointing in the same direction, there is a regular alternation of orientations. There is still only one dynamical attractor for each direction in space.

Interesting things begin to happen when both attractive and repulsive forces are allowed between neighboring atoms in the lattice. The alloy europium–strontium–sulfide has the crystal structure of ordinary sodium chloride, but it has unusual magnetic properties. In europium nearest-neighbor interactions are ferromagnetic, while next–nearest–neighbor interactions are anti–ferromagnetic. The strontium alloyed with the europium does not have a strong magnetic effect on its own, but it causes randomness in the lattice. The closest europium to a given europium atom may be its nearest neighbor, or it may be its next–nearest neighbor, if a strontium atom has intervened in the lattice. Therefore some interactions between pairs of europium atoms are ferromagnetic, while some are anti-ferromagnetic. At certain temperatures and proportions of europium and strontium, a remarkable state arises called a *spin glass* (Maletta and Felch 1979).

The force producing the spin glass state can be most easily understood in two dimensions, following a model of Villain (1977, p. 4794). Imagine a square (also called a "plaquette") with magnetic atoms at each corner, and assume that the   interactions along each edge of the square are either ferromagnetic or anti–ferromagnetic. It is possible for the ferromagnetic and anti–ferromagnetic interactions to be arranged in such a way that no alignment of the atoms satisfies all neighboring pairs; the plaquette is said to be "frustrated". Frustrated plaquettes have two states of lowest energy, although neither state is as favorable as the energy minimum of the   all–ferromagnetic or all–antiferromagnetic case. The two energy–minimizing states are said to have + and − "chiralities". Adjacent plaquettes tend to have opposite chiralities, like the red and black squares on a checkerboard.

If the ferromagnetic and anti–ferromagnetic interactions in the lattice are arranged at random so that both frustrated and unfrustrated plaquettes are present, "islands" of frustrated plaquettes with alternating   chiralities will be surrounded by unfrustrated "seas". The "seas" isolate the "islands" from each other according to Villain's model, and permit them to align themselves independently. Unlike the ferromagnet or anti–ferromagnet, no long–range order is present over the whole lattice. Vast numbers of combinations, approximately equal in energy, are possible.

4. Attractor Combinations as a Formal Language

Now we have enough background to return to the main problem: how mechanical interactions can fulfill formal laws. Imagine an array of identical dynamical systems capable of interacting with each other (identity is not essential). Initially, let the systems be uncoupled:

$$A \quad B \quad C \quad D$$

Each system is in one of its attracting states. The combination ABCD could be interpreted as a string of symbols in a formal language, whose vocabulary is the list of attractors of the members of the array. Now let an interaction be switched on between the systems. During the period of the interaction, the individual members of the array coalesce into one large system, and no longer have attracting states of their own:

$$A \leftrightarrow B \leftrightarrow C \leftrightarrow D$$

The combined system will undergo a transient motion in its own phase space, and fall into the basin of one of its attractors, which (unless the interaction is very weak) will not correspond in any simple way to the attractors of the uncoupled subsystems. Now let the interaction be switched off. The subsystems will once again become independent, and each will converge to one of its own attracting states, but not necessarily the one it started from:

$$\text{A'} \quad \text{B'} \quad \text{C'} \quad \text{D'}$$

Which basin it falls into will depend on the exact state of the combined system at the moment the interaction stopped. The sequence of attractors A'B'C'D' might be read as a second string of symbols in the formal language. Mechanical interactions have transformed one string of symbols into another.

If this process of alternating coupling and uncoupling goes on for a long time, the symbol strings can themselves be regarded as a dynamical system undergoing a motion in a phase space, which we will call the *symbol–string space*. Since, during the interaction phase, the coupled system is rapidly sampling its attractor, its exact state at the time the interaction ends is a random variable. Consequently the motion in the symbol–string space, unlike the dynamical systems we have considered so far, is not deterministic. It is a *random walk*. If we assume that each member of the array samples its attractor nearly completely in the time between coupling phases, the random walk will have the Markov property: it will not remember its past history.

States A_i of a Markov chain are either *recurrent* or *transient*, according to whether the probability that, starting in state A_i, the chain eventually returns to A_i is 1 or <1. Recurrent states always recur infinitely often; transient states always recur only a finite number of times (Karlin and Taylor 1975, Theorem 2.7.1). The random walk in symbol–string space will, therefore, (like other dynamical processes) converge to a subregion in the course of time. A *formal language* is defined by a vocabulary and an allowed set of strings from that vocabulary (Hopcroft and Ullman 1979), so the dynamical process in symbol–string space may be said to generate a formal language. A formal law (the rules which select the allowed symbol strings in the language) has arisen from a mechanical law (the interactions between the dynamical systems). There is no guarantee, of course, that the formal language is coherent or useful; that will depend on the specific interactions that generate it.

We have seen that dynamical systems sample their attractors over time. The dynamical system in symbol–string space will, similarly, run through its repertoire of strings during the course of its trajectory. It may take a long time to cover them all. Suppose, however, that there is a large *ensemble* of interacting systems, each going repeatedly through the process of coupling and uncoupling, and a corresponding ensemble of random walks in symbol–string space. At any moment of time, the symbol–string systems in their individual phase spaces will be distributed randomly throughout the region of recurrent states. Consequently the ensemble will present the entire formal language *at once*, like a parallel processing computer.

5. Attractors in Neuronal Assemblies

Since this argument is rather general, I would like to show how it might apply to the brain. To make the link I have to use uncomfortably vague expressions like "neuronal assembly". Experimentalists naturally look askance at such ill–defined phrases. I am willing to use them here because I think attractors in neuronal assemblies might someday help explain computation in the nervous system, but neuroscience has not developed to the point where these ideas can be given precise meaning. I am grateful for the opportunity to present them to this audience, because it may be that shoots too fragile for the rough winds of the laboratory will ripen in the gentler climate of philosophy.

It is not obvious what aspect of the activity of neuronal assemblies should be regarded as the fundamental computing unit. Consider, for example, a "parabolic burster" neuron modeled after cells in *Aplysia* (Rinzel 1987, Fig. 6). The interspike interval, which is smallest when the firing rate is highest, has a parabolic shape as a function of time, which gives the neuron its name. Is the computational state of a circuit including neurons like these encoded by individual spikes, by firing rates, by slow membrane potentials, by the rising–and–falling pattern of firing, or by temporal correlations between one cell and another?

Our previous discussion of attractors suggests an answer. If the length of time it takes the assembly to sample its limit cycle or its strange attractor is sufficiently short, the electrophysiological details of the system's trajectory will average out within the time it takes the cell assembly to carry out any action. The computational state of the assembly will correspond to the attractor itself.

Multiple attractors have been shown to exist in some neurophysiological systems. In the Hodgkin–Huxley model of the nerve membrane, there are conditions under which both steady and oscillatory membrane potentials coexist as possible stable states (Rinzel 1978). Bunney's laboratory has described dopaminergic neurons in the substantia nigra of freely moving animals that switch spontaneously between single spike and bursting modes (Freeman et al. 1985). These neurons seem to be organized as small assemblies of cells electrically coupled to each other (Grace and Bunney 1983).

The alternating coupling–uncoupling process that I mentioned before is reminiscent of an eloquent description by William James of the succession of slow and fast phases in our thinking. "When the rate [of change] is slow," he wrote, "we are aware of the object of our thought in a comparatively restful and stable way. When rapid, we are aware of a passage, a relation, a transition *from* it, or *between* it and something else. As we take, in fact, a general view of the wonderful stream of our consciousness, what strikes us first is this different pace of its parts. Like a bird's life, it seems to be made of an alternation of flights and perchings. The rhythm of language expresses this, where every thought is expressed in a sentence, and every sentence closed by a period" (James 1984, p. 55). When thought is "perching" it has momentarily attained an object, just as neuronal assemblies in the uncoupled phase are momentarily expressing a symbol string in the formal language. Perhaps, therefore, the couplings and uncouplings of interacting neuronal assemblies correspond to the "flights" and "perchings" of thought.

Since psychopathology is our theme, I would like to say a little about how schizophrenic thought could be accounted for from the dynamical system point of view. Earlier I remarked that the form snowflakes take depends on T_w and T_a, the temperature at which the supersaturated vapor is formed and the temperature at which it freezes. Dynamical attractors can undergo dramatic changes as their environments change. For example, a slight change in a parameter can cause a system that was restricted to a well–defined region in phase space to lose all constraint, and wander erratically over a wide region (Peitgen and Richter 1986, Figs. 10 and 13; Barnsley 1988, Fig. 7.2). It is conceivable that a change in the biochemical environment of the brain could similarly alter the dynamics of the coupled system in such a way that it would fail to restrict the subsystems properly upon uncoupling. The formal language would have too many acceptable strings. Thoughts would slip out of their normal constraints.

6. Conclusions

In order to progress toward a concrete model based on these ideas, we need to know much more about attracting states of neural circuits. I think this is an empirical research area of great promise. Too much attention has been lavished on networks made up of highly contrived "lollipop neurons" which tend to have the integrative properties that their designers expected in advance. Real neurons and real neuronal circuits are very unlike conventional computing elements, so it is likely that their principles of computation differ as well. Otherwise the head would be full of silicon. The mathematics of realistic neurons and neural circuits is very difficult, but I think it is likely to open up computational possibilities undreamed of by computer engineers. By grounding our models in the properties of real neurons we may discover interactions that are capable of fulfilling formal laws of thought, and ultimately explain *why thinking is easy*.[2]

Summary

Ordinary thinking is astonishingly easy, considering the multitude of operations involved. Normal people select from an abundance of well–formed thoughts. In schizophrenia, this preconditioning of thought is lost;

---

2 Whatever grounding in facts these speculations may have is due largely to conversations with Steven Bunney, Eugene Roberts, David Ruelle and David Turnbull. The author wishes to thank them.

patients have to struggle to filter out ill–formed thoughts. It is difficult to imagine how *mechanical laws* (interactions of neurons) can fulfill *formal laws* (syntax, logic, appropriateness). Dynamical systems theory suggests a direction in which an answer may be found. In general, any isolated dynamical system, after transients decay, will gravitate toward one of a discrete set of *attracting states*. If brief interactions are allowed to occur between isolated systems, their attracting states will undergo perturbations. These transformations are postulated to obey selection rules similar to a formal language. Study of the dynamical systems properties of actual neuronal circuits may reveal interactions that are capable of fulfilling formal laws of thought.

References

Barnsley M: Fractals Everywhere. Academic Press, Boston, 1988.

Cameron N: Reasoning, regression and communication in schizophrenics. Psychological Monographs 50: 1–34, 1938.

Chapman LJ, Chapman JP, Miller GA: A theory of verbal behavior in schizophrenia. Postscript to reprint. In: Maher BA (ed): Contributions to the psychopathology of schizophrenia. Academic press, New York, 1977, pp. 164–167.

Chomsky N: Aspects of the Theory of Syntax. M.I.T. Press, Cambridge, MA, 1965.

Freeman AS, Meltzer LT, Bunney BS: Firing properties of substantia nigra dopamine neurons in freely moving rats. Life Sciences 36: 1983–1994, 1985.

Grace AA, Bunney BS: Intracellular and extracellular electrophysiology of nigral dopaminergic neurons – 3. Evidence for electrotonic coupling. Neuroscience 10: 333–348, 1983.

Hopcroft JE, Ullman JD: Introduction to Automata Theory, Languages, and Computation. Addison–Wesley, Reading, MA, 1979.

James W: The Essential Writings. B.W. Wilshire, ed., State University of New York Press, Albany, NY, 1984

Johnston MH, Holzman PS: Assessing Schizophrenic Thinking: A Clinical and Research Instrument for Measuring Thought Disorder. Jossey–Bass, San Francisco, 1979.

Karlin S, Taylor HM: A First Course in Stochastic Processes. Second ed., Academic Press, New York, 1975.

Lichtenberg AJ, Lieberman MA: Regular and Stochastic Motion. Springer, New York, 1983.

Maletta H, Felch W: Insulating spin–glass system Eu(x)Sr(1–x)S. Phys Rev B20: 1245–1260, 1979.

Matthysse S: Schizophrenic thought disorder: a model–theoretic perspective. Schizophrenia Bull 13: 173–184, 1987.

Mill JS: A System of Logic, Ratiocinative and Inductive. 8th ed., Harper, New York, 1881.

Nakaya U: Snow Crystals: Natural and Artificial. Harvard Univ. Press, Cambridge, MA, 1954.

Peitgen H–O, Richter Ph: The Beauty of Fractals: Images of Complex Dynamic Systems. Springer, Berlin, 1986.

Rinzel J: On repetitive activity in nerve. Fed Proc 37: 2793–2802, 1978.

Rinzel J, Lee YS: Dissection of a model for neuronal parabolic bursting. J Math. Biol 25: 653–675, 1987.

Villain J: Two–level systems in a spin–glass model: I. General formalism and two-dimensional model. J Phys C 10: 4793–4803, 1977.

On the Development of Categories

Peter Klein

The title of this paper[1] when read within the horizon of "normal" history of philosophy seems to denote a contradictio in adiecto since all this history would deny categories as subjects of change. I want to show here that this impression is due to a too narrow interpretation, and that the proposed understanding offers good chances for a fruitful contact between philosophy and psychology.

1. Categories

Categories are generally defined as the *basic*, most *general* concepts in philosophy for the purpose of understanding the world, its qualities and its development. As such, they comprise as well material (like "matter", "substance", "essence") as also formal concepts (like "space", "relation", ...).

Aristotle was the first to create a system of categories as a framework of concepts apt to guide science and to be elaborated by it. Being a disciple of Plato, his system contains some platonistic basic assumptions which, due to the farreaching influence of Aristotle also in science since have continued to act as basic undercurrents in both philosophy and science: Categories through the centuries have unquestionably been supposed to denote "essential" ("ideal") and eternal, unchangeable qualities of the world. Furthermore, their Greek origin gave them the basic Greek approach towards the world which was to trust in nature's αλητεια (revelation), a belief in the tendency of nature to become manifest to the human mind, and of human mind to be attached to the truth of nature. From this trust resulted a third supposition: that human mind and the world are coordinated, that there is an isomorphic relation between them, so that those basic concepts, once gained by true philosophical reflection, do in fact express the true and basic shape of the world. The concept of categories in all epistemologically "realistic" systems (from Jungius' "Protonoetica" and Leibniz' "mathesis universalis" to those of Marx and Nicolai Hartmann) are of this kind. In speaking mainly about the *world*, however, their scientific outcome would be *physics* (though a metaphysically founded one), so they are not so relevant in the present context.

1 Contributing to this conference has been made possible by a generous gift of the *Hansische Universitätsstiftung*, Hamburg.

2. Categories and Psychology

More interesting for us, in a conference dealing with philosophical issues of *psycho*pathology (or in a wider sense: psychology) is the radical change in our understanding of categories that Kant inaugurated. He takes categories as qualities of *mind*, as structures of the human ability to think, as the precondition of getting knowledge about the world. They constitute the *formal* framework that leads to knowledge about the world only by experience, with experience giving its *material* part. Thus, the system of categories in Kant's sense does not of itself lead to knowledge about the qualities of the world as it is, but directs and sets the limits of how our mind may get knowledge about it. It thus acts as a formal filter of what may come into mind at all.

This concept is revolutionary in two respects:

—Categories are supposed as pure forms,—as the structure of knowledge. This is not completely new, because many of the classical categories had a formal character, too. But now *all* categories are declared formal, including those which classically had been assumed to be material (like "substance", "(material) causality"), whilst all material contributions to knowledge are declared a matter of experience (instead of being at least in part metaphysical[2]).

—Previously, categories meant qualities of the world, which were only reflected in our mind. Now they mean qualities of mind which direct how the world may get into our mind at all. Thus truth about the world can never be gained, and categories change their character from being structures of the world to being structures of cognition.

However, there still remains a fundamental role for the hypothetical basis of objects of cognition. Kant's saying, that "our mind dictates to nature its own laws" (Kant 1783, A 113) does not mean the view whereby Hegel exaggerated the old idea of rationalistic construction of the world, namely by mere use of the laws of mind, independent of experience; for Kant, cognition is rather a balance between experience and its formal conditions in the mind that dictate *how* these hypothetical "true" laws come into mind.

So Kant preserves the independence of the *objects* of mind (their character of standing *against* mind, as the German term "Gegen–stand" denotes, "so that our mind will not vanish into vague indefiniteness" (Kant, *Critique of Pure Reason* A 104). On the other hand, it seems only plausible to attribute the *structures* that determine how we think about objects to the side of the *medium* of thinking them. That means that we define this structure as one of the functional regions of *mind* and we declare them to be the subject of psychology.

But in spite that Kant himself derived his categories from the formal functions of mind, namely the logical laws of Aristotelian syllogistics, he

---

2 I leave out of consideration here the difficult problems exposed by Kant's *Metaphysische Anfangs-gründe der Naturwissenschaft*.

would not have called this "psychology", and his idealistic followers of course have emphasized his view by declaring it a self-consistent philosophical activity of mind itself. Especially, with respect to psychology as an empirical science, his followers would have vigorously denied that Kant's system could be understood as a result of the *empirical* study of mind. So let us first study its epistemological status and then proceed to categorical development.

3. Idealizing Empiricism in Study of Mind

In spite of its esoteric nomenclature (which however Kant chose for reasons of exactness) the system of categories basically expresses something quite simple and familiar:

If we want to think about an object of cognition we first have to organize sensual data into concepts amenable for cognitive operations. We do so by constructing them in a way that allows us to think and to speak of them by means of sentences. We construct and combine these sentences by logical laws, and the complete system of them exhausts the functions of our thinking ability. Logical laws denote the possible functions of concepts within sentences, so they must be constructed so that their structure fits into the different structures of a sentence.

Hence, these structures are not statements about the objects themselves but are structural qualities so that statements about the objects corresponding to concepts may be formulated,—a kind of grammar.

Kant now uses the different syllogisms as a guide to discover *all* functions of cognition in a systematical order[3]—he was confident that he could fulfill this demand because the syllogisms were traditionally supposed to be a complete system. This process has been misunderstood as one in which Kant had derived them merely as a self–consistent system independent of experience with our mind. But logic *is* experiential knowledge about our mind because if we study our mind we find hims to be forced to follow the logical laws (as we find a stone to follow the laws of gravitation). Kant could have gone a different way by just describing what he finds when looking at concepts. Perhaps he would not then have been sure of the completeness of his findings, but let us try to go this alternative way, and this is what probably he would have found:

—Concepts must be constructed from a continuous stream of sensory data to differentiate single objects ("Unity"), discriminated from the "Multiplicity" of other ones, all of them when seen together constituting the "Totality" of possible objects—and these are the categories of "Quantity";

---

3 This aim of Kant for a complete and systematical order of categories distinguishes his from all preceding lists of categories,—which Kant calls just "rhapsodies" (*Critique of Pure Reason* A 81; see also Kant 1783, A 118).

—concepts must allow us to attribute qualities to the objects ("Reality") and to deny others ("Negation"); now qualities are never attributed by simple "yes" or "no", but must be gradually determined by their respective opposites ("Limitation")—and this is the group of categories with respect to "Quality";

—we think objects not as isolated, but as exhibiting "Relations" to each other: with respect to themselves: qualities which endure in time (we call "substantial"), which change ("accidental"): category of "Inherence/Subsistence"; when following one after the other: did the one "cause" the other?: "Causality/Dependency"; when experienced at the same time: do they interact?: "Interaction";

—finally we have to ask for the ontological status of a concept/sentence: is it a game played with possible ideas, denoting an object of possible experience?: "Possibility/Impossibility"; does sensual experience correspond to it?: "Existence/Non-existence"; is its existence inevitable if only it is thought of?: "Necessity/Accidentality"—and these are the categories of the mode of existence ("Modality")[4].

I think it is clear that there is nothing mysterious about that scheme of Kant's; if we "look at" our concept–constructing mind we see that it really works in that way; what is lacking of course is the part played by experience, namely to fill up this formal scheme with concrete sensual experience so that knowledge will result.

"We look at" an object (here: our mind) "and then we see"—that is the language of experiential knowledge (that is turned into science by the aim of systematization); and since the object is our mind, the corresponding experiential science would be psychology, so Kant's findings should be called "psychology". Why is that opposed by Kant—not to speak of his followers—and by psychologists, too?

First Kant: He does not just *describe* what he finds out when looking at his mind or when he reconstructs the minds of others by communicating with them, but he rather constructs a systematic structure on the basis of his empirical data. To do this is called "speculation", and this term and concept since has undergone decline and distortion, currently denoting mere conceptual fantasies from the blue sky. But this in fact would be only the distorted version of what every scientist is expected to do: he is supposed not only to collect data and to describe them, but to embed them into a conceptual system that results in a well ordered theory. (Furthermore, however, Kant's system has a normative function which we will have to analyze later when speaking about development.)

---

4 The last one, "Necessity", sounds rather mysterious, and if understood as usual as a final explanation ("Letztbegründung") it would be. But Kant illustrates the true meaning by his third "postulate of empirical thinking at all" (*Critique of Pure Reason* A 218) and his commentary A 227: If we have a natural law ("possibility") and a given experience ("existence"), the empirical consequences may be derived by just applying the natural law: that in this sense they happen with "necessity" no scientist would deny. In the language of modern physics: Let a natuiral law be given by a differential equation. Its solution is an inclination field determined with the only exception of a constant factor. Given this factor by experience as a "boundary factor" the solution of the differential equation is uniquely determined.

Now psychology: To look at one's own mind in order to "describe" it is a matter of introspection, and this method seems to lack intersubjective validity necessary for science, as esp. behavioristic psychologists have emphasized. In the strict sense of orthodox behaviorism this certainly is true, but then it would apply to "hard" science like physics, too: each experience happens in the mind of each single observer; that two observers see "the same" and think on it in the same way—to assume this is always only the result of successful communication.

So, apart from that normative aspect mentioned, Kant's system of categories is true experiential psychology about the structure of the object–constructing mechanisms in mind.[5]

4. Types of Category Development

According to Kant, categories are the formal basis of cognition, they are the condition only by the use of which knowledge may be gained. If so, they must be at hand whenever cognition occurs; hence they must be "prior" to experience, must "underlie" it, antecede it, or whatever term one may choose. Kant himself uses all of them, and the usual interpretation is that his "apriori" means an antecedence in *time*, following this scheme: here is the brain and its mind; it has a certain ready structure acting as a tool to be applied to sensory data, and the result will be cognition. Our psychological analysis showed us a certain plausibility of that scheme. Kant even declares it to be universal, invariable and of general validity.

Different fields in psychology however, esp. developmental and educational psychology show that this image cannot be the full truth: children show a different, or an only rudimentary structure of "our" thinking, the same is true for the mentally sick, but one certainly cannot say that they have no cognitions at all.

Furthermore, developmental psychology shows a more or less universal sequence of the developmental process towards an adult mind, a sequence that seems to follow certain rules and laws. Although these laws are not yet known in full detail, one may at least say that the conditions of development are a mixture of innate genetic programs and environmental influences; children need contact and interaction with the environment—very often even of a *suitable* environment—so that their genetic programs will be actualized and will lead to a manifest development so that finally it will result in—why not!—Kant's system of categories as their structure of mind. But what is true now? Are categories prior to experience, or experience prior to categories? Obviously the latter, a process of development

---

5   This was so familiar to pre–Hegelian philosophers that it usually was not explicitly mentioned. (Goethe, in the *Annalen* of the year 1794, when reporting his conversation with Schiller about the "Urpflanze" characterizes Schiller's Kantian standpoint as "taking nature from the side of some *empirical human naturalities*" ("Natürlichkeiten"); Goethe 1830, p. 36.)

towards adult structure of mind by means of experience that happen to any single person.

There is another process of development to be considered; it concerns the genetic programs mentioned. Where do they come from? Man did not exist from the beginning of time, and there are different animals which certainly possess a different structure of their "minds". Since Man is considered to have evolved from animals, his mind must have acquired the structure of mind that characterizes him now at some time during his evolution, and this must have happened by fitting "mind" to environment by prolonged selective interaction, that means: by experience. Kant's epistemological a priori must be considered as an evolutionary a posteriori (Riedl 1979, pp. 54f, 181f)—that is the basic idea of "Evolutionary Epistemology".

So when speaking of a development of the formal structure of cognition showing a change of the categorical system we have to discriminate at least two different processes, both being based on experience, namely

—the "phylogenetic" development of the specific cognitive structure of a species, gained by interaction with its environment, fixed in its genotype as a disposition to become manifest during the second process,

—the "morphogenetic" development of the cognitive structure of a single creature, based on genetic dispositions and actualized by interaction with his environment during the individual development.

In biology, the last process usually, but unfortunately is called "ontogenesis", but I did not use this term reserving its use, according to philosophical tradition, to reconstruct here what Kant really meant with his aprioristic concept of cognition. For we may assume that Kant was intelligent enough to realize that these two developmental processes are seemingly contradictory to his analysis.

5. "Ontogenesis" of Cognition

If we want to avoid conflicts with Kant's terminology, we cannot use the term "experience" with respect to interactions of creatures with their environment if these are based on structures different from those that Kant denotes; instead, we have to look for different terms for all those different phases in the evolutionary and individual development, because they mean something different; whether the one or the other "exists" beyond its "meaning" does not matter. We cannot even speak of "the" specific kind of respective interaction, because this is also continuously changing in accordance with the underlying structure of cognition at each moment. In fact it is the task of developmental psychology to describe these different phases, and the well known conceptual difficulties in developmental psychology result not only from this continuous flow, but especially from the necessity to use stable terms and relate them to concepts which both *pretend* a stability that in reality does not exist, being only conceptual constructions.

This difficulty well known to psychologists has also been the problem with a correct understanding of what Kant really means. As with every scientist, Kant had to fix a flowing reality in order to apply constant concepts to it. The aim of his Critique of Pure Reason is to describe "the" structure of "cognitive reason"—not as a developing reason, but as a comparatively stable system when it has come to a comparatively terminal state in its structural development at a certain state of adulthood. This assumption, in spite of the fact that a human being usually develops till his death, is to a certain extent confirmed by cognitive psychology. At this state, Kant says, his system of categories "underlies" every experience. Obviously, this does not mean, that it is prior to experiences during development in a historical sense, but in a *systematic* sense. In describing the underlying cognitive structure, he describes the system of interrelations of its components. This is a conceptual analysis, a systematic "dissection" (in a truly medical sense: "Zergliederung") of this structure which is not a chronological succession of activities but a unity of a whole ("Synthesis", or in more detail: "the synthetic unity of apperception") which is only expressed in a seemingly chronological order because the discursive character of our mind forces us to do so. Cognition by this synthesis may be called "generated" too, but this means a systematic generation, and in philosophy this is called "ontogenesis". This certainly is something different from the biological use of the term for what we called "morphogenesis"; its mixed use certainly seriously hinders understanding[6].

In the same sense the term "experience" expresses different types of interaction between cognitive systems and their environment, depending on species, age, culture, or social system. One might use the same term for all of them, with the obligation to define exactly their different meaning in context, or one might reserve each term for a specific context. This is Kant's way, which might be called a self–referential, or even circular method, because it might be expressed this way: Kant's system of categories, and his concept of experience is valid for exactly those cognitive systems that possess these categorical and experiential structures. This self–consistent, semi-circular character of description sometimes is a little disturbing, but is well known in all sciences when coming close to axiomatization.

6. Manifestation of Formal Development

When studying the morphogenetic development of categories, their formal character has to be kept strictly in mind. Otherwise inadequacy of description will take place. This frequently happened to Piaget who might be

---

6 The difference between the ontogenetic and the morphogenetic view on human cognition may be illustrated by the analogous astrophysical resp. cosmological view on the planetary system: the one shows the inner systematic context of gravitational laws, the other, how this system developed historically.

called the developmental psychologist who most explicitly concentrated his work on the development of formal abilities of mind, i.e. categories.

The general problems that arise in studies like this are predictable; they arise from the formal character of their object: Since "mere structures" do not exist, but are bound to objects of which they are the structures, only to become manifest as the structures of those objects, they must be isolated from the study of those concrete objects, (in our case: from processes of thinking[7]).

Now Piaget continuously mixes formal categories with their concrete application. Let us study this in some detail on the basis of his opinions concerning the development of concepts of "conservation".

According to Kant, conservation is a formal structure to discriminate lasting from changing qualities of experiential objects. Since it is a biological necessity to find laws in nature which are stable, so that a creature may trust them and make use of them to run its life, one would expect "conservation" a very early, very basic formal frame of understanding the world. Nevertheless Piaget locates its development only in late childhood (age 10-12). He is not always very clear in this statement, because the concrete tests to check on conservation differ; the most representative tests are the conservation of volume and of material mass.

Now the statement of conservation of volume under deformation as Piaget uses it as an indicator of conservation is a very complicated phenomenon making use of a well developed ability to judge changes in three-dimensional space (e.g. the conservation of the length of a rope in spite of bending or winding up would be much more simple), and the conservation of mass even is a very abstract finding which in history of science became a clear hypothesis not earlier than in 18th century. We see that Piaget connects the study of his concept of "conservation" with physical magnitudes that play their role as *conservative* magnitudes only within physical theories about experiential objects, instead of investigating the formal frame by which those objects are constituted.[8] Categories are formal *questions* to nature, which are answered, perhaps in a changing manner, by the respective state of knowledge. So the small child of one year "has" the category of conservation when it is creeping under the couch—instead of weeping for his lost ball—because it knows for certain that it must be

---

7 —with the additional problem that in this case the "concrete" correlates of the structures are not concrete objects as e.g. in physics, but mental processes (see Klein 1990). Obviously, this difficulty caused the philosophical errors of behaviorism.

8 According to the traditional philosophical dignity of entities that are called "substantial" due to their conservational character, the importance of conservational laws in science may be understood; on the other hand, the search of Romantic Philosophy of Nature for "the" substance (sounds like alchymia!) is misunderstanding the problem and tends to become ideologic unless it is reformulated physically (as was the case with the law of energy conservation in 1842). It is true, however, that in highly developed, axiomatic theories it is often difficult if not impossible to discriminate between formal and material magnitudes, because it is not a favorite interest of scientists when exhibiting their science to emphasize this difference. The same holds for the difference between definitory and empirical natural laws. Both aspects have raised serious considerations in philosophy of science which we cannot discuss here; on the contrary, we have to neglect them here in order to understand its function in both, daily life and developing ("classical") science; for modern science see footnote 10.

somewhere; and it continues to learn natural laws that fulfill his search for useful stability—and so does the scientist, who since 18th century has learned to replace "mass" by energy, or who finds the laws of conservation of momentum or of baryon number on the basis of a perhaps more elaborated, but still the same formal assumption as the small child.

7. Normative Function of Categories

Kant's systematic reconstruction of the formal structure of cognition must not only be understood as a speculative systematization of empirical data, as it is normal in science (§3), nor is it only an ontogenetic reconstruction of what happens in reality by evolutionary or individual development (§5), but it has an unmistakably normative character: the outlined image of the cognitive structure of mind must not only be understood as a mere, though systematized description of the empirically existing, continuously developing minds, but as an *ideal* of cognitive structure.

This becomes obvious if we look at Kant's claim of a universal validity of his system, though he was very well aware of the existence of different cultures and languages which perhaps verbalize different formal approaches in understanding the world. In interpreting this claim for universality, one could retreat to the weaker claim, that Kant's categories were only formulated in such a basic and formal manner, that they comprise all existing human minds in a definitory sense. This view in some respect might even be correct, but it would not meet the core of Kant's problem.

Rather, Kant states that it is a quality of reason itself not to rest content with what happens in development from alone, caused only by genetic programs and environmental influence; instead he states that reason—if it is true reason—aims for ideals of development which are based on laws of reason alone, "eternal" reasonable laws. As the basic "eternal" law of reason we find its aim for "autonomy", i.e. the aim to extend individual development towards that already well known self–referential image of reason: independent of time and culture, comprising all experiental reasons, systematic and free from internal contradictions to become a habit of the individual, which nevertheless preserves and expresses its individuality.[9]

It has often been denied that it is possible to derive normative ideals from empirical data. With reason, however, it *is* possible, and this is a result of *experience* with reason itself, namely the *empirical finding* that reason

---

9 This normative function of his concept of cognitive reason is the ground for the often puzzling fact, that Kant speaks about cognition in different, seemingly unconnected writings, mainly *Critique of Pure Reason* and *Anthropology*. The first, in accordance to the other *Critiques*, is devoted to the philosophy of the normative ideal of reason, the latter to phenomena with empirical reasons. The dialectic relation between empirical and normative structure of reason later has been made the core of education and socio–cultural development by the movement of "Neo–Humanism", esp. by Wilhelm v. Humboldt (see Menze 1965, Korff 1923/30).

basically claims for ideals. We have to accept this property as an empirical fact if we intend to act as correct empirical scientists.[10]

However, we have to check (but not here) on the meaning of this normative function, and of course, its norms can only be understood as *hypothetical* norms, in a sense like: *if* reason shall develop, that and that has to occur (but nobody can be forced to aim for becoming a reasonable human being).

In this sense, Kant's view has a fourfold normative character:

—Reason itself sets an ideal of its own final aim: reason is its own ideal.

—If man, as an individual or as species, wants to be a creature of reason, he has to accept this ideal and to try to realize it.

—The intention to do so partly is innate, as a genetic disposition, but it has to be stimulated and promoted by education.

—To make reason concrete and to give it an object of activity, the cultural conditions, the values and mechanisms in culture, must accept and promote those ideals, so that they will not become rootless or ineffective, thus rather making them futile or even causing mental sickness.

8. Pathology

I can only mention some brief aspects here.

The system of categories denotes the structure of object formation, but I shall not go into details of true psychopathological disturbances of that mental function because other authors deal with them in this volume (cf. Hundert, Spitzer). A glimpse on it is necessary, however, because I believe that those disturbances to a great extent may be explained as disturbances of the connected system of factors which have to interplay correctly and in a balanced manner in order to result sane object formation ability. Instead, in case of disturbance this balance seems to be replaced by a delirious or exclusive dominance of single categories—by a dysfunction of the "censor" component in mind, as Emrich (this volume) formally describes it.[11]

---

10 It has often been stated that Kant's system of categories has been constructed in close analogy to modern European scientific thinking. This is true and sets limits to accepting certain systems of thinking as sufficient and declaring them to fulfil the normative claim of reason. This is the case, of course, for the different states of children's development or for the thinking abilities of the mentally sick (so that they are subject of education resp. therapy). But the same formal insufficiency must be stated also for the structure of thinking in different cultures, or social classes, or even with concern to the categories of running and understanding daily life as phenomenological analysis has characterized. The complicated anthropological problems resulting from this discrimination cannot be exposed here.

On the other hand it is not true that Kant's system is valid only for Newtonian physics. Extending some hints of C.F.v. Weizsäcker (1941), I have shown elsewhere (Klein 1984) that the usual criticism of Kant that his system has been proven false by modern physics (different space concept in theory of relativity, replacement of causality by statistical laws) is false itself, because Kant speaks of the formal structure of object formation in general, whilst physics deals with concrete natural laws which are formulated on the basis of this formal structure.

11 This "censor" component may be identified with Kant's "power of judgment" which, in its empirical sense (which has to be distinguished from its "transcendental" sense) is generally defined as

I would like to stress this view, because in my opinion wide spread specific disturbances in categorial development which may not yet be called "pathological" in a medical sense, may be characterized by a similar, though less marked dysfunction of a balanced and firm ability to "judge" on sensual experiences by categories.

At first glance, we would expect a far–reaching independence of the development of categories in a much greater extent than is the case e.g. for moral or esthetic values. This should be expected because the influencing environmental conditions are mainly inevitable physical conditions—if life shall not end completely. A developing child in order to gain his basic experiences, cannot, except only in very special cases, be kept from experiences with gravitation, with heat and light, with space and time, it cannot be kept from causal relations between different objects, from imagination and its difference to reality. So the basic structures of the categorical system should be universal. But its differentiation, its firmness in use, the basic trust in it depend on the *kind* of concrete experience from which the structures must be abstracted; it is well known by educators that this process may be helped or hindered by the lack, or excess, of adequate experiences.

The earliest experiential promotion seems to happen without conscious control, by an innate resp. hormonal mutual coordination between mother and child in giving and feeling signals, as psychologists like Spitz (1965, especially chapter 7), or ethologists like Eibl-Eibesfeldt (1970, especially chapter 8ff) have pointed out. A consequence would be to argue in favor of a close, and not substitutable connection between mother and child, of social control in favor of it, and of a free renunciation of pretended "freedom" and the claim for symmetry in sexual roles (cf. Hassenstein 1973, especially chapter III).

Later on, such instinctive preformations decline, and conscious educational activity, at least moderation, has to replace it. To do so, the valid laws of development should be known, and for this, the full set of categories should be taken into consideration. This is not yet the case in developmental psychology. Piaget e.g. concentrates on a very fragmentary set, neglecting esp. the categories of quality and of modality.

A sound and complete development seems to be the result of a balanced estimation and qualification of these interrelations. Thus, the neglect of some of them, or sociocultural conditions resulting such neglect in fact may raise serious disturbances of development and its final result. Looking at modern school children, I should state esp. a loss or underdevelopment of a firm feeling for reality as an opposite of mere imagination, for the acceptance and foresight of consequences of given facts, and for the

---

"the ability to think about the particular as comprized by the general" ("Urteilskraft uberhaupt ist das Vermögen, das Besondere als enthalten unter dem Allgmeinen zu denken." Kant 1790, A XXIII f; Kant specifies the "censor" function like this: "Ist das Allgemeine (die Regel, das Prinzip, das Gesetz) gegeben, so ist die Urteilskraft, welche das Besondere darunter subsumiert ..., bestimmend. Ist aber das Besondere gegeben, wozu sie das Allgemeine finden soll, so ist die Urteilskraft bloß reflektierend".)

inadequacy of mere analogies (as they are typical for arguing in new Age movement or—deplorably—widely in contemporary political life) (refer here to the categories of modality, esp. the difference between "possibility" and "reality"). Furthermore I would like to stress a lack of feeling for "nuances" in knowledge (cf. "limitation") and for the interdependence of different parameters (cf. "interaction"). As reasons for these insufficiencies I would mark specific reductions of the structure of experiences under the conditions of an age of mass media, like information gathering from two-dimensional screens or papers instead of 3-d reality; the basic replacement of concrete experiences by their symbolic surrogates; a lack of necessary activity and effort in gaining valuable experience; the growing lack of internal serious tasks for children in daily life and parental and educational neurotic efforts to protect children from difficulties and frustrations. Since all these conditions—and others—causing categorical disturbances in medically *sane* persons are part of the specific socio–cultural environment, these socio–cultural conditions are to be blamed for their insufficient results; so they have to be changed towards fitting to the necessities of sane categorial development in the interest of forthcoming generations.

In general, schizophrenia, when taken as a deep reaching disturbance of object formation touching personal identity, might be called the representative (though perhaps not the most frequent) mental disturbance of these times. This view would be corroborated by considering the change of neuroses from mainly conflicts of the ego with moral standards of the "bürgerliche" society, as in Freud's time, to narcism which might be taken as the ego–centered correlate of disturbed object formation. The transition seems to be fluent.

Kant himself, to denote a final aspect, could have even called *all* empirically given reasons "sick" (in the sense of "insufficient"), because none of them fulfills the *ideal* of reason. At least, he would have postulated that they have to *aim* for that ideal.

But what would he have called a society that does no longer see or accept reasons aim for self–augmentation, and that suppresses it in favor of usefulness—wouldn't he have said that such a society has lost its humane character?

Summary

Kant declares his categories to constitute a universally valid system of the formal structure of thinking, "preceding" every single experience. Teachers and developmental psychologists, however, know children to think in different ways; psychopathologists know the same for the mentally sick.
This fact demands careful examination what the Kantian categories are meant to describe. They are no mere description of what is just the case,

pretending: everywhere and at every age, but they are rather an idealized image of human reason. "Idealization" happens in two respects:

—it is a systematized image of the mature mind, denoting its formal structure which insofar in fact underlies every single experience, as the tool of data processing, but which has to develop to that state by innate laws of development and by the interaction with the environment;

—it is an *ideal* of mind, expressing the self–determinated aim of reason's development to realize a reasonable ideal, self–consistent and according to human dignity.

Thus, Kant's system of categories

—gives framework of comparison for the study of the developing as well as for the insane mind;

—gives a framework of criticism for a pathology of society and individual personality, insofar as physically sane minds nevertheless show typical deviations from the described ideal.

References

Eibl–Eibesfeldt I: Liebe und Haß. München, 1970.
Goethe JW v: Annalen oder Tag– und Jahreshefte. 1830 In: Cotta (ed) 1857, vol XXVII.
Hassenstein B: Verhaltensbiologie des Kindes. München, 1973.
Kant I: Kritik der reinen Vernunft. Riga, 1781.
Kant I: Prolegomena zu einer jeden zukünftigen Metaphysik Riga, 1783.
Kant I: Metaphysische Anfangsgründe der Naturwissenschaft. Riga, 1786.
Kant I: Kritik der Urteilskraft. Berlin, 1790.
Kant I: Anthropologie in pragmatischer Hinsicht. Königsberg, 1798.
Klein P: Über Räume der Erfahrung. In: Kuhn W (ed): Vorträge der Physikertagung 1984 (Didaktik). Gießen, pp. 259–268, 1984.
Klein P: Metareflexionen zur Logik des Gehirns. In: Klein P (ed): Praktische Logik. Göttingen, 1990 (Veröff. der Jungius-Gesellschaft vol. 61), pp. 335–347, part II.
Korff HA: Geist der Goethezeit. Vol. 1/2, Leipzig 1923/1930.
Menze C: Wilhelm von Humboldts Lehre und Bild vom Menschen. Ratingen, 1965.
Piaget J, Inhelder B: Die Entwicklung der physikalischen Mengenbegriffe beim Kinde. Stuttgart, 1969.
Riedl R: Biologie der Erkenntnis. Berlin und Hamburg, 1979.
Spitz R: The first year of life—a psychoanalytical study of normal and deviant development of object relation. New York, 1965.
Weizsäcker CF v: Das Verhältnis der Quantenmechanik zur Philosphie Kants (1941). In: Zum Weltbild der Physik, 10th ed 1963, pp. 80–117. Stuttgart, 1943.

Normality and Mental Illness—Dimensions Versus Categories: Theoretical Considerations and Experimental Findings

Godehard Oepen, Anne Harrington, Matthias Fünfgeld

1. Theoretical Considerations

In psychiatry one may generally distinguish two main approaches toward major psychiatric disorders: a categorical approach, which regards the concepts of "normality" and "mentally ill" as two clearly separated spheres; and a dimensional approach, which sees the two states as two poles of a continuum. It is clear to every psychiatrist that there are good and less good empirical reasons for favoring the one approach over the other. What is often less clear is the extent to which a decision for categorization or for dimensionality is *also* a decision in favor of a certain epistemological and/or ontological view of the nature of the relationship between disease and health, deviancy and normalcy, patient reality and doctor reality. In other words, the imperatives of the diagnostic enterprise ensure that philosophical considerations—usually unexamined—play a role in psychiatry from the very outset.

But that is not all. The historical record suggests that the philosophical positions represented by categorization and dimensionality may often support an implicit ethical and political agenda. Crystallizing in the classical works of Kraepelin, Jaspers and Schneider, the fundamental assumption of the categorical approach—that madness and normality share little, if any common ground—generally has had the effect of stigmatizing and ostracizing patients, especially those with the most severe disorders, the schizophrenias. In this century, the Swiss psychiatrist Manfred Bleuler would speak of schizophrenics as "strange, puzzling, inconceivable, uncanny, incapable of empathy, sinister, frightening"; all together, he concluded, "it is impossible to approach them as equals". To quote the dry words of historian Roy Porter: "in the long run, the distinction which the Greeks had drawn between [reason] and [unreason], between fully rational members of society and the sub–rational, came to weigh increasingly heavily" (Porter 1989 [1987], pp. 21, 15)

Now, almost without exception, these first *categorical* approaches to psychopathology were characterized by a *biological* model of disease etiology. In theory, the patients could be classified as sick or not sick depending on whether or not they had the twisted molecule or twisted gene (the spirochete of neurosyphilis being the paradigmatic disease model here). That is to say, biology's job in the first categorical psychiatry was to identify the "biological markers" of a disease, which could then be correlated with the nosological disease category in question. In this way (as the anti–psychiatrists have long pointed out), the mana of the biological–categorical diagnosis could be used to disempower deviancy by transforming it into "disease" (cf. e.g. Szasz 1988).

The dimensionally–oriented psychiatrists of the first decades of the 20th–century (traditionally represented by psychoanalytical and related psychogenetic traditions) were able for a time to seize the moral high ground from the categorizers by abandoning biology and attempting to give psychosis a human meaning rooted in the biography of the individual (for a critical historical overview, see Fullinwider 1982). Yet this approach would also turn out to be ethically problematic. By the 1970s, it was becoming clear that the end effect of the first experiment in psychiatric dimensionality had been to institutionalize an attitude of "blaming the victim" (either the patient himself or his confused and long–suffering family) for the fact of psychosis. At the same time, the mentalistic and developmental assumptions that had formed the foundation of this first dimensional approach to schizophrenia were increasingly rejected as inappropriate for dealing with the severe psychoses.

Today, the general consensus seems to be swinging back towards a biologically–oriented approach that would reaffirm the status of schizophrenia as a "real disease" (so "Mother is not to blame"). Research into the possible neurochemical, neuroanatomical, neurophysiological and genetic "markers" of schizophrenia expands exponentially every year. Not surprisingly, this revival of the biological orientation has been accompanied by an equal revival of the tendency to categorize. We see this, for example, in the tireless attempts of the DSM–III and DSM–III–R to define criteria for categorical classification of disordered behavior, using cut–off–scores that tell practitioners the precise number at which "normality" stops and "pathology" begins.

It might seem, having taken our reflections up to this point, that we are now stuck between a rock and a hard place. On the one hand, the Freudian and post–Freudian non–biological dimensional approach to the severe psychosis has been effectively rejected on empirical, conceptual and ethical grounds. On the other hand, the dominant categorical orientation of the new biological psychiatry seems to be leading to a revival of the old stigmatizing attitudes of the past—witness Daniel Koshland's recent suggestion at the First Human Genome Conference in San Diego (October, 1989) that the United States tackle its problem of homelessness by searching for the genetic basis of the mental disorders from which homeless people are obviously all suffering (Michael Fortun, personal communication).

The question now arises: *must* a biological orientation in psychiatry be categorical? We do not think so. We recall that there is in fact another important philosophical tradition in the bio–medical sciences—going back at least to the work of the French physiologist Claude Bernard—that has always attempted to conceptualize biological concepts of disease and health in terms of dimensions or a continuum. What might be the effect of using this alternative approach to explore the neurobiology of schizophrenia and the other major psychoses? A pilot research project recently completed in our laboratory in Freiburg, West Germany attempted to find out. In other words, we undertook to combine a commitment to a *neurobiological* model of schizophrenia with a *dimensional* approach to disease and health. The results were surprising, underscoring the empirical fruitfulness of this neglected "third way" in psychiatry. The results also—as will be seen— raised for us a number of new questions on the nature of abnormal versus normal experience and the proper role of the psychiatrist in society.

The Freiburg project involved an attempt to induce and monitor the beginning stages of a schizophreniform psychosis in "normal" people. Mescaline was used to achieve the desired effects. Phenomenologically, there is no single cross–sectional feature or symptom that might allow one to distinguish mescaline–induced psychosis from the beginning states of a paranoid–hallucinatory psychotic episode; mescaline–induced psychotic states may therefore serve as a useful clinical model of schizophrenic psychoses (Hermle et al. 1988, Stockings 1940).

Our goal, however, was to go further than earlier researchers, and see how far mescaline–induced neurometabolic and neuropsychological altered functioning might resemble the sorts of abnormal functioning that had been found in schizophrenic patients. Our working hypothesis—based on several years of neuropsychological research with schizophrenic patients—was that the experiences associated with a mescaline–induced psychosis (florid hallucinations, disordered thinking, etc.) would be corre- lated with two factors:

(1) abnormally heightened metabolic activity in right hemisphere subcortical regions of the brain;

(2) changed performance in a recognition task associated with normal right hemisphere functioning (a tachistoscopically–presented face recog- nition task).

That, then, was the basic structure of our experiment. We then intro- duced a final variable or twist. To make the study "dimensional", we turned the concept of "normality" into a *relative* one—i.e. we set up a "sliding scale" of "normalness"—by requiring all our subjects to fill out a questionnaire that assessed the number of so–called "schizotypical" personality traits each possessed—the traits having been selected according to DSM–III criteria (Claridge and Broks 1984).

Our final hypothesis, then, was that the *general* expectation of finding a parallelism between psychopathological experience and RH metabolic and neuropsychological changes would express itself in a sliding scale relationship with the individual personality traits of our subjects. In other words, we assumed that clinical, neuropsychological and neurometabolic changes would be most pronounced in subjects with high schizotypal features (high STQ) and lower in subjects further down on the schizotypal scale.

2. Method

12 male healthy volunteers with a mean age of 35.3 years and without any history of psychiatric diseases were studied before (t_0) and after ingestion of 0.5 g mescaline-sulfate. Psychiatric symptoms were assessed throughout the experiment using the Brief Psychiatric Rating Scale (BPRS, Overall and Gorham 1976) and the Paranoid-Depressivitäts–Skala (PDS, v. Zerssen 1976) after 0.5 hour (t_1), 1.5 hours (t_2), 3 hours (t_3), and 7 hours (t_4) following drug intake.

After psychopathological rating, subjects performed a face/nonface decision task (face test, FT with known right hemispheric (RH) superiority (Regard and Landis, 1986) in a visual half–field experiment on a 3–channel–tachistoscope. Standardized faces and nonfaces were presented simultaneously on each side of the fixation point. Exposure time was 60 ms. The subjects had to press a lever ipsilateral to the target stimulus (face) with their index–fingers as fast as possible. Two runs were presented at each testing. The first run consisted of 36 cards: 12 targets in the left visual field (LVF), 12 in the right visual field (RVF) and 12 bilateral non–targets. In the second run, three additional cards with emotionally–arousing material (a naked woman, a spider, and Rorschach ink blot no. 10) were added. Each stimulator was presented once in each hemi–field with a target or a non–target in the other hemifield. Our earlier studies with schizophrenic patients had shown that lateralized cognitive functioning of this sort can be selectively disturbed through such emotional stimulation (Oepen et al. 1987).

At the peak of the experimental psychosis, brain metabolism for each subject was investigated using 99m–Tc–HMPAO SPECT with a rotating gamma–camera. The results were then compared with earlier scans of the same subject produced under pre-testing or control conditions.

Several weeks after the experiment, but before evaluation of the data, subjects completed the Schizotypy Questionnaire STQ (Claridge and Broks 1984). Test results were used to dichotomize subjects in a group of subclinically schizotypy low (ST–low) and subclinically schizotypy high (ST–high) subjects. Separate MANOVA's for repeated measurements were calculated for SPECT results in different regions of interest with and without mescaline, and for neuropsychological performance at fixed times after drug intake, using ST–low vs. ST–high as a group factor.

3. Results

3.1 Psychopathological

For both groups, mescaline led to an increase of psychopathological symptoms in all external ratings (BPRS) and self–ratings (PDS), especially the

BPRS–subscales Thought Disorders (THOT), Activation (ACTV), and the PDS–subscales Paranoid Ideas (P) and Depression (D). Converging results of external rating and self–asssessment found that the peak of the experimental psychosis was reached at t_3, approximately 3 hours after drug intake.

Prior to drug–intake, ST–low subjects (ST–scores: 2–7) and ST–high subjects (ST–scores: 8–17) could not be distinguished from each other using the BPRS or the PDS, except for a tendency of ST–high subjects to report more symptoms of depression. After drug intake, at the peak of the experimental psychosis, ST–low subjects showed—*contrary to expectations*—larger gains and higher absolute values in the BPRS–subscale Thought Disorders (THOT) and in the PDS subscale Paranoid Ideas (P) than ST–high subjects. Results, however, did not achieve significance.

3.2 Neuropsychological

Over repeated tachistoscopic testings, RH–performance in the LVF deteriorated steadily after drug intake in both groups. At the same time, LH–performance in the RVF improved to a level of performance even exceeding that seen prior to drug intake. That is to say, mescaline–induced psychosis led to a practical reversal of normal hemifield asymmetries for the RH–specific face/nonface decision task (table 1: FT). Most interesting of all were the group differences in reaction to the tachistoscopically–presented emotional stimulation (see table 2): while ST–low subjects tended to show a deterioration of performance in the LVF (RH), ST–high subjects showed deterioration of performance predominantly in the RVF (LH).

3.3 Neurometabolic

As expected, mescaline led to an increase in the metabolic rate in the subcortical structures of both hemispheres. More interestingly, ST–high subjects showed larger absolute increases of tracer substance uptake in both hemispheres than the ST–low group; i.e., ST–high subjects had lower tracer uptakes without mescaline and surpassed the ST–low subject uptake levels when under the influence of mescaline (ST x MESC). As predicted by our beginning assumption that mescaline mimics a true schizophreniform psychosis, the SPECT scans of both ST–low and ST–high subjects (figure 1, table 3 – MESC) revealed that more marker substance was taken up in subcortical—presumably striato–limbic—regions of the RH (table 3 – HEM). As further predicted by our hypothesis that schizotypy level would be related to degree of pathology experienced in the mescaline psychosis, SPECT scans also revealed that RH asymmetric metabolic increases were more pronounced in ST–high subjects than in ST–low subjects (ST x HEM) in the transversal slice.

Tab 1: Changes of tachistoscopic hemi–field advantage for face/nonface decisions in mescaline–induced psychosis. Right hemisphere (RH) performance in the left visual field (LVF) at t_0 (without mescaline) deteriorates under mescaline (t_1 to t_4) with onset of psychotic symptoms as assessed by BPRS. At the same time left hemisphere performance in the right visual field (RVF) increases. At the peak of psychosis significant increases of RH blood–flow in the striato–limbic areas of the right hemisphere (RH) as compared to LH are found using SPECT scans. Neuropsychological alterations begin to normalize again at t_4.

TRIALS	FT mean freq correct LVF RVF	BPRS	SPECT
t_0	8,0 — 5,5	$\bar{X} = 19\ 7$ $Sx = 1\ 4$	$\emptyset$
t_1 40- 60min	8,0 — 5,5	$\bar{X} = 27\ 0$ $Sx = 6\ 0$	$\emptyset$
t_2 95-115 min	8,0 — 5,5	$\bar{X} = 32\ 0$ $Sx = 9\ 3$	$\emptyset$
t_3 225-245 min	8,0 — 5,5	$\bar{X} = 335$ $Sx = 102$	sign r CBF - increase in basal ganglia of the RH (p < .050)
t_4 430-450 min	8,0 — 5,5	$\bar{X} = 27\ 3$ $Sx = 5\ 4$	$\emptyset$

Tab. 2: Results from the comparisons of tachistoscopic face/nonface decision tasks without mescaline and four subsequent trials with mescaline. Only main effects are listed and interactions with significance levels of less than .15

	Face/Nonface Decision	
Effects	F (1,10)	Signif
ST	.96	.350
SEQU	.73	.578
STIM	.04	.850
VF	2.07	.181
ST x STIM	2.85	.122
SEQU x VF	1.96	.119
ST x STIM x VF	2.91	.119

legend: ST = ST–low vs. ST–high subjects
VF = left vs. right visual field
SEQU = without vs. with mescaline
STIM = effect of additional emotional stimulation

Tab. 3: SPECT results in coronal and transversal slices comparing data without mescaline with data from the same subjects three to four hours after ingestion of 0.5 gram mescaline–sulfate. Only main effects are listed and interactions with significance levels of less than .15

	Coronal		Transversal	
Effect	F(1,9)	Signif	F(1,9)	Signif
ST	1.00	.343	.61	.455
MESC	38.25	.000	35.67	.000
HEM	40.89	.000	79.61	.000
ST x MESC	10.20	.011	12.69	.006
ST x HEM	.82	.387	7.43	.023

legend: ST = ST–low vs. ST–high subjects
HEM = left vs. right hemisphere
MESC = without vs. with mescaline

Fig. 1: 99m technetium HMPAO–uptake in the cerebral SPECT scans of 11 male volunteers (one scan is missing for technical reasons), subdivided into low and high schizotypia (ST) groups. Note that the asymmetric metabolic increase is more pronounced in ST–high subjects.

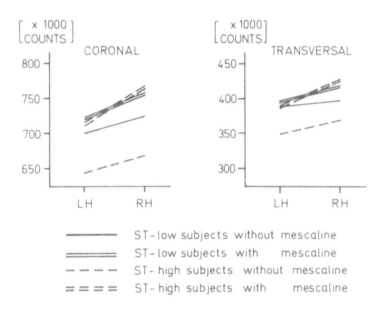

4. Discussion

First of all, as expected, our results pointed to a covariation of heightened RH subcortical metabolic activity with deterioration of RH cortical performance in the face/nonface tests in all subjects under the influence of a mescaline–induced psychosis. This relationship of neuropsychological and neurometabolic features was most pronounced at the peak of the mescaline–induced psychotic experience; i.e., while subjects suffered from thought disorders, loosened associations, feelings of depersonalization and visual and auditory hallucinations. The RH performance decline during experimental psychosis ($t_1 - t_4$) closely parallelled results in patients with schizophrenia taking the same test under additional emotional stimulation. (Oepen et al. 1987).

Our SPECT results did suggest—as expected—a tendency towards RH, presumably striato–limbic, hyperactivity during the mescaline–induced psychotic state; an earlier SPECT study we carried out on a small group of schizophrenic patients had produced similar results (Oepen and Botsch 1987). Thus our general expectation of finding neuropsychological and neurometabolic similarities between schizophrenia and mescaline–induced psychosis was not disappointed.

The surprise, however, came when we proved unable to find the expected parallels between psychopathological experience (as assessed through tests) and neurophysiological parameters—our "biological markers". This showed itself on a number of dimensions:

(1) Contrary to expectations, our high–STQ subjects failed to show higher initial metabolic activity in relevant brain regions before drug–intake than low STQ subjects; indeed, their brain metabolism was lower than the brain metabolism of our low STQ subjects. Under mescaline, however, their brain metabolism, especially in the RH, shot up to levels above those of our low STQ subjects. This piece of data was more in line with our expectations, but raised problems of its own because—

(2) Under mescaline, our high–STQ subjects—in spite of all this heightened neurometabolic activity—did *not* as a group experience more psychotic symptoms on the average than low STQ subjects (an exception must be made for two individuals). In general, they coped better where we had predicted they would cope worse than low STQ subjects.

(3) This disparity between clinical and neurometabolic findings had a parallel in the neuropsychological performance test results. Contrary to all expectations, the peculiar instability of RH performance that we had previously been inclined to see as a "marker" of the acute schizophrenic state when under emotional stress (Oepen et al. 1987), emerged in the mescaline situation mainly in our *STQ–low subjects*, and not in our ST–high subjects.

The first conclusion we can draw from all this is that categorical concepts of "normal" and "pathological" are completely inadequate to deal with the data being given. The second conclusion, no less important, is that psychiatry's traditional dependence on "biological markers" to define the objective borders of clinical categories are more problematic than has usually been realized. We can say this because the "biological markers" we selected for study (neurometabolic and neuropsychological processes) did *not* parallel subjective pathological experience in the way we had expected. We found no linear relationship in our subjects between physiological (neurometabolic) disturbances and mental (neuropsychological and esp. psychopathological) disturbances. In some strange way, it seems that the working philosophical assumption of the overwhelming majority of neuropsychiatrists today—that there is an uncomplicated "identity" between mind and brain processes—cannot stand up to close scrutiny.[1]

To explain our unexpected results, we have now speculated that, because the low STQ–subjects were relatively unfamiliar with the more extreme ends of the spectrum of "normality", they tended as a group to

---

1 Although there is obviously very strong evidence of a general dependance of mental functioning on the functioning of the brain, it has still to be shown that the correspondence is so exact that observation of a person's brain functioning could ever allow one to arrive at a knowledge of his or her experiences in every detail (in a manner reminiscent of the old dream of the early naturalist philosophers of reading a person's thoughts from his brain as if from a "book").

experience a more radical reaction to the mescaline experience than was experienced by the high STQ–subjects. We suppose that this second group possessed higher "tolerance levels" and/or more sophisticated coping strategies for dealing with abnormal perceptual, cognitive and affective experience. The question then arises: if the relationship between biological indicators of abnormality and subjective experience of pathology is so dynamic and individual for our so–called "normal" subjects, what is to justify our supposing that matters are so different for our schizophrenic patients?

All this leads us to reaffirm the value of a *dimensional* approach in biological psychiatry over one that places psychopathology in a categorical relationship to selected biological markers. Psychiatry must realize that the human brain is apparently capable of producing a broad spectrum of psychological, behavioral and neurophysiological combinations.[2] Recognition of such dynamic individuality even at the brain level might help the new biological psychiatry avoid many of the ethical ambiguities and much of the conceptual rigidity that so weakened the first biological psychiatry. The new biological psychiatry, benefitting from the conceptual flexibility afforded it by the dimensional approach, might instead want to focus its research and therapeutic energy on behavior associated, *not* with "pathology" (understood in the old sense), but with personal *suffering* and/or larger social risk. Such a shift in orientation would imply that a certain descriptive diagnosis would not implicate an automatic reaction ("therapeutic reflex"), unless careful individual evaluation suggested an individual requirement for some form of intervention. In other words, the new biological psychiatry—oriented towards dimensions rather than categories—might come to understand the state of being "mentally ill" in a manner similar to how modern neurology understands the state of "being in pain"— with all the varieties of etiologies, potential for individual defensive coping responses, and range of appropriate therapeutics that this comparison implies.

Summary

The paper examines the problematic historical relationship between psychiatric categorization ("normality" and "disease" as distinct spheres) and psychiatric dimensionality (the two conditions as poles of a continuum). The association is noted between categorization and biology on the one hand, and between dimensionality and psychodynamics on the other hand. While the stigmatizing dangers of rigid categorization in psychiatry are stressed, the importance of a biological approach to explaining psychosis is no less affirmed. It is proposed that psychiatry could

---

2   This said, it must also be said that dimensional differences might at some point lead to categorical, i.e. qualitative changes at the phenomenal level; catastrophe theory offers us a model for conceiving the mechanics of this kind of nonlinear process.

explore the potential of combining biological approach to psychosis with a dimensional approach to deviancy and normalcy. A pilot research project on schizotypy and mescaline–induced experimental psychosis in healthy volunteers is discussed as an example of the empirical fruitfulness of such an approach. The upshot of the results is that there is a dynamic and from person to person varying relationship between biological indicators of abnormality and subjective experience of pathology. Ethical conclusions are drawn from these results.

References

Claridge G, Broks P: Schizotypy and hemisphere function (1). Theoretical considerations and the measurement of schizotypy. Person individ Diff 5: 633–648, 1984.

Fortun M (Department of the History of Science, Harvard University): Personal Communication, October 5, 1989.

Fullinwider SP: Technicians of the Finite: The Rise and Decline of the Schizophrenic in American Thought, 1840–1960. Contributions in Medical History, No. 9, Greenwood Press, Westport CT, 1982.

Hermle L, Oepen G, Spitzer M: Zur Bedeutung der Modellpsychosen. Fortschr Neurol Psychiatr 56: 48–58, 1988.

Oepen G, Botsch H: SPECT bei Schizophrenie. In: Oepen G (ed), Psychiatrie des rechten und linken Gehirns. Deutscher Ärzte Verlag, Köln, pp. 147–155, 1987.

Oepen G, Fünfgeld M, Höll T, Zimmermann P, Landis T, Regard M: Schizophrenia—an emotional hypersensitivity of the right cerebral hemisphere. Int J Psychophysiol 5: 261–264, 1987.

Overall JE, Gorham DR: Brief Psychiatric Rating Scale. In: Guy W, ECDEU Assessment Manual for Psychopharmacology, Rev. ed., Rockville, Maryland, pp. 157–169, 1976.

Porter R: A Social History of Madness: The World Through the Eyes of the Insane (1987), E.P. Dutton, New York, 1989.

Regard M, Landis T: Affective and cognitive decisions in normals. In: Ellis HD, Jeeves MA, Newcombe F, Young A (eds): Aspects of face processing. Nijhoff, Dordrecht, pp. 363–369, 1986.

Stockings GT: A clinical study of mescaline psychosis, with specialreference to the mechanism of the genesis of schizophrenic and other psychotic states. J Ment Sci: 29–47, 1940.

Szasz T: Schizophrenia: The Sacred Symbol of Psychiatry. Syracuse University Press, New York, 1988.

Zerssen Dv: Paranoid–Depressivitäts–Skala (PDS) Klinische Selbstbeurteilungsskalen aus dem Münchner Psychiatrischen Informationssystem. Weinheim, Beltz, 1976.

Transcendental Philosophy
And Its Relevance to the
Foundations of Psychopathology*

Paul Hoff

1. Introduction

One of the topics of this symposium is the way in which psychopathology
sees itself as a science. This way is by no means homogeneous. At one end
of the scale there is the view of psychopathology as a nomothetic science,
based upon the principles of natural sciences, especially logical empiricism.
In extreme contrast, others hold the position, that psychopathology has to
understand the individual human being ideographically. Discussion about
the appropriate position of psychopathology within the scientific community has considerably increased in recent years.

After the "linguistic turn", which had already challenged classical
philosophical concepts, "Analytical Philosophy of Mind" has gained much
influence and is being widely discussed with regard to psychopathology
(Bieri 1981, Möller 1976, Mundt 1984, Schwartz and Wiggins 1988,
Spitzer et al. 1988). Not pretending to become a philosophical system,
whose emphasis lies on creating a link between empirical sciences and
philosophical reflexion by such concepts as "physicalism" (Nagel 1965),
"identity theory" (Smart 1981), "intentionality" (Searle 1983), and
"emergence" (Hastedt 1988).

In this paper, I want to argue in favor of a transcendental approach,
although I know that the term "transcendental" has a lot of negative connotations not in American philosophy only. But as a clinical psychiatrist, I
think that dealing with transcendentalism is more than a mere reminis-
cence of 19th century philosophy: With respect to the multitude of epistemological and methodological aspects in our field of research, it may
serve as an undogmatic link. And such a link is urgently needed to keep
different scientific methods in touch with each other. Even if all theoretical concepts, that have been developed in recent years, are taken into
account, our basic epistemological problems are far from being solved. For
example, if voting for "identity theory" (Smart 1981) or "eliminative materialism" (Churchland 1981), one has to ask oneself, by which means are

---

*) This paper is dedicated to Professor Hanns Hippius on the occasion of his 65th birthday.

statements about "reality" made, what is considered "identical" with what, or which kind of "object" is to be "eliminated". A dualistic theory will be criticized for defending the existence of two substantially different classes of objects, in the face of an obvious unity of human self–perception.

With this as background, the present paper has two main intentions:

1. I want to argue that a transcendental foundation of epistemology can be of substantial value for contemporary philosophy.

2. Transcendental philosophy is particularly interesting for psychopathology, which more than other sciences needs an undogmatic epistemological framework, if it is to avoid being split up into many unrelated subunits.

2. Transcendental Philosophy

First, some principles of transcendentalism are briefly summarized, in the form in which they were understood by its founders—Immanuel Kant and Johann Gottlieb Fichte. As a consequence of Kant's critical comments and his somewhat harsh rejection of Fichte's arguments, it is quite unusual to bring these two philosophers as close together as I am suggesting here. However, many basic transcendental hypotheses were in fact accepted both by Kant and Fichte, and Fichte's *Wissenschaftslehre* was explicitly intended not to reject, but to develop Kant's "critical philosophy"; consequently, both approaches may with good reason be regarded as the most seminal representatives of transcendentalism. From that point of view, it is unjustifiable to divide the so–called "German Idealism" into Kant on the one side and Fichte, Schelling and Hegel on the other. As for the strict application of transcendental positions, the dividing line should rather be drawn between Kant/Fichte and Schelling/Hegel (Hoff 1989b, Lauth 1984, 1989).

With regard to epistemology, transcendental philosophy seeks to overcome the traditional distinction between subject and object. But it does not ignore one or other of the two, as realism and idealism tend to do. It focuses on the whole process of cognition itself: We cannot recognize something completely unrelated to ourselves, but make use of preexisting "apriori" patterns of thinking—which may be called "categories". These categories do not depend on individual environmental conditions; this statement does imply an important issue, namely that Kant's "transcendental deduction" is in no way a procedure placed within a kind of "empirical psychology", it is not an "empirical deduction". On the contrary, it had been Kant's starting point, in dealing with Hume's position, to insist, that empirical data do not "lead" us to more complex constructs such as natural laws or causality, but that we already have these constructs "prior" to all empirical evidence, the latter not being possible without them.[1]

---

1 The dispute about the role of introspection and of empirical psychology in general was going to be especially controversial between the original Kantian position and the philosophical school founded by Jakob Friedrich Fries (1773 - 1843). The main argument against Fries was that he was misunder-

We apply these patterns to what we perceive by our sense organs. Only such a process can constitute nature or reality as having a meaningful structure. Kant calls nature "the synthetical unity of the multitude of phenomena, standing under certain rules" (Kant 1781, p. 186a).

And the human mind is—again according to Kant—"the source of natural laws and therefore of the formal unity of nature" (Kant 1781, p. 187a).

If nature was nothing else but a mere composition of various sensory perceptions, any kind of regularity would be inexplicable: Nature would be a chaos of unconnected perceptions.

But Kant had gone one step further, a step later called the "Copernican turn": Apriori categories do not only make cognition possible formally, but they have a significant impact on the contents of knowledge, relating to what we *can* know. This has often been misunderstood. It should therefore be emphasized that categories will never be able to replace empirical data. They will not bring forward any piece of knowledge unless applied on what Kant calls "Anschauung" ("intuition").

According to Kant and Fichte, transcendental epistemology rejects "blind empiricism" as well as "empty idealism".[2]

To illustrate this problem, we should have a look at two completely different concepts, realism and idealism.

3. Realism and Idealism

Realism postulates the existence of objects, which are truly independent from the person recognizing them. Even so-called "critical realism" (Putnam 1975) remains a realism. According to this concept we have access only to "images" and not to "things themselves". But these "things" are still supposed to have an existence independently from ourselves.

In natural sciences, the most widely accepted epistemological approach is "positivistic empiricism". Scientific data have to be obtained "positively": Conditions of obtaining data must be clearly defined, the object has to be—at least indirectly—observable and measurable. Therefore the empiricist relies on sensory perception, which he believes to be "valid".

However, there are some objections from a transcendental point of view:

There is no such thing as a "pure empirical fact". No field of research can proceed "atheoretically". The empiricist must have an idea about what he is looking for and by which means, otherwise he will not be able to develop general concepts such as "natural laws". According to Fichte, an

---

standing Kant in a "psychologistic" way (Hoff 1989b, Lauth 1989). But nonetheless there has been a considerable influence of Fries's concept on modern psychopathology by the philosopher Leonard Nelson (1882 - 1927) and the psychiatrist Arthur Kronfeld (1886 - 1941).

2 This refers especially to Kant's apodictic statement, that "thinking without intuition is empty, intuition without thinking is blind" - "Gedanken ohne Inhalt sind leer, Anschauungen ohne Begriffe sind blind." (Kant 1791, p. 95).

empiricist, applying his concept sensu strictu, can only count, but not reorganize or interpret his data. In recent years, research in experimental psycho(patho)logy has confirmed this philosophical point of view, by showing that sensory data are by no means "pure" or independent from ourselves, but the product of highly complex information processing (Emrich 1988).

The opposite position—idealism—considers any experience to be completely dependent on apriori ideas and to have no significance of its own. This philosophical concept, as represented for example by Schelling (Schelling 1843), did not gain much influence on psychopathology apart from the era of "romantic medicine" in Germany. Absolute idealism cannot be an adequate framework for practical sciences. The main reason is that it disregards the most intriguing discovery of Western philosophy since Descartes: The fact that we do not *find* concepts, reasons and theories by simply watching the external world or passively relying on metaphysical forces, but that we *produce* them by our own mental acts. Hume, Kant and Fichte—in that order—held this position despite the fundamental differences between their philosophical theories in general (Fichte 1804, Hume 1748, Kant 1781/1787, Lauth 1989).

Kant and—particularly—Fichte presented their concepts in such a difficult and sometimes ambiguous language, that even contemporary German philosophers gave rise to a number of profound misunderstandings: For example, transcendentalism has been misinterpreted as "subjective idealism", even as "solipsism", as being antagonistic to empirical sciences, or as being a "mere philosophy of consciousness" ("bloße Bewußtseinsphilosophie"). Lauth has dealt with some of these misconceptions in his comprehensive study of Fichte's transcendental concept of nature (Lauth 1984).

4. Relevance to Psychopathology

What is the connection between these philosophical reflections and psychopathology?

Although many authors agree that psychopathology is a "basic science" for psychiatry, others like Janzarik (1976) state a "crisis of psychopathology". According to the most influential criticism, psychopathology is operating with too many poorly defined concepts, which tend to be mutually exclusive. Under these circumstances, psychopathology is in danger of being more and more restricted, while the scientific importance of specialized approaches like neurobiology, sociology or experimental psychology is increasing. In my point of view, this is indeed going to take place, unless psychopathology will realize the harmful influence of philosophical prejudice. This issue had been emphasized as early as 1913 by Karl Jaspers in his "General Psychopathology" (Jaspers 1913, Hoff 1989a).

As for these prejudices, we should take a closer look at two examples:

A psychopathologist might define a mental illness only by certain observable clinical symptoms, the assessment of which he considers to be valid and reliable. Moreover, he may believe that these symptoms epistemologically constitute scientific data, that are completely independent from himself, from his own mental activity. In this case, the psychopathologist will be overcome by a "realistic prejudice". By identifying directly observable symptoms with mental illness or—even worse—with the ill person, he will close his mind to the inner experience of the patient, to his personality, his interpersonal relationships and so on—an unjustified truncation.

But that is only one side of the coin. The opposite direction leads to a prejudice, too, an idealistic one. Any dogmatic nosology is such a prejudice, because all clinical data will only be interpreted in the light of the preexisting concept, which itself may not be questioned. Different kinds of mental illness are then believed to be distinct, invariable, "ontological" entities. It should be mentioned, that Emil Kraepelin has been misunderstood as opting for such a dogmatic point of view. But we cannot go into details about his position here, which has been critically discussed elsewhere (Hoff 1988, Mayer–Gross 1929).

If psychopathology intends to remain a basic science for psychiatry, it will have to meet with the following demands:

—It has to be epistemologically undogmatic.

—It has to be open to different research strategies for empirical studies.

—It must provide a comprehensive anthropological framework ("Menschenbild"), thus preventing its disintegration into several unconnected subunits.

These demands have in fact always been substantial parts of transcendental philosophy, which in my view is therefore especially qualified for application on psychopathology.

To illustrate this judgement, we should consider how concepts of illness are created in psychiatry:

We can at present differentiate between three levels of data collection and interpretation: the empirical one, the teleological one and the level of "free reason".

On the empirical level, physiology may be compared with physics. Strictly speaking, psychopathology is not amenable to such an approach. But it is justifiable to speak of the empirical level when talking about observable clinical symptoms, especially if operationalized systems like DSM–III–R (1987) are applied. There is no doubt that validity and reliability of empirical data are much more questionable in psychopathology than in biology or physics. But nonetheless we must insist that the empirical level is an indispensable point of reference for psychiatric research and therapy. If it is neglected, dogmatic and fanciful concepts will result, and will be harmful for the patients. But, on the other hand, the same harm will be done to them, if these operationalized concepts are used uncritically, for example under the unrecognized influence of the above mentioned "realistic prejudice". To avoid misunderstandings, it should be stressed of course that recently developed diagnostic systems do not necessarily lead to a realistic prejudice. But they can do so, if the psychiatrist does not realize their epistemological limits.

On the teleological level, organic structures are regarded as oriented on purposes. The concept of teleology has been examined very critically in recent decades (Möller 1976, Nagel 1979). It has been accused of impeding empirical research and relying on purely speculative, "metaphysical" concepts. Of course that critique was not completely without reason. However, regarding the transcendental position towards teleology, it rejects—just as positivism claims to do—any "metaphysic speculation". But contrary to positivism, it does not deny the scientific dignity of teleological argument in general. It considers teleology as a limited, but necessary part in creating knowledge. For reasons of space, we cannot go into details about the significant philosophical differences between Kant's and Fichte's concepts of teleology. This issue has already been examined intensively (Hoff 1989b, Lauth 1984, 1989; see also Rychlak, this volume).

Practical examples are self–regulating biological systems such as the control of blood pressure, of metabolism of neurotransmitters or hormones. In fact, terms like "steady state" or "set point" cannot be understood without teleological assumptions. And these do not at all exclude or discriminate empirical research.

Many scientists avoid to comment on the third level. Its topics— freedom of the will, free reason, self–consciousness—are often said to be intractable to scientific research. We do not want to evaluate the complex philosophical debate on this issue here. But from a practical point of view, any psychiatrist is familiar with psychotic patients who are severely suffering from their restricted freedom of decision making and acting. Some psychopathologists as Henri Ey apply the term "pathology of freedom" to psychotic disorders (Ey 1969, 1975).

A transcendental concept of mental illness holds the position that the level of free reason and self–consciousness is a necessary, but not sufficient attribute of human beings, as are the two other levels, regardless whether a person is healthy or psychotic.

To summarize, what is the main reason to apply transcendental ideas on psychopathological topics?

It is the obvious failure of specialized theories to deal with the phenomenon of mental illness without uncritical overgeneralization and without creating new prejudice and dogma. Many concepts are unidimensional. They interpret psychopathological data on a physiological, biochemical, sociological or psychoanalytical basis. This is adequate, unless the particular concept is broadened uncritically.

In philosophical terms, neither strictly realistic nor strictly idealistic approaches are suitable. Psychopathology needs a theoretical framework which accepts the scientific competence of different disciplines within their well–defined limits. And it has to insist on the fact, that a mentally ill person is a unity as is any other person, even if this unity does not fit into preexisting scientific frameworks.

In my view, a transcendental theory is the most appropriate one for that purpose: It is considering human beings as self–conscious, able to make decisions and responsible (level III). But they also function on a material basis (level I), and they can be described by means of teleology (level II).

Mental illness interferes with all of these levels. And there will be no comprehensive "explanation" of psychotic phenomena within just one level.

The main intention of a transcendental concept is in contrast with any kind of dogma. It does not presume to be competent for practical questions of empirical research, but wants to provide a critical philosophical link. Different approaches to psychiatric research are accepted within their epistemological limits, thus preventing them from becoming dogmatic.

In my view, it is unacceptable, that—depending on the theoretical orientation of the psychiatrist—a psychotic patient is considered to be *nothing but* a group of observable symptoms or a destabilized system of neurotransmitters or a victim of adverse psychosocial circumstances.

A transcendental concept will take into account all these different aspects and nevertheless insist on the unity of the person. And it will do that not just as a compromise, but on a sound philosophical basis.

Philosophical reflection in psychiatry has been criticized as being too abstract, as having no practical consequences. This position is not justified. Looking at all the competing psychiatric theories, there is one important conclusion: The scientific respectability of psychopathology is not threatened by philosophical arguments, but by its own theoretical assumptions if they are uncritically overgeneralized.

Finally, more recent psycho(patho)logical concepts shall be mentioned briefly, not in order to comment on their special contents, but to point out their compatibility with a transcendental background.

In cognitive psychology, although mainly oriented on experimental designs (Hoffmann 1988), the epistemological framework is sometimes called "constructivism". According to Rusch (1987), the main point in this theory is, that "the world's nature is not the starting point of cognition, but its expression." (Rusch 1987, p. 205)

This is clearly in accordance with Kant's and Fichte's view.

Another example is the well–known controversy between Piaget's structuralism and Chomsky's innatism within his concept of "Generative Grammar" (Chomsky 1968, Piaget 1977, Piattelli–Palmarini 1980). This debate is of course more important for neuropsychology. But as for our present context, it is relevant that both Piaget and Chomsky reject empiricistic theories of cognition. Chomsky is particularly close to transcendental arguments by emphasizing the influence of preexisting ("inborn") mental structures.

The concept of emergence postulates that mental phenomena will only take place if there is a material background in the form of complex neuronal systems. But these mental acts are asserted to represent and to create something new, and not to be just "copies" of neurophysiological processes. Some authors state that not all facts about mental acts will be sufficiently described by logical empiricism. For example, Hastedt (1988) stresses, that the human mind is not only an object of its own scientific interest, but plays the active part in this process. He calls this phenomenon the "perspective of a participant", as opposed to the "perspective of a spectator". The "perspective of a participant" is regarded as the superior one (Hastedt 1988).

In my view, a concept such as "emergence theory" can be more suitable for the complex matter of psychobiology than a strictly materialistic position (Churchland 1981) or identity theory (Smart 1981) or even functionalism (Fodor 1983). By laying emphasis on the activity of the human mind when it is considering itself, emergence theory applies an important transcendental thought: To know something, always implies to know about this knowledge as a knowledge, as a mental act.[3] From Kant's and Fichte's point of view, this is the essential meaning of the term "reflection".

Finally, what should not be forgotten in this context, is the long standing controversy about the different epistemological status of natural vs. social sciences. When critically reflecting, for example, upon the positions of Dilthey (1958), Weber (1922), Jaspers (1913), Wittgenstein (1922), Gadamer (1975), Habermas (1968), Ricoeur (1970), these appear to be centered around one question: What is the relationship between the social scientist as an active subject and the surrounding world or society as a complex object, of which the scientist himself is a part. Debates on the hermeneutic approach often draw heavily on transcendental concepts, even if these are developed in directions differing from those of their founders.

In conclusion, one issue should be emphasized again: This paper does not plead for an uncritical adoption of Kant's and Fichte's transcendental positions. But on the other hand, it is not true, that recently developed theories have made it unnecessary to consider questions and answers arising from so–called "classical" philosophical theories. Neopositivism, critical realism and several theories within the analytical philosophy of mind explicitly object to a transcendental point of view. To evaluate these controversies without severe misunderstandings, the basic transcendental framework has to be pointed out clearly and reflected upon through examination of primary sources.

In my view, this kind of undogmatic link between philosophy and psychopathology will not only have theoretical, but practical consequences, especially for the way we deal with our patients.

---

3 Especially Fichte insisted on cognition being an active process, an "act" of the transcendental I ("Tathandlung des Ich", Fichte 1804).

Summary

In this paper two hypotheses are discussed: (1) Transcendental philosophy, as defined by its two founders Kant and Fichte, represents a body of knowledge which proves to be of value not only from a historical point of view, but for present day philosophical discussion as well. Transcendental reflection holds the position that neither pure realism nor pure (absolute) idealism constitute an adequate epistemological framework. (2) For two reasons psychopathology is especially qualified for transcendental reflection: First, any kind of dogmatism will be fatal for psychopathology as a scientific discipline, and the basic intention of transcendentalism is an antidogmatic one. Second, transcendentalism is regarding philosophy as an unity; it therefore may serve as a philosophical connection between different specialized scientific approaches.

If psychopathology does not succeed in defining its identity as "field of basic research for psychiatry" (Janzarik), pessimistic assumptions in recent literature might turn out to be correct: Psychopathology could then easily be replaced by related disciplines such as neurobiology, psychoanalysis, sociology, and experimental psychology.

Transcendental reflection may help to meet with the following basic demands in psychopathology: (a) Psychopathology has to be epistemologically undogmatic. (b) It has to be open to different research strategies for empirical studies. (c) In order to prevent its disintegration into several unconnected subunities, it should be grounded on a comprehensive anthropological framework ("Menschenbild").

Some of the recent developments in theoretical psychopathology actually make use of transcendental concepts, sometimes without recognizing it. This is illustrated by the examples of "constructivism", "structuralism" (Piaget), "generative grammar" (Chomsky), and the concept of "emergence" within the philosophy of mind.

References

Bieri P (ed): Analytische Philosophie des Geistes. Hain, Königstein/Ts., 1981.

Chomsky N: Language and Mind. New York, 1968.

Churchland PM: Eliminative Materialism and the Propositional Attitudes. J Phil 82: 8–28, 1981.

Diagnostic and Statistical Manual of Mental Disorders. Third Edition, revised (DSM-III–R). American Psychiatric Association, Washington DC, 1987.

Dilthey W: Der Aufbau der geschichtlichen Welt in den Geisteswissenschaften. Gesammelte Schriften. Vol. 7. 2nd ed. Berlin, 1958.

Emrich HM: Die Beziehung zwischen Philosophie und Psychiatrie, vom Standpunkt einer systemtheoretischen Konzeption produktiver Psychosen aus betrachtet. In: Spitzer M, Uehlein FA, Oepen G (eds) Psychopathology and Philosophy. Springer, Berlin, Heidelberg, New York, London Paris Tokyo, pp. 57–70, 1988.

Ey H: La Conscience. 2nd ed. Presses de Univ de France, Paris, 1969.

Ey H: La psychose et les psychotiques. Evol Psychiat 4: 103–116, 1975.

Fichte JG: Die Wissenschaftslehre (1804). Zweiter Vortrag. Lauth R, Widmann J (eds), Meiner, Hamburg, 1975.

Fodor JA: The Modularity of Mind. Cambridge/Mass, London, 1983.

Gadamer HG: Wahrheit und Methode. Grundzüge einer philosophischen Hermeneutik. 4th ed. Tübingen, 1975.

Habermas J: Erkenntnis und Interesse. Suhrkamp, Frankfurt/Main, 1968.

Hastedt H: Das Leib–Seele–Problem. Suhrkamp, Frankfurt/Main, 1988.

Hoff P: Nosologische Grundpostulate bei Kraepelin. Zschr Klin Psychol Psychopathol Psychother 36: 328–336, 1988.

Hoff P: Erkenntnistheoretische Vorurteile in der Psychiatrie. Fundamenta Psychiatrica 3: 141–150, 1989a.

Hoff P: Der Begriff der psychischen Krankheit aus transzendentaler Sicht. Campus, Frankfurt/Main, 1989b, in press.

Hoffmann J: Kognitive Psychologie. In: Asanger R, Wenninger G (eds): Handwörterbuch der Psychologie. 4th ed. Psychologie Verlags Union, München Weinheim, pp. 352–356, 1988.

Hume D: An Enquiry Concerning Human Understanding. London, 1748.

Janzarik W: Die Krise der Psychopathologie. Nervenarzt 47: 73–80, 1976.

Jaspers K: Allgemeine Psychopathologie. Springer, Heidelberg, 1913.

Kant I: Kritik der reinen Vernunft (1781 A, 1787 B). JF Hartknoch, Riga. Reprint, Meiner, Hamburg, 1956.

Lauth R: Die transzendentale Naturlehre Fichtes nach den Prinzipien der Wissenschaftslehre. Meiner, Hamburg, 1984.

Lauth R: Transzendentale Entwicklungslinien von Descartes bis zu Marx und Dostojewski. Meiner, Hamburg, 1989.

Mayer–Gross W: Die Entwicklung der klinischen Anschauungen Kraepelins. Arch Psychiat 87: 30–42, 1929.

Möller HJ: Methodische Grundprobleme der Psychiatrie. Kohlhammer, Stuttgart, 1976.

Mundt Ch: Der Begriff der Intentionalität und die Defizienzlehre von den Schizophrenien. Nervenarzt 55: 582–588, 1984.

Nagel E: Teleology revisited. Columbia Univ Press, New York, 1979.

Nagel Th: Physicalism. In: Feigl H, Sellars W, Lehrer K (eds): New Readings in Philosophical Analysis. New York, pp. 408–417, 1965.

Piaget J: The Development of Thought: Equilibrium of Cognitive Structures. Viking Press, New York, 1977.

Piattelli–Palmarini M (ed): Language and Learning. The Debate between Jean Piaget and Noam Chomsky. Harvard Univ Press, Cambridge/Mass, 1980.

Putnam H: Mind, Language and Reality. Philosophical Papers. Vol 2. Cambridge/Mass, 1975.

Ricoeur P: Freud and Philosophy: An Essay on Interpretation. New Haven, 1970.

Rusch G: Erkenntnis, Wissenschaft, Geschichte–von einem konstruktivistischen Standpunkt. Suhrkamp, Frankfurt/Main, 1987.

Schelling FWJ: Philosophie der Offenbarung (Paulus–Nachschrift). CW Leske, Darmstadt, 1843.

Schwartz MA, Wiggins OP: Perspectivism and the methods of psychiatry. Compr Psychiat 29: 237–251, 1988.

Searle JR: Intentionality. An Essay in the Philosophy of Mind. Cambridge Univ Press, London, 1983.

Smart JJC: Physicalism and Emergence. Neuroscience 6: 109–113, 1981.

Spitzer M, Uehlein FA, Oepen G (eds): Psychopathology and Philosophy. Springer, Berlin Heidelberg New York, London, Paris, Tokyo, 1988.

Weber M: Wirtschaft und Gesellschaft. Mohr, Tübingen, 1922.

Wittgenstein L: Tractatus logico–philosophicus. London, 1922.

Final Comments
and Reflections

Synopsis and Critical Remarks

Manfred Spitzer, Brendan A. Maher, Friedrich A. Uehlein

A synopsis of the contributions contained in this volume seems to be indicated for several reasons: (1) the contributions in this volume are heterogeneous. (2) There are no established "schools of thought" in the field of psychopathology *and* philosophy. (3) Philosophers, psychologists, and psychiatrists may each need a somewhat bigger picture in order to make sense out of the various lines of thought offered in this volume. (4) Furthermore, it is not always self–evident what kind of problems are addressed by each contributor and how the proposed solutions are related to clinical practice. We will try to approach some of these issues by, first, providing a general conceptual framework of possible relations between philosophy and psychopathology, and second, by commenting on what may be regarded as some common threads that can be found in the articles, specifically aspects relating to certain features of experience, of rationality, of the self, and of schizophrenia.

1. Philosophy and Psychopathology

Collaboration between psychopathology and philosophy requires some initial understanding of the goals of each of the two disciplines and the problems that beset their achievements. When the psychiatrist and the clinical psychologist ask, "What can philosophy contribute to psychopathology?"[1] this can mean at least two quite different things. One relates to the manner in which the philosopher can help the psychopathologist solve problems that have already been defined by the psychopathologist. The other relates to the manner in which the philosopher might encourage the psychopathologist to examine the basic premises of his discipline. We will look at each in turn here.

What Europeans term "Anglo–American" psychopathology has evolved historically in ways that reflect an abiding concern with pragmatic aspects of mental illness. From this point of view an oversimplified picture

---

1 The question can of course be asked the other way: "What can psychopathology contribute to philosophy?", and there are interesting aspects to this question (cf. Castañeda 1988 and this volume, Hundert 1989 and this volume, Spitzer et al. 1988). Psychopathology, for instance, can provide philosophy with certain cases which may broaden the spectrum of phenomena to be included by any theory of experience. In the main text, however, we are interested in the contribution of philosophy to psychopathology.

of the ideal outcome of psychiatric investigations of, let us say, schizophrenia would look something like this. A pathological entity (or set of sub–entities) would be defined with such precision and reliability that any two clinicians with sufficient training and experience could agree that a given patient does or does not exhibit symptoms of the entity in question. Patients diagnosed as possessing the entity would prove to have similar etiologies, similar pathologies, similar prognoses, and would respond similarly to specific treatments. Etiologies might turn out to be genetic, environmental, or some combination of both, but whatever the etiology might be, it would be the same for cases presenting the appropriate defining symptoms. A measure of sophistication is added by the recognition that prognosis may be affected by uncontrollable events in the patient's post–morbid environment, and hence "similar prognosis" means "similar given that the patients are returned to similar environments".

Fulfillment of this kind of outcome is severely hampered by several factors. Two of them are of major importance. Clinical realities are such that by the time a patient comes to the clinician it is generally too late to make direct observations of the etiological processes that led to the morbid condition. Nor is there yet any way in which genetic factors can be confirmed directly by karyotyping or other first–hand observation of genetic material. Environmental factors are inferred from the retrospective accounts of sometimes unreliable informants, including the patients themselves. Genetic factors are inferred from the record of similar pathologies in family members past and present; these too are subject to the unreliabilities that typically plague such records. In brief, the ideal of a well–established etiology is very difficult to achieve in practice. Matters are a little better when we turn to the observation of current clinical condition, prognosis, response to therapy and the like, but even these observations are often far from satisfactory.

The sanguine psychopathologist would readily admit to the importance of these difficulties, but could justifiably claim that they are only practical, meaning thereby that with technological and methodological advances they can be overcome. Thus in the past three decades the use of high–risk prospective studies has diminished the problem of the unreliability of retrospective accounts of etiologically relevant experiences. Similarly, refinements in the structured ratings of current clinical phenomena reduce the judgment bias that enters into less formalized methods of observations, and so on.

However, a more serious problem remains. This is the fact that quite similar patterns of behavior may arise on the basis of rather different etiological sequences. In essence the belief that similar clinical pictures should have similar etiologies is an article of faith rather than a demonstrably self–evident principle (see for example Mundt's discussion of the problem in his chapter in this volume). Differential diagnosis has a long history in psychiatry, and this testifies to the fact that quite different etiologies and pathologies may have many clinical features in common, sufficiently so to make correct diagnosis dependent on rather precise inspection of the subtle clinical features that do discriminate between them. We may perhaps retain our faith in the notion of a linear determination between cause and effect in psychopathology by recognizing that the classification of clinical syndromes requires a far greater scrutiny of the details of a case than has hitherto commmomly been undertaken. The fact that all hallucinations are classed as hallucinations regardless of individual differences between them, may mislead us into thinking that two patients who both have hallucinations are, in that respect, similar. The same applies to all general symptomatic descriptions, such as delusion, anhedonia, withdrawal, and the like.

It is no exaggeration to say that the core of clinical observation and procedure consists of asking the patient to describe his or her conscious processes. Most of the time, for example, our conclusion that a patient is deluded is based upon the fact that the patient has expressed certain (often false) beliefs about the external world, beliefs which we define as delusional because we judge that these beliefs possess the particular kind of certainty and incorrigibility that we typify as delusional. The same applies to hallucinations, to anhedonia, to depressed ideas of worthlessness, to manic ambitions, and so on. Another way to put this is to point out that it is very difficult to diagnose a patient who has been mute from birth, or even a patient of whose language the clinician is totally ignorant; in brief, a patient whose conscious processes are inaccessible to us.

One of the many unfortunate consequences of the former intellectual hegemony of psychoanalysis was the practice of regarding the statements of psychotic patients (and everybody else as well, for that matter) as material to be interpreted rather than as communications to be largely understood in the terms in which they were conveyed. The framework for interpretation was already in place, consisting mainly in certain assumptions about intrapsychic entities and their interactions, and the outcome putatively known in advance, hence the effect was to transform variegated descriptions of conscious experience into more or less uniform patterns of allegedly unconscious experience. One consequence was the predictable impoverishment of the concept of differential diagnosis. Another was the demotion of the study of consciousness to the study of disguises. Fine-grained analysis of the reported conscious experience of the patient was regarded as not merely unnecessary but, unless interpeted dynamically, downright misleading.

With the decline of psychoanalysis came an accompanying decline in doctrinaire interpretations and a revival of interest in diagnosis. However, there has not been a corresponding interest in the detailed study of consciousness through the phenomenological description of psychopathological states. Moreover, in respect to interpretation the baby has been thrown out with the bathwater, and it has been overlooked that some form of interpretation is always at work in any attempt to understand another person. The problem is not, therefore, "How can we describe without any theory?", but rather "What is the best (i.e., most useful, most reliable, most adequate, etc.) conceptual framework for the purposes of psychopathological description?". As indicated in the introduction, this problem already motivated Jaspers in his attempts to find a "phenomenological" solution, and it still can be traced in contemporary textbooks and manuals such as the *Diagnostic and Statistical Manual of Mental Disorders* (DSM–III–R).

2. Frameworks of Interpretation

For the reasons already adumbrated above, the fine–grained analysis of conscious experience is an important, perhaps crucial, component in the development of a system of symptom description that will permit the kind of differential diagnosis that is essential to progress in psychopathology. This is not to say that conscious experience is the only realm in which fine–grained analyses are required. Language utterances, motor behavior, social interactions, and other phenomena that are open to the inspection of a clinical observer demand similar scrutiny if valid and reliable differential diagnosis is to be achieved—and with it a thorough understanding of the psychopathologies that underlie different conditions.

The analysis of conceptual schemes or frameworks is, of course, one of the major tasks with which the philosopher is concerned. Philosophers focus on the necessity for detailed analysis of such concepts as perception, consciousness, thought, self, etc. Through the use of such clarified concepts, psycho-pathologists can produce clearer and more accurate descriptions of how the minds of mentally ill patients appear from the "inside". Clearly this approach does not tell the whole story; nonetheless it provides information that is generally lacking in formulations of psychopathology that are based exclusively on reports of "outside" clinical observers.

In this volume several contributors provide examples of the way in which this can be applied to problems of psychosis. Wiggins, Schwartz and Northoff present a Husserlian framework for understanding the incipient development of schizophrenia. They contend that a basic, normal certainty in the stability of fundamental features of the self and the world around us or to use Husserl's term, *Urdoxa,* is shaken in schizophrenia. They do not focus on an even earlier etiology for this, being concerned instead with the concurrent conscious experience of the patient, rather than with the physiological events that brought these experiences into being. Their fine–grained analysis is carried out in the best Jasperian spirit and sheds light on the various stages of psychotic mentality as viewed from the "inside".

Mundt takes up a similar theme, but with an important difference. Rather than ascribing a mere loss of certainty to the core of schizophrenic psychopathology, he suggests that the normal individual in fact lives with a balance of certainties and uncertainties. This balance is lost in schizophrenia, with a major tilt towards uncertainties and a resultant disorganization of the patient's connectedness with the world around him; this disrupted connectedness is reflected in instability of meanings of words and other symbols used by the patient.

In keeping with the general emphasis upon the organization/disorganization of the experience of the psychotic patient, Hundert turns to the role of categories in the organization of perception (and hence of knowledge), and the consequent possibility that schizophrenia may be understood as involving a loss of the categorizing function in the patient. Madness, he suggests, consists of experience "produced by mental faculties whose categories manifest structural defects" (p. 64). Here again, Hundert does not propose a physiological etiology for these defects, i.e., he is not concerned with any "outside view", but he is rather interested in the kinds of structural defects in patients' categories that may provide a core framework for understanding psychopathology "from the mind's point of view."

Spitzer provides a Kantian approach to the proper understanding of a certain subgroup of schizophrenic symptoms. He argues that only with a theory about the experiencing subject, and of its basic features in mind it is possible to diagnose disturbances of experience, "Ichstörungen" (as these are called in the German psychiatric literature). Without an understanding of those general features of any normal experience (unity, mine–ness, distinctness between me and not–me, reflexivity, identity, etc.) utterances of patients such as "my thoughts are controlled" and "there is no boundary between me and reality" can only be interpreted as false, nonsensical and/or mad. with such an understanding, however, they can be treated as valid descriptions of disturbances regarding various features of experience in general.

If considerations of the stability of the relationship of self to the world and, second, the integrity of categories of experience, provide two philosophical approaches to the definition of psychopathology, delineations of the condition of the self of the patient provides another. Contributions on this topic were made by Casatañeda and by Margulies. We will focus on some problems of self in a special section below.

3. External Validity

How is the psychopathologist to link the reports of patients' experience to other relevant sets of data? Such a link is absolutely essential if psychopathology is not to remain a purely descriptive matter, based upon reports of individual experience but leading nowhere in the quest for etiology, prognosis, therapy or other concurrent pathologies of a biological or behavioral nature. There is, of course, a significant recent history of work on biological aspects of schizophrenia and other psychoses: It has been confined, however, to studies of biological factors that are associated with overt behavioral manifestations of psychosis, including patient reports as behavioral indices and not as direct measures of conscious experience. Oepen Harrington and Fünfgeld report an investigation in which psychotic–like experiences were induced pharmacologically in normal subjects, who were then studied with psychiatric symptom rating scales, laboratory measures of face recognition, and scans of brain metabolism. Their data lead them to conclude that psychotic experience is indeed inducible in normal subjects, and that category distinctions between the "normal" and the "mentally ill" might be replaced with concepts that place individuals along a continuous dimension, their position on the dimension being amenable to change with alterations in brain functioning.

Emrich also relates subjective psychopathology to objective measures of the perceptual capabilities of schizophrenic patients. While his objective measure consists of a sophisticated device that attempts to index the capability of normal subjects and patients to cope with perceptual stimuli that contradict their prior experience, his measures on the subjective side are less fine–tuned and consist merely of the dichotomic variable of productive versus non–productive psychosis. His theory of perception, however, suggests that a more precise analysis at the subjective level, i.e., an analysis of single symptoms and their aspects, should yield higher correlations between "inner" (subjective) and "outer" (objective) aspects of what is, presumably, the same pathology.

4. Experience and Its Features

It is striking that several authors in this volume (coming from different countries, and from various backgrounds and fields of research and study) emphasize the fact that experience is not simply "given" but rather the result of some active constructive process (cf. Emrich, Hundert, Maher, Rychlak, Spitzer, Wiggins et al.). What the nature of that process is, how and in what terms it can be understood, what the appropriate methods to its study are—these questions are anything but solved, and in fact are related to the most puzzling questions that philosophy faces up to the present day.

It is no wonder that most of the authors mentioned address the problem of experience in an idealist, and broadly speaking, Kantian framework. Contrary to the Anglo–American Empiricist tradition of philosophy, wherein it is held that all knowledge can only be derived from either sensation or inductive and deductive reasoning, Kant claimed that, in addition, we have knowledge about ourselves—i.e., the *presuppositions* of any given experience—by means of reflection. We cannot undertake the attempt here to answer the questions whether such knowledge may rightly be called, as Kant claimed, "synthetic apriori" or "transcendental", and we are not in the position—200 years after Kant—to build an epistemological "machine" like the one he had built, without addressing all the problems inherent in such an enterprise which philosophers have pointed out in the meantime. Moreover, when we use a Kantian approach to conceptualize basic features of experience (and what may be wrong with them in the case of disordered mentality), we have to confront ourselves with the charge of doing merely "armchair psychology", i.e., of making empirically unjustified assumptions about how the mind works. However, even the tradition of analytic philosophy, which is considered to be agnostic in respect to positive statements about the human condition, has provided us with arguments about necessary presuppositions.[2] The so–called private language argument, for example, tries to establish a necessary link between the use of meaningful concepts and the communicative aspect of a language, or, in other words, between truth and falsity and intersubjectivity.[3] To give another example, one prominent figure in analytic philosophy, Peter Strawson—while trying to preserve Kant's insights without adopting the parts of Kantian philosophy that are rejected by most present philosophers as no longer tenable—argues for a necessary link between the objectivity of experience and a specific form of self–consciousness[4], as well as for a necessary link between the "mine–ness" of our experiences and the existence of other minds (Strawson 1966). However, while philosophers try to assess the possibility of reflective and reflexive knowledge–claims about the presuppositions of any experience, Hundert (1989, p. 25) points out, that the "seemingly innocent assumptions about experience, 'as we know we have it' may be called into question when we begin to consider psychotic experience". This again could prove to be the case where the absence of apparently necessary presuppositions of experience might render patients' talk meaningful (and not just non–sensical) and illuminating in the course of differential diagnosis.

Given the fact that schizophrenics frequently report experiences in which very basic features such as "mine–ness", "reflexivity", "objectivity", or "intersubjectivity" are somewhat disturbed, it may be no wonder that the three authors in this volume who happened to be educated in philosophy as well as in psychiatry, *independently* chose the same philosophical background to account for or interpret the phenomena in question (cf. Hoff 1988, Hundert 1989, Spitzer 1985).

To the Anglo–American reader who might be accustomed to construing German idealism and transcendental philosophy as the prototype of dogmatic thinking, the thesis of Hoff's paper—that transcendental philosophy is the remedy for the contemporary danger that psychiatric practice may become dogmatic—may sound strange. Hoff argues that in the absence of a clear fact–theory distinction, the concepts that lead us to "construct" reality have to be taken into account, especially in such a complex area as psychiatry. Some critical remarks have yet to be made: Does

2 Methodologically speaking, analytic philosophy may help to keep the arguments of psychopathologists clear and to avoid unwarranted fanciful thought about the human mind. That is to say that we highly respect the way of arguing in the analytic tradition without necessarily accepting the kind of reductionistic view of the mind that some analytic philosophers seem to pursue.
3 The private language argument is generally attributed to Ludwig Wittgenstein (*Philosophical Investigations* 1952), although there might be as many versions of the argument as there are Wittgenstein scholars.
4 That is, the capability of the "I think" to accompany all the perceptions of a single subject of experience (cf. Strawson 1966, p. 102).

230 M. Spitzer, B.A. Maher, F.A. Uehlein

one really need to go back to a transcendental approach to experience in order to justify an undogmatic and "multi–level" interpretation of facts? While Hoff seems to be right in saying that "specialized theories" suffer from the danger of "uncritical overgeneralization" and "prejudice and dogma," his claim that transcendental philosophy is the *only* way out is questionable. Although it is historically true to some extent, it need not be the case that an empiricist's view of human nature must always be reductionistic. Rather, the undogmatic empiricist could maintain that the human being must not to be reduced to a body (which ultimately has to be described and accounted for in terms of physics), but must be viewed from as many different angles as possible to achieve the most comprehensive picture possible. However, has the empiricist not already developed a kind of theory about man, i.e., about the different possible (or at least feasible) approaches to man as his "subject matter"? Or is this most comprehensive picture merely the outcome of an unreflective pragmatic stance, warranted only by the fact that it "works" somehow? Moreover, how does the empiricist delineate the boundaries of such a view? Hoff's notion that existing nosological entities tend to become unquestioned prejudices could be viewed as a typical example of what can ensue if the empiricist's stance is not taken seriously enough.

One further, brief critical remark on Hoff's account of idealism has to be made: Schelling's version of idealism is misconstrued if we say that he did not consider experience to have any significance. How could ideas and experience be distinguished (and the idea of absolute ideas be developed) without a distinction being made between experience and ideas in the first place? Schelling's idealist position, like that of many other "idealist" philosophers since Plato, does not disregard the empirical or factual or even replace it by "metaphysical forces," but rather attempts to account for necessary presuppositions, the possibility and the objectivity of experience, as well as for regularities, invariances, and generalities within experience. A short quotation from Schelling's *Introduction to the Project of a System of Philosophy of Nature (Einleitung zu dem Entwurf eines Systems der Naturphilosophie)* may not only clarify the point, but may also shed some systematic light on the relationship between experience and (a priori) presuppositions of experience.

"We do not only know this and that, rather we do not know anything originally by any other means than experience. Hence, all our knowledge consists of empirical statements. These statements may become statements a priori only by way of considering them as necessary by means of reflection. Thus any statement, regardless of its content, might be elevated to this dignity, because the difference between a priori and empirical statements does not, as some might have thought, ultimately inhere in the statements themselves. This difference, rather, exists *only in respect to our knowledge,* and the kind of our knowledge of these statements. Therefore, any statement which happens to be a historical, contingent statement for me, might become a statement a priori, as soon as (and only if) I understand—immediately or indirectly—its necessity" (Schelling 1799, p. 278, italics in the original, transl. by the author, M.S.).

5. Rationality

As presumably "normal" individuals, we tend to ascribe our capability for functioning adequately to our ability to relate to reality as it is (versus the mentally ill patient who, we think, relates to reality as it is misconstrued by him or her). The clinical notion of "reality testing" seems to imply that we *do* something in order to have that special contact with reality that some unfortunate others (the ones with "impaired" reality testing, as the clinical jargon tells us) lack. It is pointed out by Maher that this picture is grossly oversimplied. On purely empirical grounds he argues that the human nervous system has not evolved to provide an isomorphic representation of the world, but rather, to convey information about the probabilities of various stimuli. However, it is conceptually unclear, first, what such an isomorphic representation could be, and, secondly, how the notion of a stimulus can be generalized to make sense within the argument (the concept of a stimulus only makes sense in a specific framework, e.g., within an experiment; there are no "stimuli as such", which seem to be presupposed by the argument). A way of rephrasing the problem is to say that human beings always act in a world which is already an interpreted one: whether there are (supposed to be) tables and chairs or particles and energy–fields or numbers in a multi–dimensional mathematical space—in all these cases reality is interpreted according to specific rules, practices and actions (which we may conceive as having evolved[5]). There is no "reality as such" with which we may come in contact in some absolutely "better" or "worse" way.

If rationality is equated with logic and certain inductive statistical methods widely used in a scientific context, it turns out that such a rationality is almost useless for the purposes of managing the decisions of everyday life. As everyday life functioning is highly disturbed in psychotics, it follows, as Maher convincingly argues, that there is much more to the distinction of normalcy and pathology than rationality.

While it is hard to delineate a concept of rationality that matches the psychiatrists' needs when they distinguish between the rational and the irrational by means of something other than mere statistical norms (which are rarely applied clinically), an accurate, convincing, and consistent reconstruction of what happens when such clinical distinctions are made is far from being fully developed at present. As pointed out by Döring, irrationality can only be ascribed to another person against a background of rationality.[6] To put his argument somewhat simply, there is always a tradeoff

---

5 The notion of evolution is tricky: if it is meant to guarantee any further contact to reality, it is misleading, as we do not know what "reality–as such", i.e., prior to all out attempts to conceive it, means. Saying that the rules, practices and actions according to which we interpret reality have evolved according to reality is circular because the study of evolution itself is such an interpreting activity. While the concept of evolution is a powerful empirical concept, it does not—contrary to what so–called evolutionary epistemologists believe—provide us with *any further* reason to believe that, what we think is real, is, in fact, real.

6 In the fourth paragraph of his paper, Döring tries to confirm that one cannot ascribe contradictory beliefs. There arise some questions concerning method. Ascribing beliefs, Döring states, involves

between the reasons for ascribing irrational thoughts, feelings, motives and so forth, and the reasons for saying that one has simply not understood what is going on in the patient. Whereas normally, if someone we know behaves somewhat strangely, we are inclined to admit that we do *not understand* what is going on, in the set and setting of a clinic, as psychiatrists, we tend to opt for the construal that we have *understood irrational* thoughts, feelings, motives etc." Although in practice there may not be too many cases where this arises as a clinical problem, Döring's argument shows that the grounds for difficulties that sometimes actually occur clinically are deeply rooted in our concepts of understanding and of rationality.

The arguments of Maher and Döring depend on a "strong" version of the concept of rationality, which neither includes nor allows irrational acts or behavior. Nevertheless, a concept of rationality does not have to be this strictly or narrowly defined. Plato and Aristotle, for example, and the various traditions that adopted and transformed their ideas, developed a different conception of rationality. For Plato man is a *synamphoteron*, i.e. a "both–together" of two heterogeneous parts: soul and body (Timaios 87 c). Rationality is a part of this composite whole, viz. "soul in the primary and most essential sense" (Timaios 90 a). This means—to state one instance only—that "man forms a general conception *by collecting into one* the many perceptions of the senses by means of reason" (Phaidros 249 b/c). Reason being the primary, most essential and preferably leading part does not exhaust the nature of soul, let alone that of the whole man. According to the emblematic account of the *Phaidros* (246 a – 249 d), soul can be

---

behavioural considerations. And he concludes rightly that no action or any action whatsoever would be appropriate to follow from a person's contradictory beliefs. Does the strategy of behavioural considerations work towards the intended aim? Do behavioural considerations elucidate contradictory beliefs? One must have understood beforehand—so it seems—whether those mental states simultaneously held are mutually exclusive or consistent. From these (at least allegedly) understood and estimated beliefs we do then interpret the behavior of the person in question and end up with the judgement that any action or none might follow from that situation. The whole strategy amounts to this: We cannot ascribe mutually exclusive mental states because they are logically exclusive, and not, as is suggested, because a person is unable to behave in a way that was appropriate for both states and hereby persuading us to conclude she is holding contradictory beliefs. Why is she unable to act appropriately? Since "nothing (or everything ...) is appropriate in an impossible situation". But why is the situation impossible? Since the mental states simultaneously held in that situation are mutually exclusive. The behavioural considerations appear to argue in a circle. The whole argument dwindles down to logic: there is no set of beliefs that can be determined by p and non–p at the same time and in the same relation. Since such a belief cannot be identified it hence cannot be ascribed to a person.

A similar slight objection to method might be presented—mutatis mutandis—against the "language of thought" and against "the course of explaining and predicting an agent's behaviour". A strong, rigid and at the same time rather vacuous version of the concept of rationality forbids the ascription of such a non-entity as a set of contradictory beliefs.

The concept of "ideal rationality" appears to be hampered by a prima facie innocuous but truly ambiguous and inflated use of the word *belief*. *Belief* is to cover knowledge of necessary truths and of convictions whose reasons can be given and whose range and consequences can be surveyed, as well as intuitions received on the spur of the moment, opinions on slight or proven empirical grounds, inferences, and conclusions (Döring, this volume, pp. 92–93), hypotheses etc. Consequently, the belief that 2+2=4 need not, for example, imply any correct belief about the number of primes, since they may belong to different *kinds of belief*, that latter founded in a thorough knowledge (*episteme*) of arithmetic, the first being a true opinion (*alethes doxa*) gleaned from everyday occurrences in childhood. Döring's elucidating analysis of "ideal rationality" can thus be supported by ordinary analysis of the crucial word *belief* and the way it is used.

likened to a pair of horses and a charioteer: "The charioteer of the human soul drives a pair of unequal horses, one noble and of noble breed, the other quite the opposite in breed and character" (246 b). The charioteer personifies reason, or soul in the primary and most essential sense, the horses embody the drives, appetencies, desires and fears, emotion, sensation, the imagining part, phantasy etc. Human perception and understanding of the world, and man's action and behavior (in the most inclusive sense) are therefore always and in each case a delicate balance of his rational and irrational (but nevertheless psychic) powers and his body within the composite whole of heterogeneous parts. Plato adds dryly: "Therefore in our case the driving is necessarily difficult and troublesome" (246 b).

This conception leaves a wide range or dimension for irrational thinking and acting *within* the bounds of human rationality. The latter are marked off by divine intelligence which "sees what is [*to on*] and beholds truth [*alethea*]' (247 d) and a possible kind of prehension which is neither rational nor irrational, but having no charioteer, as it were, falls outside the sphere of rationality. Plato elaborated this conception in various dialogues, especially in the second part of the *Timaios* (69 ff). In Aristotle's ethical writings as well as in *De anima* and the second book of the *Rhetoric* a rather similar and (for our present concern) equivalent conception is to be found. In the last century, Hegel expressed a similar view:

"The truly *psychic* treatment of derangement therefore holds firmly to the view that it is not the abstract loss of reason, neither in respect of intelligence nor of the will and its responsibility, but that it is literally derangement, i.e. not the absence but a contradiction within rationality; just as physical illness is not an abstract, that is to say an entire loss of health (which would mean death), but health involving a contradiction. ... By presupposing the patient's rationality, this human, i.e. benevolent as well as reasonable treatment can take as firm a hold of him spiritually as one can of his bodily nature by treating his vitality as the presupposition of his physical health" (Hegel, *Encyclopedia*, § 408).

The problem of how to deal with *teleology* as a feature of rational thinking remains a passionately discussed theme in philosophy. It was emphasized by Kant that we can only determine the organic nature of living organisms by applying teleological categories. If these were omitted, we would only be able to state causal relations between "things" rather than accounting for the particular unity which an organism builds up out of its organs, and noticing its life–process and purposeful behavior. Causal explanations of an organism's behavior, therefore, can only be detected in a teleological framework, i.e., by the attempt to make sense out of a specific organ or function. Whether the question "what is this for" is ultimately (i.e., by the time when all the causal connections of an organism have been scientifically established) superfluous, as Francis Bacon held, or is a necessary constituent of our knowledge, remains a matter of dispute. It cannot, however, easily be dismissed, as even the concept of an organism itself (as well as the concepts of an "organ" or a "system", respectively) depends on a teleological framework and in no way can be construed only by the conceptual means of causality and substance. As we have not achieved a state of an "ideal" science, the point for teleology has to be made anyway, and Rychlak is right in laying emphasis on it. No matter how one decides at present about the range and validity of final explanation in the field of organic nature and life–processes, teleology is certainly valid for all kinds of intentional phenomena, such as drives, wishes, motives and overtly intentional acts like perception, experience, speech (dialogue), action, and behavior. Rychlak goes back to the most elaborate framework of final explanation, to Aristotle's teleology and attempts to develop a "language" appropriate to the description of the "telosponsive" and not simply responsive character of human behavior.

6. Self

The term "self" obviously has two quite different meanings which must not be confused. Psychologists use this term with a different meaning than that employed by philosophers.

In psychology and especially in psychotherapy, the meaning of "self" may be described somewhat like "a set of a person's features (character aspects, dispositions to behave, qualities—to name but a few terms that have been used to capture what is at issue here) as known or experienced by that person", in short, "the person (or personality) as known to that person". The problem encountered in many psychotherapies may then be rephrased by saying that such features can be more or less consistent with one another or with what the person feels or thinks that these features should be like. Through understanding and interpretation, such inconsistencies may be brought to the attention of the person and may be worked through in a way that results in a more consistent set of features or a better match between what is actually there and what is wanted. (That is, of course, just another way of saying that "unconscious conflicts" are made conscious and are somehow "resolved".) Moreover, in psychotherapy, "self" also may refer to a specific subset of features (as in ordinary language: there may be good or bad selves, critical ones and foolish ones) or to a specific age of a person (the childhood–self, the boy–self etc.). The paper of Margulies illustrates many of the different uses of the term "self" in psychotherapy. It also shows that these selves are not simply the result of discovery but also of construction. Needless to say, such construction takes place in an intersubjective framework, in a dialogue, which takes into account other persons and their opinions (Margulies refers to this process as "empathy with oneself through another"; Mundt, having about the same concept in mind, talks about "referential systems of third order").

However, there is nothing conceptually opaque or even paradoxical when one wonders who one "really" is: one is just referring to what one knows about one's dispositions, thoughts, feelings etc. and may do so by thinking of some episodes in the past. Just as I have two hands whether I see them or think about them or not (they don't come into being by my thinking about them or feeling them), so also my self (in the psychological meaning of the term) is there whether I think of it or not (as others can easily tell, who watch me acting, reacting, and behaving in some more or less consistent way). Of course, by way of reflecting about those features of mine (e.g., their relations or desirability), I may decide to attempt some improvements (which actually may turn out to be all but easy, and oftentimes impossible to *do*), but although such changes are the result of reflexive acts there is nothing special or intrinsically problematic to those acts: I do the same thing when worrying about other problems, I discover inconsistencies (which may just be a result of my way of seeing things), and make some efforts at correction.

Even in the extreme case when I think about features of mine and wonder which ones "really" belong to me, while the very same features I am wondering about may contribute to the decision ("am I 'really' a happy person?") the "paradox" seems to be only the result of a misconstrual: there is no general trait of happiness that makes me happy whenever I may feel so, but rather there are feelings of happiness which—if occurring frequently—make me think that by and large I am a happy person. By the same token, the question of how to relate my goal to be more reliable, communicative, and open to change to my desires to sometimes do foolish things, to my tendency not to talk to people and if I do, to disregard what they say, is not decided by reflecting endlessly about presupposed respective traits or even their origins, but rather by specific actions. By their very character of continuity (not acting is just a special way of acting), those tiny real life actions will tell me what and who I am without any paradox. Only by the unwarranted assumptions of the existence of "traits" ("I am happy because I have much happiness in me") and of rationally establishable emotions ("I want to be happy because that's better") do problems bearing a paradoxical flavor arise ("if I want to be happy, is this because I happen to be happy right now and thus I am biasing my decision which should be made independent of any bias and on purely rational grounds"). Of course, we are not saying that actions are, or should be, irrational. We rather claim that the construal of our thoughts, feelings, motivations etc. as at our constant rational disposal amounts to overshooting the mark by far.

Bearing this in mind, we can easily account for some clinical phenomena related to the consistency of personality traits (the different selves of clients in therapy): the fact that some substances have effects on mental life is not at all new.[7] When we get drunk, we rarely do so as a result of a rational decision about how we are like when drunk compared to how we are like when we are not drunk—we mostly simply get drunk (and any decision has to be invented afterwards). By the same token, a patient under

---

7 Even the fact that material substances, or "psychic molecules", as Margulies calls them, restore some function that had been present and has been affected by an illness is not new. Alcohol was known for thousands of years to provide some relief for insomnia, and certain pain killers have also been known for a long time. Modern psychoactive drugs are thus merely extreme cases of what mankind for long could handle without great puzzlement.

lithium may feel some deprivation of huge swings of his emotions[8] but may ordinarily accept that as a minor drawback compared to the serious and disabling consequences of being manic or depressed. In other words, the patient may know that taking the drug results in certain changes in his emotional life. As a matter of fact, many patients with major affective disorder from time to time discontinue lithium medication and many of them, indeed, again become ill. Although this is frequently presented by the patients as a result of choice, we don't think that any rational choice has been at work. From clinical experience it seems much more likely that the discontinuation of therapy was the result (rather than the cause) of the new manic or depressed episode, and that there was a different way of acting involved in the process rather than a different way of evaluating carefully the pros and cons of the therapy.

Even the case of Dostoevsky loses much of its puzzling flavor once the general question of personal identity ("who is who?") is distinguished from the question who Dostoevsky may have wanted to be ("do I want to suffer from epilepsy and one of its symptoms, hypergraphia, because in this way I may become a famous writer?"). The question of who Dostoevsky was if he had not suffered from epilepsy (or if he had been treated as patients with seizures are presently treated) has to be answered along the lines of possible worlds and their properties (and thus is of no more interest than the case of Caesar had he not crossed the Rubicon, Eve had she not picked the apple, or us had we not become interested in psychiatry and philosophy). The question of who (or how) Dostoevsky may have wanted to be is hard to answer as we cannot ask him. One may assume that he may have acted somewhat analogously to some manic patients such as those discussed above. We can be quite sure, however, that had anticonvulsive treatment been available a hundred years earlier, the question of who really is Dostoevsky may hardly have ever occurred to Dostoevsky himself. By simply being and acting, he always already had solved that question before he had been able to choose.

The meaning of "self" as just outlined is different from the meaning of the term as used and mentioned in philosophical contexts. In philosophy, "self" (or "the I") denotes a *general structure* rather than a set of idiosyncratic features. Although different philosophical approaches vary in their account of the self, most will agree that this structure is unique: there is no way to reduce it to other structures, regardless of whether one has a semantic, epistemic or ontological structure in mind. As Castañeda has pointed out in many of his works (cf., for example, Castañeda 1966, 1967, 1968, 1988), from a semantic point of view, the first–person pronoun "I" is unique in its referential features, i.e., it cannot be replaced by any other word salva propositione. "A correct use of 'I' cannot fail to refer to the entity to which it purports to refer..." (Castañeda 1968, p. 261).

From the point of view of the philosophy of subjectivity, the I is the active, unifying, identical center of any possible experience. It should be

---

8 Artists, in particular, complain about that side effect.

noted that such a philosophical notion of "self" is useful and even necessary to clearly interpret clinical cases like the ones in Margulies' paper: If there is change, there has to be an *identical* subject of such change, otherwise we (i.e., the patient as well as the doctor) could not recognize the change as such. Therefore, whereas the talk of two selves may be convenient clinically sometimes, it has the drawback of blurring the picture: Only from the point of view of the changed person knowing that his identity with himself has undergone some changes, can those changes be experienced as such. Thus the changed person has somehow integrated the old features; he knows about them and may appreciate them (even if they are not only for the good of the person).

7. Schizophrenia, Thought Disorder, Hallucinations, and Delusions

Although not explicitly stated in any of the contributions, schizophrenia is *the* case in question when it comes to psychopathological theorizing. As the contributions of Emrich, Jaynes, Hundert, Matthysse, Mundt, Oepen et al., Spitzer, and Wiggins et al.—in various different ways—point out, the symptoms of schizophrenia are poorly understood. Note that the problem is *neither* the fact that we do not know the causes of the illness (let alone how to treat it properly), *nor*—as tacitly assumed by many psychiatrists— the difficulty in knowing how to combine different symptoms in such a way that a reliable diagnosis can be made. The problem is, rather, that on the very basic level of symptoms it is far from clear how to put into appropriate terms what is going on in the patient. Psychiatrists commonly approache the "mental state" of a patient by referring to the "faculties" of the mind, but the question of how to justify this approach has remained.[9] In fact, as it is now commonly accepted in psychology that there are no such things as mental faculties comprised of nicely assorted capabilities with underlying separate structures, the question of how to justify a faculty approach to the mind becomes more urgent that it was when it was first introduced to psychiatry in the last century. This problem is not solved by simply adopting another approach, as every such approach has to be justified in some way. Thus, the question of what concepts to use in order to make sense out of mental disorder at the very basic level of symptomatology is far from solved and has to be addressed in psychiatry as long as it wishes to be a science.

---

9 As early as 1830, Hegel (*Encyclopaedia*, § 379, addendum, transl. by the author, F.A.U.) approached this problem as follows: "Empirical psychology takes up spirit in general, as well as the particular faculties into which psychology divides it, as these are given in presentation... in empirical psychology, it is the particularizations into which the spirit is divided which are regarded as being rigidly distinct, so that spirit is treated as a mere aggregate of independent powers, each of which stands only in reciprocal and therefore external relation to the other."

One way to be more specific than the faculty approach seems to consist of abandoning "mental talk" completely, replacing it with "cognitive" talk about data and their processing. By now we are so used to such an approach that we hardly see the problems that are necessarily involved in it. What is frequently overlooked, for example, is the fact that we only understand these notions because we *already* know (implicitly) what thinking, perceiving, sensing, etc. means. Moreover, if thought is believed to consist of some raw material (which is not conceived as thought) the problem of how the peculiar qualities of thought "emerge" is not solved. This fact is frequently overlooked by cognitivists who stipulate and model processes in order to simulate some features of what we call thinking, especially when it comes to the proper interpretation of such experimental work.

From the different approaches to schizophrenia that are contained in this volume, it seems clear that there is no general unifying view of the subject matter. However, it seems to be better to have competing, and maybe even mutually fertilizing, views of the mental aspect of schizophrenia rather than to exclude research and study of that aspect altogether.

When we asked *"Why philosophy?"*, we started out from Jaspers' question of "what one knows, how one knows it, and what one does not know" (Jaspers 1957/1981, p. 19, cf. this volume, p. 8). These questions are still valid, and we, the psychopathologists, should not conceal the blind spots in our knowledge about what is really going on in the minds of the mentally ill, either by means of talking about their brains, or by disregarding the question of validity (while only allowing questions about reliability) in our inquiry. Psychiatry seems to be particularly prone to losing either its field of inquiry or its status as a science, i.e., it is prone to "lose the mind" (Reiser 1988) and to forget about "truth" (cf. Wallace 1988).

> "Psychiatry is a medical discipline, but it shares with psychology and other behavioral sciences a set of intriguing questions. How can we know about mental life? And how can we explain it? In our search for agreement over these fundamental issues lies much of psychiatry's fascination and much of its discord... It seems to us that the best hope for a resolution of such difficulties lies in an understanding of the strengths, limitations, and appropriate uses of the most basic concepts in psychiatry, in a definition of what we know and how we know it."

In their book on *The Perspectives of Psychiatry*, McHugh and Slavney (1986, p. 1) rightly ask the very same question as Jaspers. Although the answers may differ, and although at times it may seem as if there is little progress in the psychopathologist's struggle for knowledge, it is important to *ask* the questions. This will keep our inquiries intellectually honest, our attitudes modest, and our approach to the patient human.

References

American Psychiatric Association: Diagnostic and Statistical Manual of Mental Disorders, Third edition, Revised (DSM–III–R). American Psychiatric Association, Washington, D.C., 1987.

Castañeda HN: 'He': A study in the logic of self–consciousness. Ratio 8: 117–142, 1966.

Castañeda HN: Indicators and quasi–indicators. American Philosophical Quarterley 4: 85–100, 1967.

Castañeda HN: On the phenomeno–logic of the I. Akten des XIV. Internationalen Kongresses für Philosophie, Wien, 2.–9. September, Herder, Wien, 1968.

Castañeda HN: Persons, Egos, and I's: Their Sameness Relations. In: Spitzer M, Uehlein FA, Oepen G (eds): Psychopathology and Philosophy, pp. 210–234, 1988

Hegel, GFW: Hegel's Philosophy of Subjective Spirit, ed and transl. with and introduction and explanatory notes by Petry MJ, in three volumes, comrising the Einleitung, Anthropology, Phänomenologgie und Psychologie. Reidel, Dordrecht, 1979.

Hoff P: Der Krankheitsbegriff in der Psychiatrie aus transzendentalphilosophischer Sicht. Phil. Diss, Munich, 1988.

Hundert E: Philosophy, Psychiatry, and Neuroscience. Three Approaches to the Mind. Clarendon Press, Oxford, 1989.

McHugh PR, Slavney, PR: The Perspectives of Psychiatry. Johns Hopkins University Press, Baltimore and London, 1986.

Reiser MF: Are Psychiatric Educators "Losing the Mind"? Am J Psychiat 145: 148–153, 1988.

Schelling FWJ: Einleitung zu dem Entwurf eines Systems der Naturphilosophie (1799). In: Sämtliche Werke, Stuttgart und Augsburg, 1858.

Spitzer M: Allgemeine Subjectivität und Psychopathologie. Haag & Herchen, 1985.

Spitzer M, Uehlein FA, Oepen G (eds): Psychopathology and Philosophy. Springer, Berlin, Heidelberg, New York, London, Paris, Tokyo, 1988.

Strawson PF: The Bounds of Sense. Methuen, London, 1966.

Wallace ER: What is "Truth"? Some Philosophical Contributions to Psychiatric Issues. Am J Psychiat 145: 137–147, 1988.

Wittgenstein L: Philosophical Investigations, transl. Anscombe EM, Blackwell, Oxford, 1952.

Name Index

Subject Index

Made in United States
North Haven, CT
01 December 2024

61301080R00143